# Clinical
# Disorders
# of Memory

CRITICAL ISSUES IN PSYCHIATRY
An Educational Series for Residents and Clinicians

*Series Editor:* Sherwyn M. Woods, M.D., Ph.D.
*University of Southern California School of Medicine*
*Los Angeles, California*

Recent volumes in the series:

ADULT DEVELOPMENT: A New Dimension on Psychodynamic Theory
and Practice
Calvin A. Colarusso, M.D., and Robert A. Nemiroff, M.D.

CLINICAL DISORDERS OF MEMORY
Aman U. Khan, M.D.

CLINICAL PERSPECTIVES ON THE SUPERVISION OF
PSYCHOANALYSIS AND PSYCHOTHERAPY
Edited by Leopold Caligor, Ph.D., Philip M. Bromberg, Ph.D.,
and James D. Meltzer, Ph.D.

CONTEMPORARY PERSPECTIVES ON PSYCHOTHERAPY WITH
LESBIANS AND GAY MEN
Edited by Terry Stein, M.D., and Carol Cohen, M.D.

DIAGNOSTIC AND LABORATORY TESTING IN PSYCHIATRY
Edited by Mark S. Gold, M.D., and A. L. C. Pottash, M.D.

DRUG AND ALCOHOL ABUSE: A Clinical Guide to Diagnosis
and Treatment, Second Edition
Marc A. Schuckit, M.D.

EMERGENCY PSYCHIATRY: Concepts, Methods, and Practices
Edited by Ellen L. Bassuk, M.D., and Ann W. Birk, Ph.D.

ETHNIC PSYCHIATRY
Edited by Charles B. Wilkinson, M.D.

EXTRAORDINARY DISORDERS OF HUMAN BEHAVIOR
Edited by Claude T. H. Friedmann, M.D., and Robert A. Faguet, M.D.

MARITAL THERAPY: A Combined Psychodynamic–Behavioral Approach
R. Taylor Segraves, M.D., Ph.D.

MOOD DISORDERS: Toward a New Psychobiology
Peter C. Whybrow, M.D., Hagop S. Akiskal, M.D., and
William T. McKinney, Jr., M.D.

THE RACE AGAINST TIME: Psychotherapy and Psychoanalysis
in the Second Half of Life
Edited by Robert A. Nemiroff, M.D., and Calvin A. Colarusso, M.D.

SCHIZOPHRENIA
John S. Strauss, M.D., and William T. Carpenter, Jr., M.D.

TREATMENT INTERVENTIONS IN HUMAN SEXUALITY
Edited by Carol C. Nadelson, M.D., and David B. Marcotte, M.D.

# Clinical
# Disorders
# of Memory

## Aman U. Khan, M.D.
*Southern Illinois University School of Medicine*
*Springfield, Illinois*

PLENUM MEDICAL BOOK COMPANY
New York and London

Library of Congress Cataloging in Publication Data

Khan, Aman U.
  Clinical disorders of memory.

  (Critical issues in psychiatry)
  Includes bibliographies and index.
  1. Memory, Disorders of. 2. Memory, Disorders of—Etiology. 3. Memory, Effect of
drugs on. I. Title. II. Series. [DNLM: 1. Memory—physiology. 2. Memory Disorders. WM
173.7 K45c]
BF376.K33   1986                              616.8                              86-18708
ISBN 0-306-42259-X

© 1986 Plenum Publishing Corporation
233 Spring Street, New York, N.Y. 10013

Plenum Medical Book Company is an imprint of Plenum Publishing Corporation

Printed in the United States of America

# Preface

Memory is essential for the retention of learning. In the presence of memory deficits, new learning is impaired and performance of previously learned habits deteriorates. What is the nature of memory? Where does it reside in the brain? What biological events are associated with the formation and retrieval of memory? These questions are explored in the first chapter of this volume. The answers are not final, but we have learned a great deal about memory processes during the past few decades.

Memory is influenced by most of the pathological processes that influence the brain such as infection, trauma, cerebrovascular disorders, and metabolic and degenerative diseases. The nature and course of memory impairment are unique for each of the disorders and are fairly distinguishable. More than fifty conditions are known to cause dementia, which now affects several million Americans. In Alzheimer's disease, memory disorder predominates for two to three years before other intellectual functions are affected. Many neurological diseases, such as Huntington's disease, Friedreich's ataxia, and multiple sclerosis, are associated with progressive memory deficits.

Forgetting is a problem that becomes progressively worse with age. Most individuals in their forties begin to experience some difficulty in quick recall of past events. By age sixty definite changes are evident in the process of registration, storage, and recall of memory. At this age the material that is to be remembered is processed more slowly, stored less firmly, and poorly recalled.

Functional disorders of memory have fascinated psychologists for centuries. Posthypnotic amnesia has been attributed to functional separation or dissociation in different types of mental processes. Hypnotically induced age regression highlights selective activities of childhood and does not involve total reinstitution of childhood mental processes and memories. The dissociative disorders of memory, such as psychogenic amnesia, fugue, depersonalization, and multiple personality, have moved up to the forefront of scientific investigation. Better understanding of memory impairment in depression and schizophrenia has led to innovative therapeutic interventions.

A large number of drugs have been shown to influence memory. Clinicians need to become more aware of the memory-impairing effects of various drugs, especially in the treatment of the elderly with marginal memory functions. Chronic use of alcohol, even in small amounts, appears to have an accumulative effect on the nervous system, producing progressive impairment of intellectual and memory functions.

The treatment of memory disorders is just beginning to receive the attention of clinicians and researchers. Memory clinics have been established in various medical centers. A large number of drugs, such as cholinergic drugs, stimulants, and nootropic drugs, are being experimentally employed in an effort to improve memory deficits. Other methods of treatment, such as surgical procedures to improve brain blood supply and rehabilitation methods to help older people better organize their daily activities, have become important tools in the management of memory disorders.

ACKNOWLEDGMENTS. Jean Brown and Kathy Ruffer contributed greatly to the preparation of this book with their organization and typing skills. I am also very grateful to Joseph Cataio, who spent a great deal of time in library research and in the editing of the manuscript.

                                                              Aman U. Khan
*Springfield, Illinois*

# Contents

*1. Nature of Memory* ........................................... 1

A. Psychology of Memory ....................................... 1
B. Neurobiology of Memory .................................... 12
C. Summary ................................................... 33
D. References ................................................ 35


*2. Memory Assessment* ........................................ 41

A. Single Tests of Memory (Verbal) ........................... 41
B. Single Tests of Memory (Nonverbal) ........................ 45
C. Test Batteries for Memory ................................. 50
D. Neuropsychological Test Batteries ......................... 51
E. Questionnaires to Assess Memory ........................... 56
F. Clinical Examination of Memory ............................ 57
G. Specific Rating Scales and Inventories .................... 58
H. Summary ................................................... 60
I. References ................................................ 63


*3. Drugs Influencing Learning and Memory* ................... 67

A. Introduction and Historical Overview ...................... 67
B. Drugs Impairing Memory .................................... 68
C. Drugs Facilitating Memory ................................. 74
D. Summary ................................................... 84
E. References ................................................ 86

*4. Alcohol and Memory Impairment* ............................... 89

A.  Social Drinking ................................................. 89
B.  Acute Alcoholic Intoxication ................................ 91
C.  Chronic Alcoholism ......................................... 94
D.  Summary ...................................................... 99
E.  References ................................................... 101


*5. Role of Neuropeptides in Memory* ........................... 105

A.  Noradrenaline and Dopamine System ....................... 105
B.  Serotonergic System ........................................ 107
C.  Cholinergic System ......................................... 108
D.  Opioid Peptides ............................................ 110
E.  Hormones .................................................... 111
F.  Summary ..................................................... 116
G.  References ................................................... 117


*6. Memory in Degenerative Diseases of the Nervous System* .......... 121

A.  Alzheimer's Disease ......................................... 122
B.  Pick's Disease .............................................. 129
C.  Progressive Supranuclear Palsy ............................. 131
D.  Huntington's Disease ....................................... 132
E.  Wilson's Disease ............................................ 135
F.  Hallervorden–Spatz Syndrome ............................... 137
G.  Parkinson's Disease ......................................... 137
H.  Amyotrophic Lateral Sclerosis and Parkinsonian Dementia
    Complex of Guam ........................................... 141
I.  Idiopathic Calcification of Basal Ganglia ................... 141
J.  Spinocerebellar Degenerations ............................. 142
K.  Summary ..................................................... 143
L.  References ................................................... 144


*7. Memory in Cerebrovascular Disorders* ......................... 149

A.  Chronic Ischemia of the Brain .............................. 150
B.  Transient Ischemic Disorder ................................ 151
C.  Large Cerebral Infarctions ................................. 152
D.  Multi-infarct Dementia ..................................... 154
E.  Summary ..................................................... 155
F.  References ................................................... 156

### 8. Memory in Chronic CNS Infections ........................... 157

A. CNS Syphilis ................................................ 157
B. Chronic Viral Infections ...................................... 158
C. Subacute Sclerosing Panencephalitis ......................... 159
D. Progressive Multifocal Leukoencephalopathy .................. 159
E. Transmissible Spongioform Encephalopathies ................. 160
F. Long-term Sequelae of Bacterial Meningitis in Children ......... 161
G. Summary .................................................. 162
H. References ................................................. 163


### 9. Memory in Chronic Diseases ................................ 165

A. Chronic Anoxia of the Brain ................................. 165
B. Cardiac Diseases ........................................... 165
C. Lung Diseases ............................................. 166
D. Anemias .................................................. 166
E. Chronic Renal Failure ....................................... 166
F. Chronic Liver Diseases ...................................... 168
G. Fluid and Electrolyte Disturbances ........................... 169
H. Endocrine Disorders ........................................ 170
I. Summary .................................................. 176
J. References ................................................. 177


### 10. Memory in Head Trauma ................................... 179

A. Severity of Injury ........................................... 180
B. Focal versus Diffuse Brain Damage .......................... 180
C. Nature of Disability ......................................... 182
D. Recovery of Physical and Mental Functions .................. 183
E. Memory Disorders from Head Trauma ....................... 184
F. Recovery of Memory ........................................ 188
G. Nature of Impaired Memory in Head Trauma ................. 192
H. Summary .................................................. 194
I. References ................................................. 195


### 11. Functional Disorders of Memory .......................... 199

A. Memory Functions in Depression ............................ 199
B. Memory Functions in Schizophrenia ......................... 201
C. Memory Dysfunction in Autistic Children .................... 202
D. Memory Impairment in Dissociative Disorders ............... 203

E.  Other Dissociative Disorders .................................. 205
F.  Dream Memory and Dream Amnesia ......................... 209
G.  Hypnosis and Memory Dysfunctions ....................... 212
H.  Memory Loss Induced by Electroconvulsive Therapy ........... 214
I.  Summary ............................................... 215
J.  References ............................................. 216

12. *Memory Changes with Aging* .................................. 219

A.  Psychological Aspects of Memory Changes with Aging .......... 219
B.  Other Factors Affecting Memory in the Elderly ................ 228
C.  Biological Aspects of Aging and Memory ..................... 229
D.  Summary ............................................... 235
E.  References ............................................. 236

13. *Treatment Strategies for Memory Disorders* ................... 239

A.  Pharmacological Treatment ................................ 240
B.  Memory Skill Training ................................... 249
C.  Psychiatric Treatments .................................. 252
D.  Environmental and Reality Orientation Program ............... 252
E.  Other Therapies ........................................ 253
F.  Summary ............................................... 253
G.  References ............................................. 253

*Author Index* ..................................................... 257

*Subject Index* .................................................... 265

# Clinical
# Disorders
# of Memory

# CHAPTER 1

# Nature of Memory

## A. PSYCHOLOGY OF MEMORY

### Introduction

The ancient Greeks portrayed memory in their mythology as the goddess Mnemosyne. Zeus was the supreme god of the ancient Greeks and through Mnemosyne he fathered nine daughters who were called the Muses and who were the patron saints of the various arts. Plato (427–347 BC) described memory as a block of wax, which was of different sizes in different men and which also differed in hardness, moistness, and purity. Aristotle (384–322 BC) assigned the memory function to the heart. From Aristotle we still have the expression "learned by heart." Erasistratus (310–250 BC) doubted Aristotle's ideas about memory. He performed the first dissections of the brain and concluded that the brain was the seat of mental functions, including memory.

Ebbinhaus (1850–1909) laid the groundwork for the objective study of human memory. He evaluated the effects of practice and rehearsal on the amount of retention and forgetting. Ribot's book on the "diseases of memory" and Korsakoff's paper (1889) on memory deficits focused attention on the pathological aspects of memory disorders. William James (1890) devoted a detailed chapter to memory in his book, *Principles of Psychology*.

Memory, however, remained a peripheral interest of psychologists for about 80 years after Ebbinhaus's early work. Psychologists focused instead on the parameters of learning, and memory was treated as one of the many intervening variables. The learning process was equated with the attachment of responses to stimuli. The repeated simultaneous occurrence of stimuli and responses strengthened the association beween them. Forgetting was considered the result of the weakening of the associations. However, a temporary failure to remember was considered the result of competition between responses attached to the same stimulus. The weakening of association was referred to as "extinction." In the late 1950s interest in memory per se surfaced with the focus being on short-term verbal retention. This was influential in

1

opening up other lines of memory research such as research on visual memory and auditory memory.

## Definition of Memory

Learning is concerned with the operations that place a relatively stable behavioral potential in memory. From this point of view, memory may be defined as the storage of learned behavioral potentials over time. Memory may also be defined as a persistent change in the central nervous system brought about by environmental input and by the activities of the organism (including the self-generation of an image, idea, or thought that is retained as memory).

The operational definition of memory derives from the results of laboratory testing of individuals for memory processes. The individual is provided some input and then tested for the amount of retention with memory being measured by determining how closely the output matches the input for various types of materials.

A variety of theories have been advanced to explain the various memory processes. Atkinson and Shiffrin (1968) divided the structure of memory into three components: the sensory register, the short-term store, and the long-term store. The information received by the sensory register may be lost or transferred to the short-term store from which it may also be lost or transferred to long-term store.

## Psychological Concepts of Memory

### Sensory Memory

The first stop an incoming stimulus makes is called sensory memory. All sensory modalities (visual, auditory, tactile, olfactory, and kinesthetic) are involved in receiving these first impressions. These impressions are either lost with time or processed further for later remembering. It is not clear whether the sensory memory is a peripheral phenomenon, a central phenomenon, or some combination of the two. The duration of sensory impression or memory is very short and it varies in time for different sensory modalities: visual sensory memory (iconic memory) may last from 250 msec to 500 msec; auditory sensory memory (echoic memory) from 2 to 10 sec; tactual memory about 4 sec and motor memory (kinesthetic) as long as 80 sec.

### Iconic Memory

Sakitt (1976) suggested that iconic memory is predominantly a retinal phenomena. Meyer and Maguire (1977), however, came to a different conclusion indicating a more central locus of iconic memory. Sakitt's view of iconic memory as an afterimage was further challenged by DiLollo (1977) who proposed that iconic memory can more properly be regarded as an ongoing feature extraction process than as the decaying of a sensory impression. An active process of feature extraction includes continuous processing of the input until sufficient information is extracted from the visual display, then the iconic memory ceases.

## Echoic Memory

Auditory sensory memory is assumed to store literal copies of auditory information for brief periods of time. Recent research has focused on clarifying the characteristics of auditory memory. Two common areas of research include "suffix effect" and "modality effect." The suffix effect is defined by reduced recall, especially in the last part of a list, when an extra word (suffix) is presented after the final item of the list and the subject is told to ignore the extra word. The reduced recall of the latter items is explained on the basis of the masking effect of the suffix. However, the exact way in which auditory memory operated in suffix experiments has not been resolved.

The modality effect refers to the superior recall of items that are presented auditorially compared with items presented visually. The auditory sensory memory lasts much longer than the visual sensory memory. This may increase the recall of the latter items in a list when presented auditorially rather than visually.

## Short-term Memory

There are several terms for short-term memory (STM): primary memory, immediate memory, span memory (Kelly, 1964), and short-term store. There has been a gradual acceptance of the distinction between STM and long-term memory (LTM) by psychologists. It was found that individuals with hippocampal lesions may have an intact STM with severe impairment of LTM (Scoville and Milner, 1957).

An item can always be recalled if tested immediately after its presentation, but it may be lost within a very short period of time, 20 to 40 sec (Norman, 1973; Shiffrin, 1973), unless it is placed in a "rehearsal buffer," which constitutes the essential part of the STM. The STM is a system of limited capacity in which information is maintained by continued attention and rehearsal. The format of the information is predominantly phonemic, but probably also visual and possibly semantic. The information in STM may be lost through displacement by new incoming information or simply lost by decay with time. The item in STM may also be transferred into LTM with a probability that is proportional to the length of its stay in the rehearsal buffer.

Research has focused on determining the capacity of the STM and on the relative importance of the displacement and decay processes. The estimates vary with the definition of functional capacity and the methods of measurement. Miller (1956) operationally defined STM as capacity that can retain seven items plus or minus two. There has been little progress in the understanding of the relative role of displacement and decay in the loss of material from STM.

Short-term memory is considered to be equivalent to "working memory" (Shiffrin and Schneider, 1977) whose principal function is the active control of thinking, problem solving, and general memory processes. At the initial input all features of the incoming information are analyzed and are represented as active elements in STM. Attentional processes select important information for maintenance by rehearsal or transfer them to LTM. Unattended information is lost rapidly from STM.

The working memory may also contain items recalled from LTM. Watkins (1977) suggested that word span reflects components from both STM and LTM. He concluded that the initial items on the list of a word recall task are drawn from the LTM whereas the latter items on the list are still in STM.

There are many factors that influence the retention of verbal material in STM such as the type of information, the relatedness or the unrelatedness of the material, and the order in which the material is presented. Murdock (1976) showed that recall of items is enhanced when the items are drawn from the same category, but that recall of order is poorer in categorized than in non-categorized lists of items. It appears that categorization helps item information but not order information.

Much recent evidence points to the probability that the memory record of an event contains several qualitatively different kinds of information. We remember not only what occurred, but also when, where, and how frequently. Different sensory inputs seem to communicate and influence each other through some common abstract code.

*Research Methods*

The psychological study of STM involves a broad range of techniques organized on the basis of theoretical issues concerning the nature of memory. The major source of information about STM is a set of recall tasks in which the subject is presented with a sequence of items to be recalled. This basic design is modified in various ways to determine different aspects of STM: free recall, serial recall, probe recall, and distractor recall. In the "free recall" technique, a sequence of words is presented to the subject who is then asked to recall as many of the words as possible. In "serial recall" tasks, the experimenter presents a sequence of items, such as numerals, letters, or words, and has the subject repeat the items in the same order. In the "probe recall" tasks, the subject is required to recall particular elements in a sequence of elements. A common example of this technique is paired-associates probe, in which the subject is presented with several paired associates and is then given the cue item as the probe for the response item of the pair. In the "distractor recall" task, the subject is presented with a sequence of items to be recalled, followed by a rehearsal-blocking or distractor task that is continued for varying periods of time.

Other techniques utilized in the study of STM include "recognition paradigms," rehearsal and repetition, and measures to determine modality effects and storage capacity of STM. Two recognition paradigms are used to study particular aspects of short-term storage: (1) Sternberg's scanning paradigm and (2) differential probe paradigm. The scanning tasks include a set of digits, one to six, which are presented sequentially at a rate of one digit every 1.2 sec. A test item is presented 2 sec later. The test item either is one of the previously displayed digits or not. The subject's task is to indicate whether or not the test item was a number of that set. The main measure is the latency of the subject's response. The theoretical analysis of the task and the type of data it yields (a straight line) make it possible to determine various stages in the processing of input information. In differential probe tasks, the subject is shown a list of words followed by a letter that indicates one of three response conditions: is the probe word identical with a list word; is it a homonym of a list word; or is it a synonym? Then a probe word is shown to get the response. These tasks are used to determine the content or the form of the storage in STM.

One major concern of any experimenter or theorist is what the subject is doing while the material to be remembered is being presented. Subjects may report doing nothing or may report rehearsing the items. The rehearsal usually refers to the covert repetition of items. This concern has led to the use of techniques in which the experimenter specifies the type of rehearsal the subjects are to carry out. This provides better control over the covert activities of the subject and reduces the number of variables to be considered in the analysis of STM.

The presentation of recall tasks through different sensory modalities has somewhat different effects on recall. This leads to a complex theoretical question—whether there are different types of codes in memory for different sensory modalities, i.e., visual, auditory, and so forth. Early work emphasized the dominant role of acoustic factors in STM. Visual information was considered to require translation into a verbal code in order to be held in STM and in order to be processed further. More extensive research led to the demonstration that the information from auditory, visual, and other sensory modalities was encoded distinctly in STM and that the distinct information could be carried through and stored in LTM. The idea that semantic information was represented only in LTM was contradicted by several studies (Shulman, 1970).

### Long-term Memory

This implies a permanent record of events and learned material. Several synonyms include "long-term store," "secondary memory," "delayed memory," and "distant memory." Long-term memory begins within about 0.5 sec from the time an item enters attention (Zangwill, 1969). There is some overlap between STM and LTM. Thus the test requiring subjects to recall a list of words will include the assessment of both STM and LTM. Words at the end of the list will be in STM, while words from the initial portion of the list would have entered into LTM. Tulving (1972) distinguished between two major forms of LTM contents: episodic memory and semantic memory. The episodic memory consists of the events that have been given a temporal and spatial coding—where and when something happened. The semantic (or categorical) memory contains stores of learned words, verbal symbols, and semantic relationships. There are no temporal and spatial contexts. Norman (1976) suggested an expanded semantic memory containing other nonverbal concepts that are attached to a particular time and space context. Most of the items in semantic memory are learned with some context of time and space, but the context gradually drops out and only the item relationship to various coded categories is remembered.

Research methods employed in determining the characteristics of LTM contents use subjects who are presented with tasks requiring semantic or lexical decisions. In one variant the subject is presented with one word. In the semantic decision task, the subject decides if the word is a member of a particular semantic category. In a lexical decision task, the subject decides if the presented string of letters is a word. Other common semantic tasks may include presentation of a simple English sentence such as "Rubies are gems" and then asking the subject to decide if the sentence is true or false. The theoretical goal of most of this research is to make inferences about the organizational structure of semantic knowledge and the processes that operate on that structure.

Little research has been carried out on LTM of the distant past. We speak of LTM if the retention interval exceeds 30 sec and the bulk of the articles on memory deal with intervals of a few seconds to minutes. Since all performance measures have to be obtained under the controlled conditions of the laboratory, the methods studying LTM reflect these constraints.

## *Encoding*

This implies that input information is somehow selectively processed or transformed before it is stored in LTM. The transformations may include additions, subtractions, substitutions, and elaborations (Underwood and Erlebacher, 1965). Substitution coding refers to the replacement of the input stimulus by another symbol, the code, together with a general decoding rule, for example, the translation of telegraphic signals into words, numbers, and phrases. Elaboration coding refers to the storage of additional nonredundant information with the input stimulus to be remembered, for example, recalling a word with its initial letter or recalling other information with the help of a cue. Temporal coding is perhaps the most common one, at least initially, since most items to be remembered include some time reference. The time tags frequently drop out over time.

Bower (1967) has described various other processes involved in encoding: (1) selection process—a component is selected out of a complex pattern of the input, (2) rewriting—an input is translated into another format, e.g., a sequence of visual symbols may be transformed into a verbal description; (3) componential description—a nominal item such as a word is registered as a list or complex of attributes or features; and (4) elaboration, additions, and so forth are made to the nominal input in order to transform it or render it more memorable.

Tulving (1973) has raised an important issue about the nature of encoding: whether memory of a stimulus is stored by marking or tagging a preexisting node or nodes in the memory, or as a distinct episodic trace (i.e., each unique episode is represented by a unique constellation of nodes, contexual elements, and associative links). The notion of tagging of new events in the preexisting nodes appears unsatisfactory since it does not provide any specific context in which the events occurred or of the subtle shades of meaning placed on a word during comprehension. The context issue was further elaborated by Tulving and Watkins (1977) in studies showing that subjects are able to recognize a word better when presented in the context of a sentence or phrase than when presented singly.

Arbuckle and Katz (1976) suggested that different learning tasks may not induce qualitatively different memory codes. For example, a nonsemantic task may simply yield a weaker semantic trace. This suggestion is in contradiction to Tulving's encoding specificity hypothesis which indicates that the effectiveness of a particular type of retrieval cue is strongly dependent on the type of encoding induced at input.

## Retrieval Processes

Reactivation of stored memory is called retrieval. A distinction must be made between an item that is available in the memory but not necessarily accessible. Having an item in the memory and being able to use it are two different things, just as a book that may be available in the library but is not accessible to the reader because its card is missing from the catalogue. Although retrieval from memory can occur in the absence of any apparent stimulus, most psychological studies on retrieval have utilized various types of cues to enhance retrieval. The research in this area has focused on multiple issues such as finding a relationship between encoding processes and retrieval, determining the effectiveness of cues, differences between recognition and recall, and recognition failure.

The fate of the information copied into the LTM from STM depends upon the mechanism responsible for transfer. Some information enters the LTM as a consequence of rehearsal in the buffer. In that case the information would be in a relatively weak state and easily subject to interference. Alternatively, rehearsal operations may be replaced with various encoding mechanisms that increase the strength of the stored information. There is growing agreement that retrieval processes are quite similar to encoding processes in many respects (Flexner and Tulving, 1978). Effective retrieval cues may resemble the original events at the time of encoding in its entirety or may represent only a fraction of the original episode.

Jones (1976) advances a "fragmentation hypothesis" in which the memory trace in LTM is viewed as a fragment of the perceived situation and retrieval cue is effective to the extent that it is stored in the fragment. Several studies appear to support this hypothesis (Flexser and Tulving, 1978). The effectiveness of a cue has been demonstrated to depend on several characteristics. A cue is more effective, for example, if it acts as the identifying property of the total unit. Dimensions of classification (i.e., shape, color) are better cues for unitary patterns.

Retrieval processes are constrained and inhibited in certain lawful ways. Graesser and Mandler (1978) suggested that retrieval from natural categories involves a sampling system that is limited by the span of apprehension. Once the sample limit is reached, there is a pause while the system seeks a new point of entry into the category. A similar limit on the span of apprehension appears to constrain encoding processes as well (cue overloading).

How do we know that we have not experienced a particular event? Brown *et al.* (1977) suggest that the subject assesses the "memorability" of an event presented to him for possible recognition. Well-known events are high on the memorability scale and can be rejected confidently, whereas false alarms and intrusions are low on the scale and require a longer time to reject. The memorability involves some form of operation to analyze salient features. The notion of an exhaustive search or matching procedures in finding false alarms is rejected by most authors.

In retrieval research, recogniton and recall are considered distinct processes. Recognition memory has at least two different meanings. In one sense, it refers to an act of recognizing someone or something, such as a familiar face, a familiar piece of music, a scene, and so forth. Second, it refers to a method of testing memory that presents one or more alternatives and asks for a judgment of familiarity. The distinction between recall and recognition involves whether or not alternatives are presented to the subject. For example, if a person is asked, "What is the capital of X," recall is being tested. But if the subject is asked, "What is the capital of X," and is given several possible answers, then recognition is being tested.

The nature of the recognition process continues to be a topic of interest. Mandler (1980) proposed a dual-process model of recognition that is based on (1) familiarity and (2) retrieval. The familiarity is the result of intraevent integration of sensory and perceptual elements. The events become more familiar the more often they are encountered. Retrieval is the result of interevent integration. Thus the retrieval processes involved in recognition are presumably the same as those involved in recall.

The phenomenon of failure to recognize previously presented items which are subsequently produced in cued recall continues to provoke controversy both on experimental and theoretical levels. Generation-recognition theory assumes that recall begins by implictly generating potential target items and then recognizing those items that were previously studied. The theory considers recall and recognition to involve similar processes, although the criteria employed during the recognition phase of the two tasks may be different. Watkins and Gardner (1979) conclude that while this model is useful in integrating some facts about recall and recognition, it fails as a theory to account for the majority of the empirical findings.

Tulving (1982) has proposed a model of retrieval called the "synergistic ecphory model of retrieval." According to this model, information available in the environment and information in the memory trace interact through a process of "ecphory" to jointly produce what Tulving calls "ecphoric information." The ecphoric information in turn gives rise to a "recollective experience," or what the individual is aware of remembering. They begin to differ when the recollective experience and the ecphoric information jointly, through the process of conversion, are translated into memory performance. In recall, conversion requires a description of some aspect of the target event (such as its name), whereas recognition requires identification of the target event (as "old") based on similarity with the originally experienced event.

## Forgetting

Forgetting is said to occur when a performance loss is observed in some memorized items after a retention interval. It may be that the material disappears with time, or that the learning of new responses interferes with the to-be-remembered items. It is also noted that an item may exist in full strength in memory, but the person may not be able to recall it on the first attempt. These observations have given rise to several theories of forgetting: trace decay theory, interference theory, and cue-dependent theory.

As discussed earlier, input information is retained in STM for a few seconds. Some of this information is transferred to LTM through rehearsal and encoding. The rest of the information is lost from the STM. Information is also lost from LTM. Postman (1969) reported that the loss of well-learned verbal material was 15% to 20% in the first 24 hr. The primary mechanisms assumed to play a major role in forgetting include decay, displacement, and interference.

## Trace Decay Theory

This is a passive theory. Forgetting is assumed to occur regardless of the subject's experience. Trace decay is spontaneous degeneration of the memory with time. Time alone in the absence of other variables is sufficient to produce forgetting. Sensory memories in various sensory modalities are said to be lost through the mechanism of trace decay in a very short period of time. Forgetting of material from STM and LTM is difficult to explain with trace decay theory. Empirical tests of this theory have been few. A strict test of the theory would require empty time, free of all mental activities after a period of learning in which the memory trace can spontaneously decay and this is obviously impossible to achieve.

*Interference Theory*

This theory dictates that events occurring between learning and recall may induce interference in retention and a decrement in recall. Forgetting depends upon the nature and frequency of interfering events. The interference may be retroactive or proactive. Retroactive interference is defined as decrement in recall produced by events between learning and recall. Proactive interference is defined as a decrement in recall of a criterion activity produced by events that occurred before learning of the criterion activity.

Several hypotheses have been advanced to explain the underlying mechanism of interference in causing forgetting. (1) The independence hypothesis suggests that interfering responses compete at recall and the strongest one in the competition (learning or interference) is the one that occurs. (2) The unlearning hypothesis (Melton and Irwin, 1940) suggests that at least some of the decrement in recall (forgetting) is attributable to unlearning, a kind of permanent weakening of the learned material caused by interference. (3) The differentiation hypothesis asserts that forgetting of the original material occurs because it is not sufficiently differentiated from the interfering items. Thus, recall depends on discriminability or differentiation.

*Forgetting in Long-term Memory*

There are those who believe that once information is processed to be included in LTM, it is permanently available and remembering is entirely a matter of retrieval problems; everything is remembered indefinitely and in principle can be retrieved. The evidence available at present supports more of an intermediate position. There is no evidence that all forgetting is nothing more than a failure to retrieve. Forgetting probably represents some combination of changes in the stored information with time and some loss of retrieval cues. In most cases, however, appropriate cues may help recall the apparently lost information (cue-dependent forgetting).

## Psychological Theories of Memory

Although a large number of theories and models have been advanced (Norman, 1970), two of the theories (dual-process theory and levels of processing theory) have remained influential in most of the research work carried out on memory.

## Dual-Process Theory

There are several versions of this theory, differing in details. Atkinson and Shiffrin (1968) first advanced this theory. A large number of details have since been added through the research efforts of many psychologists. The theory distinguishes three types of memory: sensory memory, STM, and LTM. The sensory memory is an afterimage or a temporary sensory persistence after stimulation has ceased. Short-term memory is different from afterimage and lasts a little longer (for a period of a few seconds) and makes us aware of the "just past." Short-term memory is a temporary store of limited capacity but not as temporary as sensory memory. The LTM holds the stable behavioral repertoire of a lifetime of experience.

This model of memory and a digital computer have a number of similarities. A computer has an input and an output, a working memory of limited capacity, and a central memory of large capacity. The information is transferred from one type of memory to the other. The STM may be regarded as the limited working memory of a computer and the LTM as the central storage memory of a computer.

Voluminous research has been carried out in support of the dual-process theory in spite of the obvious objection that it postulates a discontinuity of functions. The conviction that there are separate memory stores was founded on indications that STM and LTM had different properties and that the establishment of the latter was dependent on the survival of the former. Criticism of dual-process theory centers around the processes involved in the transfer of information from STM to LTM such as the processes of rehearsal and encoding. In contradiction to the prediction of dual-process theory, studies show that long-term retention of information is not determined by either the sheer amount of rehearsal or the duration of an item's stay in STM. Rather what is critical is the type of rehearsal or processing that takes place at input. Rehearsal activities can vary in effectiveness since maintenance rehearsal has only momentary effects and fails to influence recall even a few minutes later (Woodward, 1973).

## Level of Processing Theory (Craik and Lockhart, 1972)

This is an alternate model based on levels of processing and does not rely on a computer analogy. It is assumed that the presentation of any stimulus initiates a hierarchy of processing stages that can be graded along a continuum of depth. The basic idea of the theory is that the more the subject uses the data and processes them, the less he will forget. This theory hypothesizes several levels of processing. The first level is a preliminary stage where the processing is concerned with the sensory and physical features of the stimulus input. At a somewhat deeper level of processing the stimulus might be recognized as a whole. At the deepest level of processing, the stimulus can engage and interact with the mature and more sophisticated knowledge of the perceiver. There is a hypothesized mechanism called the "central processor," which is free floating and which can be directed to any processing level. The items in the central processor, which is regarded to be receiving attention, are in the consciousness and are in a kind of STM of limited capacity. There is no forgetting so long as the items are in the central processor, but once the central processor is diverted from them, the rate of forgetting is determined by the level of processing the new material has undergone.

The level of processing approach has been strengthened by research on sentences and prose memory. Dooling and Christiaansen (1977) demonstrated the multilevel nature of memory for prose, showing that surface details are lost relatively rapidly whereas higher-level processing was more durable. Similarly, Goldman and Pellegrino (1977) found that multiple encoding of an input was additive to some extent and repetitions of deeper-level encodings were more beneficial for later retention. More processing effort to achieve comprehension was associated with higher levels of retention.

The level of processing theory has been criticized by a number of researchers on both theoretical and empirical grounds. Nelson (1977) demonstrated that, contrary to level of processing expectations, repetitions of an encoding at the same level were associated with an increment in retention. The level concept continues to be plagued by the lack of an independent definition of depth and by continued demonstrations of context dependencies. Comparison of research on semantic and nonsemantic tasks tends to support the level of processing position. However, some findings in this area also contradict the theory. For example, Hunt and Elliot (1980) have shown that nonsemantic processing sometimes results in more durable memory traces than the level of processing view would predict.

## B. NEUROBIOLOGY OF MEMORY

The studies have been concerned primarily with the neurobiological nature of memory. The same questions asked by psychologists have been investigated in biological terms such as: Are there single or multiple types of biological processes underlying the various types of memory? What is the nature of these biological processes? How localized or generalized are these processes in the central nervous system? How is the stored information retrieved in terms of neural processes? What happens in neural terms when information cannot be retrieved on one occasion, although it can be retrieved on a subsequent occasion?

External and internal stimuli that impinge upon an organism constitute an experience, image, or sensory memory. This experience is somehow converted into a neural representation which may be stored in some electrical or molecular form within the CNS and constitutes LTM. During recall or remembering, the stored memory must somehow stimulate or create a similar neural configuration as was created during the intial experience.

There are several models based on neurobiological studies of memory. The most popular model of memory has been a two-phase model that recognizes a labile phase and a stable phase during the consolidation of memory. Recently a four-phase model has been advanced on the basis of neurotransmitter studies.

## Two-Phase Model of Memory

### Labile Phase

A great deal of experimental evidence has accumulated to support the contention that there is an early phase, immediately after an experience, during which the representation of that experience is mediated by a labile process. During this period, disruption of ongoing activity by various types of intervention interferes with the consolidation of that experience in more permanent storage. As time elapses after the actual experience, these various interventions gradually lose their ability to prevent consolidation.

Physiological evidence for the existence of a labile phase arises from the studies of retrograde amnesia in individuals suffering a head injury. Russell and Nathan (1946) surveyed 1000 cases of head injury. Over 700 cases in this study reported amnesia for events occuring up to 1/2 hr before the injury and 133 reported retrograde amnesia for the events during a period longer than 30 min. The authors concluded that the loss of memory for recent experiences was due to interference with a preservative process.

There are a variety of perturbations of the CNS that cause interference with the registration of recent experiences. These include electroconvulsive treatment, heat narcosis (Cerf and Otis, 1957), cerebral ischemia (Baldwin and Soltysik, 1965), anoxia (Ransmeier and Gerard, 1954), anesthetics, and convulsant agents.

Interference with registration of recent experience has also been obtained by electrical stimulation of many areas of the brain, including parts of the various major functional systems. Similarly, interference with learning has been obtained by "spreading depression" (SD) of various areas of the brain. The SD is a reaction displayed by neural tissue to a variety of agents, varying from electrical stimulation to topical application of KCl. The reaction seems to consist of a gradually spreading potential change accompanied by a flattening of the EEG, a disappearance of evoked responses, and impedance changes apparently resulting from a marked intracellular chloride shift and massive extracellular potassium shift. These changes result in a massive depolarization of involved neurons (Bures and Buresova, 1965).

Substances that increase neural excitability seem to facilitate registration even when injected after the experience; e.g., systemic injection of anticholinesterases and intraventricular potassium facilitate registration.

*Mechanism of the Labile Phase of Memory.* The assumption most frequently encountered as an explanation or mechanism of the labile phase of memory is that it depends upon the ability of specific neuronal circuits to sustain a reverberatory activity. This hypothesis originated from the anatomical studies of Lorente de No (1938). It was explicitly proposed by Hilgard and Marquis (1940) and by Hebb (1949) who suggested that the neural representation of the events to be memorized may be maintained by reverberation of electrical activity in the appropriate neural networks until permanent structural or chemical storage has been accomplished. This reverberation hypothesis (also called trace theory) remained purely theoretical until the 1950s when it was shown that impulses do not simply reverberate along circular loops, but form complex matrices moving in a highly organized fashion in complicated, multilane, thalamic and cortical pathways.

The experimental evidence accumulated during the last 20 years (Verzeano, 1972) indicates that spontaneous neuronal activity occurs in thalamic and cortical networks in the absence of an external stimulus and is modified by incoming sensory information. This neuronal activity can be recorded by means of multiple microelectrodes from all regions of the cerebral cortex and from all the thalamic nuclei during relaxed wakefulness and deep sleep. The activity circulates at velocities varying from 0.5 to 9 mm/sec along a series of loops of diameters of 0.1 to 0.2 mm whose locus shifts continually through the neuronal network (Verzeano and Negishi, 1960). This activity is greatly modified by incoming sensory information. Specific changes in the characteristics of the sensory stimuli (such as frequency or intensity) cause specific changes in the patterns of circulating activity.

Although the existence of neuronal activity and its modification by sensory information is well established, the mechanism on which they are based is not entirely known. Verzeano *et al.* have suggested that the circulating matrices of neuronal activity serve as carriers that, modulated by incoming information, transport the neural representation of events to be stored over the networks in which it would ultimately be retained.

Burns (1958) studied the electrical activity of cortical slabs that were isolated neurally from the rest of the brain while retaining an intact blood supply. Such slabs display a marked diminution of spontaneous electrical activity. However, Burns has observed that a single electrical stimulus can intiate bursts of electrical activity in these slabs that last for 30 min or longer and seem to involve reverberatory circuits. Some characteristics of reverberatory activity may be better understood through an analysis of the normal physiological activity of neurons.

Hebb (1949) suggested that a set of cells, perhaps in the appropriate association areas, act as a closed system in which activity continues to circulate for a brief period of time after stimulation. The association of activity between two adjacent cells causes alterations in membranes in such a way that the influence of one cell upon the other is facilitated. In this fashion, the activity of each cell is enhanced. Integration of several cell assemblies, constituting a superordinate structure or organization, is mediated by mechanisms such as physical continuity, as suggested by Hebb (1949), and temporal continuity, suggested by John (1967).

At the instant of arrival of a specific afferent stimulus, certain cells in the population are refractory while others are responsive. The initially responsive set now propogates the disturbance in the available set of pathways. Certain of these possible routes are blocked due to refractoriness, while others are momentarily facilitated or inhibited by the ongoing activity. The cumulative effects of these constraints plus the inhibitory consequences of the input itself act to terminate the propagation of the disturbance along certain of the possible paths, while other paths sustain propagation long enough to succeed in becoming reentrant. Only cells in pathways that become reentrant can participate in reverberatory activity. Multiple reentrant pathways undoubtedly exist in parallel and may be thrown into activity at different times. However, all cells that do not belong to such reentrant pathways or receive its influence would seem to be necessarily excluded from participation in the reverberatory activity.

### Stable Phase of Memory

Since memories are extremely resistant to erasure, persisting through sleep, unconsciousness, excitation, and seizures once consolidation has been completed, it is reasonable to assume that during the consolidation phase durable changes must occur. Although reverberatory neural activity may be the basis for STM during the labile phase, LTM cannot be attributed to enduring reverberations.

Whether the information is stored by the actual growth of new connections between nerve cells or the synthesis of substance inside neurons or glial cells, or whether the responsible mechanism operates in a deterministic or a statistical manner, these processes must require changes in the brain's structure and composition. Biological mechanisms for the stable phase are discussed in the section on molecular and structural changes.

### Four-Phase Model of Memory

Frieder and associates (1982a,b) have carried out several experiments on rats that indicate that consolidation of memory may occur in four phases. In one experiment, 30 min prior to training in an active avoidance task, rats were injected intracisternally (IC) with 3 mg of diethyldithiocarbamate (DDC), a norepinephrine (NE) synthesis inhibitor. The rats showed a complete retention of task memory for about 10 min after the training. Subsequently, memory decayed to the naive level over the next 80 min but reappeared later. The brain NE level fell to 50% of its normal level 30 min after the injection; 90 min later it recovered to 85% of its normal level. The dopamine level did not change. This DDC-induced transient amnesia could be prevented by injecting 10 mg NE IC 30 min prior to training. These findings indicated that NE was needed shortly after the training to form medium-term memory (MTM).

Another group of rats were injected IC with 4 mg ethacrynic acid 30 min prior to training. These rats showed complete retention of memory 2 min after training, amnesia developed 10 min after training, and complete recovery occurred 15–90 min after the training. There was a partial amnesia 3.5 hr later. These results indicated that ethacrynic acid interfered with STM formation.

In a second experiment, rats were subjected to hypoxia (2% oxygen in nitrogen) for 30 sec following an active avoidance task. They showed a transient MTM amnesia for that task. The occurrence of this transient posthypoxic amnesia was prevented by treating the animals with hyperoxia (100% oxygen for 2 min), provided this was done within 1 to 5 min following the hypoxia.

In view of the rapid recovery of normal brain functions with air following hypoxia, the ability of hyperoxia to reenable MTM formation even if it were given 1.5 min after hypoxia suggests the existence of a "very short-term trace" that normally gives rise to MTM formation. The authors suggest that there are separate biochemical mechanisms that operate in parallel and give rise to four overlapping phases in memory consolidation.

1. Very short-term memory (VSTM): decays in 1–5 min.
2. Short-term memory:
   a. Formation—1–5 min.
   b. Plateau—5–10 min.
   c. Decays—10–90 min.
3. Medium-term memory:
   a. Formation—0–30 min.
   b. Plateau—30–180 min.
   c. Decays—180–300 min.
4. Long-term memory:
   a. Formation—90–240 min.
   b. Plateau—?
   c. Decays—?

### Localization of Memory

Investigations to determine the sites of memory traces (engram) have progressed on several parallel lines. The most common methodologies have included (1) brain lesions, (2) electrical stimulation of the brain, and (3) molecular changes at the cellular and intercellular levels.

### Brain Lesions

Ablation and destruction of various areas of the brain have been carried out to identify specific loci in the brain that may be related to the storage and retrieval of LTM. The literature in this field is enormous. Animal studies constitute the major portion of these studies. With this technique, animals are trained to learn certain tasks. They are then tested to show that they have learned the task well before a brain lesion is made. The animals are tested again after the lesion to determine decrement or loss in learning, presumably caused by the lesion. Unfortunately, lesions of the brain destroy not only the site of the lesion, but they also disrupt various networks of distant neurons. Thus a deficit in learning and memory produced after a lesion reflects the function lost by the lesion site as well as the disrupted functions of the rest of the brain. Brain lesions may also impair motor functions, motivation, emotions, and sensory-perceptual capacities which themselves may produce a decrease in the performance of learned behavior.

There are many other problems that have plagued lesion studies. The laboratory tasks utilized by different studies are not strictly comparable in terms of what they test. Interspecies differences are also frequently ignored in the interpretation of the findings. Lesions produced by different methods (surgical, electrical, and chemical) are likely to produce different consequences and are therefore not easily comparable. In spite of these pitfalls of the lesion method, a great deal of knowledge has been accumulated from this methodology.

*The Cerebral Cortex.* The pioneering work of Lashley (1950) on various types of learning in rats was hailed by those holding a holistic theory of brain function in general and memory function in particular. By removing various cortical areas and testing the retention of learned discriminations afterward, Lashley found that the lesions only impaired memory in a general way. The degree of impairment was, on the whole, proportional to the volume of cortex removed (the principle of mass action). Although there is no doubt that the mass-action effect can be demonstrated in certain maze-learning situations in rats, it occurs in only a fraction of the total spectrum of laboratory tasks on which the brain-damaged rat has been examined. In many other laboratory tasks such as visual discrimination problems (Horel *et al.*, 1966), vestibulo-kinesthetic discrimination problems (Thompson, 1976a,b), tactile discrimination problems (Simons *et al.*, 1975), and latch-box problems (Spiliotis and Thompson, 1973), it is the locus of the lesion rather than its size that is the critical factor in determining retention deficits. Consequently, the mass-action effect cannot be offered as a principle for all types of learning or for the distribution of memory.

Studies showing that some decorticate animals can learn certain laboratory tasks favor the existence of the engram at subcortical levels. Alternate views locate the engram (1) at both cortical and subcortical levels, and (2) at several levels of the brain axis. Several authors (Lashley, 1935; Glendenning, 1972) support the notion of two distinct levels of the engram—neocortical and subcortical. It is hypothesized that in normal rats subcortical mechanisms are suppressed by the neocortical functions. However, in a decorticated animal, subcortical mechanisms are released from cortical inhibitions and become independently functional.

Rozin (1976) and others have suggested that the engram is located at several levels of the brain axis. The lowest level may be conceived at the level of the brain stem and corpus striatum, the middle level might involve the limbic forebrain areas and the higher level would include the neocortex. The learning of simple tasks such as simple visual discrimination may be mediated by the mechanisms at lower levels (Bauer and Cooper, 1964) whereas more complex tasks would involve mechanisms at all three levels (Thompson, 1974).

In lower mammals, connections between regions of the cortex are fairly direct with little association cortex in between. Association cortex, however, increases in size and complexity as one moves up the phylogenic scale. Research with primates and humans indicates that damage to even small cortical areas of the brain may cause impairment of learning and memory. Extensive destruction of the visual association cortex in a macaque monkey led to the loss of a previously learned visual discrimination task (Geschwind, 1965). But if the operation were carried out in stages with practice between the serial ablations, the learning was retained. It appears that simple tasks can be learned after partial ablation of the association cortex and that there is a great deal of flexibility and overlapping of functions in the association cortex.

The understanding of the functions of the human cortex has been derived primarily from the pathological destruction of the cortex resulting from occlusion of blood supply, tumors, injuries, and by surgical removal of certain areas to treat uncontrollable seizures. The natural pathology frequently involves wide areas of the brain and is rarely restricted to small, discrete areas. However, any damage to the cortex results in some loss of learning and memory. Disorders such as aphasia, apraxia, alexia, agraphia, acalculia, and agnosia result from cortical damage.

Alexia is defined as an acquired inability to comprehend written language as a consequence of brain damage. Two major clinical syndromes have been described: alexia without agraphia and alexia with agraphia. Dejerine (1891) described alexia without agraphia resulting from destruction of fibers connecting the calcarine region to the angular gyrus with the central site of damage being in the white matter of the lingual lobule. Subsequent studies have emphasized a combination of lesions in the lingual and fusiform gyri of the dominant occipital lobe and in the splenium of the corpus callosum (Sperry and Gazzaniga, 1967). Dejerine (1891) also found that cortical–subcortical lesion affecting the angular gyrus caused alexia with agraphia. Most other authors agree that a dominant angular gyrus lesion may cause alexia with agraphia (Hecaen and Kremin, 1977).

A variety of writing disorders (agraphia) have been associated with cortical damage. These disorders often accompany disorders of oral language (aphasia) and reading disorders. Lesions of the frontal lobe appear to be responsible for most cases of writing disorder.

Henschen (1925) found that some globally aphasic patients with extensive left-hemispheric disease had an impaired ability to perform numerical operation (acalculia). Subsequently, left angular gyrus lesions have been implicated for alexia and agraphia for numbers in patients who are not globally aphasic.

An aggregation of symptoms including agraphia for words, finger agnosia, right–left discrimination problems, and acalculia was described by Gerstmann (1940) arising from left parietal lobe disease. This syndrome has been recognized by subsequent neurologists as resulting from damage to the posterior parietal region of the dominant hemisphere. There is, however, no concensus with regard to the type of acalculia associated with the syndrome.

*Basal Ganglia.*   The lesion studies in animals suggest that the basal ganglia participate in memory functions of one kind or another. The basal ganglia are elements of the extrapyramidal motor system and their lesions impair retention of such learned responses as pushing aside a stimulus card (Thompson, 1976a), operating a bolt latch (Spiliotis and Thompson, 1973), and active avoidance responses (Kirby and Kimble, 1969). In addition to motor responses, some nonmotor responses are also affected by lesions of the basal ganglia, such as brightness and pattern discrimination.

*Brain Stem Reticular Formation (BSRF).*   The BSRF is a complex system having an abundance of intercellular connections and projections to all areas of the cortex. The role of the BSRF in memory retention has been controversial since lesions in the BSRF have failed to provide consistent support for such a function. Discrete lesions in the BSRF at mesencephalic levels have been reported to have little effect on learned responses in rats (Kesner *et al.*, 1967), cats (Chow and Randall, 1964), or monkeys (Thompson and Meyers, 1971). In contrast, Meyers (1964) found that ventrally placed lesions within the midbrain BSRF of cats produced greater disruptive effects on visual discrimination performance than the dorsally placed lesions. Similar findings have been reported in rats. It has been suggested that the decrement in the performance of certain tasks arising out of the lesion in the BSRF may be due to a reduction in the "tonic" or "energizing" effect of the BSRF on the neocortex.

*Ascending Raphe System.*   The raphe nuclei contain serotonergic neurons that project to widespread regions of the forebrain; some of the hypothalamic, thalamic, and basal ganglia; and the neocortex. Discrete lesions of the raphe nuclei have been reported to impair retention of a variety of learned tasks in rats such as visual discrimination (Thompson, 1976b), a vestibulo-kinesthetic discrimination, and a maze habit. Some of the impairment is attributed to hyperkinesia produced by the lesion. The hyperkinesia impairs learning of discrimination tasks but promotes learning of active avoidance habits (Thompson, 1978). Thus the ascending raphe system, which is predominantly inhibitory, has been viewed as regulating those inhibitory processes that are involved in the storage and retrieval of information.

*Locus Coeruleus (LC).*   The LC is a major nuclear area giving rise to norepinephrine-containing cells. The projections of the cells in the LC are widespread, terminating in the cerebral cortex, the cerebellum, the thalamus, the hypothalamus, the amygdala, and the hippocampus. The LC appears to be strongly involved in the initiation and maintenance of rapid eye movement (REM) sleep (Jouvet, 1972). One recent line of speculation concerning REM sleep is its possible importance in information processing, specifically its role in consolidation of recent memories into permanent or long-term memories (Dallett, 1973). A great deal of recent evidence suggests that REM sleep is very important for memory processes.

Damage to the LC alters either the temporal aspects of the susceptibility period of newly formed memory to disruption or the retrieval of such memories. This suggests that the LC may be involved in an extended neuroanatomical memory system involving both the cerebral cortex and brain stem regions.

Both the dentate gyrus and the LC independently project to the hippocampal pyramidal cells. The synaptic action of the former is almost exclusively excitatory while the synaptic action of the LC is inhibitory upon the pyramidal cells. Zornetzer *et al.* (1976) suggested that the dentate gyrus and LC work in concert, possibly exerting a reciprocal action on the hippocampal pyramidal cells. One of the normal functions of the dentate gyrus in the mouse appears to be related to the transfer of at least some types of newly formed memories.

*Limbic System.* This system includes all the components of the Papez circuit (the cingulate cortex, the hippocampus, the fornix, the mammillary bodies, the mammillothalamic tract, and the anterior thalamus) together with the olfactory bulb, the septum, the amygdala, the medial forebrain bundle, the habenulopeduncular complex, the mesencephalic central gray area, and Gudden's nuclei. This system has been conceived as the anatomical substratum for emotional behavior. Some parts of this system such as the hippocampus appear to be involved in memory processes. Selective lesions in the limbic midbrain area (the ventral tegmental areas, the interpedunculo–central tegmentum, and the median nuclei) have been reported to impair retention of such tasks as a passive avoidance habit, visual discrimination, an incline plane discrimination, latch-box problems, and a complex maze learning (Thompson, 1982).

*Temporal Lobe.* Augusto Fernandez-Guardiola (1976) studied 18 uncontrolled epileptic patients who were chronically implanted with eight electrodes each in the temporal lobe from the cortex to the hippocampus, passing through the amygdala and the periamygdaloid areas. The stimulation of these electrodes produced memories, reminiscences, hallucinations, verbalizations, aggressive conduct (in rare occasions), and emotional change in most cases. Most interestingly, stimulation of the contralateral temporal lobe (opposite the epileptic focus) produced a great number of reminiscences. Deep sagittal stimulation produced most of the responses that were of a personal and affective type, related mainly to situations causing anger and fear. Stimulation of superficial leads led to intensely pleasant and happy experiences. Categorical memories, related to learned abstract concepts, were elicited extremely rarely.

Stimulation of the periamygdaloid region always provoked very elaborate reminiscence phenomena and the old memories were always related to infantile experiences. These evoked infantile memories were never of experiences earlier than 5 or 6 years of age. No patient was capable of recalling his memories during the first months or earliest years of life. Despite the large numbers of patients, no reminiscences of recent happenings were provoked.

Scoville and Milner (1957) described the severe memory disorder of a young man (H.M.) who had undergone bilateral medial temporal lobe ablation to treat an uncontrolled form of epilepsy. Upon recovery from surgery, H.M. manifested a severe inability to learn new information and was even unable to recall many events that had occurred prior to surgery. Scoville and Milner later described the memory disturbances of eight psychotic patients who had received similar surgery to improve their psychotic thought disorder. Severe anterograde amnesia was noted in those patients whose surgery included the anterior sector of the hippocampus, but was not evident when the hippocampus was spared and only the uncus and the amygdala were removed. On the basis of the findings in these nine patients, the investigators concluded that the hippocampus was necessary for the consolidation of new memories and for the retrieval of some of the old memories. H.M. has been studied extensively. There has been no change in his IQ and personality from the surgery. He has, however, suffered from severe impairment of STM and he is unable to acquire new information although his immediate recall is unimpaired. He cannot learn the names of new friends or new addresses.

## Electrical Stimulation of the Brain

This technique has played a significant role in the elucidation of the neuroanatomical circuits associated with simple and complex behaviors such as sleeping, fighting, vocalization, drinking, and fearlike responses (Delgado, 1964; Kaada, 1972). The technique is criticized for its unnatural mode of action since electrical stimulation of the brain does not stimulate the naturally triggered valleys of nerve impulses. The electrical stimulation of the brain disrupts the ongoing neural activity not only at the site of stimulation, but affects brain activity at distant sites.

Kluver and Bucy (1937) demonstrated that bilateral ablation of the anterior temporal lobe changed the aggressive rhesus monkey into a tame animal. Such operated-upon animals also demonstrated hypersexuality and visual agnosia. It was later found that the removal of the temporal lobe neocortex did not produce tameness (Akert *et al.*, 1961). However, stimulation of the amygdala produced a ragelike response and its ablation produced a tame animal. On the other hand, stimulation of the septal regions produced an apparently pleasant state in which the animal stimulated itself without additional reward (Olds, 1958), whereas septal lesions produced a ragelike state (Brady and Nauta, 1955).

Electrical stimulation of the human brain has been carried out at the time of surgery and through stimulation of implanted electrodes.

Penfield and Rassmussen (1950) found that electrical stimulation of the primary motor cortex of the human brain produces motor movements of various parts of the body, but the motor movements are very crude such as those performed by a baby and manifest no skill. Similarly, stimulation of the primary sensory cortex produces crude sensations of touch. Stimulation of some parts of the frontal, the parietal, and the temporal areas produced vocalization of speech arrest. The vocalization, as produced in the somatic sensorimotor area of either side, is usually a continuous cry. That which is produced in the superior frontal region is often rhythmic or interrupted. Interference with speech was produced by stimulation in three cortical areas of the dominant hemisphere—frontal, parietal, and temporal.

Stimulation of the temporal cortex before surgical removal in patients with seizure disorder shows that stimulation of the left temporal lobe (but not right) leads to a variety of anomias, or naming errors. Two distinct areas have been located in the temporal lobe: stimulation of the anterior sector of the left temporal lobe resulted in anterograde amnesia while stimulation of the posterior (temporoparietal) region produced retrograde amnesia. The investigators (Fedio and Van Buren, 1974) suggested that structures in the anterior portion of the left temporal lobe (e.g., the hippocampus) may play a role in the consolidation or the storage of verbal material, while sectors of the left posterior temporal region may be important in the retrieval of previously stored verbal information. Corsi (1969) has reported similar findings in patients who had left temporal lobe ablation with extensive hippocampal damage. The patients showed impairment on STM tasks and in learning superspan digit sequences. On the other hand, maze learning and recognition of faces and photographs were impaired only with extensive lesions of the right hippocampus.

Sem-Jacobsen (1968) has reported a comprehensive study on depth-electrographic stimulation of the human brain. Several patients with mental and neurological disorders were implanted with deep electrodes to record and produce lesions for therapeutic purposes. Most electrodes were placed in the frontal lobe in mental patients and near the third ventricle in Parkinson's disease patients. The electrical stimulation of the electrodes produced single and multiple responses as well as no responses in all sections of the brain with great consistency. The memory patterns elicited in response to electrical stimulation as reported by the patients were of two types: recollection of simple memory in which the patient suddenly and vividly remembered a certain past episode ("recollective memory" by Penfield) and flash-back memory in which there was a sudden transfer back in time, always to the same specific point or moment.

In one patient, electrical stimulation elicited one recollection from the right temporal lobe, another from the area left of the third ventricle. In a second patient, a recollection was elicited by stimulation in the anterior part of the frontal lobe on the left side, whereas a flash-back memory was elicited from the posterior part of the right frontal lobe, medial to the top of the temporal lobe.

The primary response of flash-back was associated with "afterdischarge." The afterdischarge was associated with an outpouring of thoughts. That is, in response to each stimulation, the past experiences seemed to be "played back" to the patient as from a tape recorder. When the electrical stimulation was maintained for a prolonged period, the sequence continued, uninterrupted, until the stimulus was removed. The next time the stimulus was turned on, the patient exclaimed, "Here we go again. Here we are again." The patient described how his memory returned to the same point in time, yet he also realized that he was in the examining room.

## Molecular and Structural Changes

Perhaps the first suggestion in the literature that information storage might involve macromolecules was made by Von Forester (1948) who pointed out the large information capacity that might be afforded by variations in the base sequence in macromolecules. Several years later, Katz and Halstead (1950) proposed a set of hypotheses suggesting that changes in brain nucleoproteins might be the basis for memory. However, most scientists at present believe that memory coding is accomplished not through the synthesis of some hypothetical "memory molecule," as was first speculated, but in the form of "patterns" specific for each act of memorizing, of neuronal assemblies uniting different brain areas.

The creation of such assemblies during training, that is, during memory consolidation, could be accomplished with the help of some specifiable proteins causing the action of essential synaptic contacts, namely membrane proteins.

Although the search for brain-specific proteins has existed for more than 100 years, it is only recently that new biochemical and immunochemical methods have made it possible to recognize some of the new brain-specific protein fractions. Bogoch (1968) reported the discovery of a new brain-specific antigen, BE, which is a water soluble protein causing an experimental encephalomyelitis. Moor (1973) discovered two other brain-specific proteins, S-100 and 14-3-2. The content of S-100 in the brain is $10^4$ times greater than in other organs. The content of S-100 rises rapidly postnatally after the 10th day as the brain functions develop. The protein is contained in the cytoplasm of the glia, the neuronal nucleus membrane, and the synaptic membrane. The protein is mostly concentrated in the hippocampus, in the area $CA_3$.

The brain specificity of protein 14-3-2 has been established by immunochemical methods. Its role in the membranal processes of neurons appears to be similar to that of S-100. The content of 14-3-2 in the brain is 100–200 times greater than in other organs. It is present in neurons and most of all in synaptosomes and can be transferred into membrane form like S-100. In mice it appears about the 7th day postnatally.

Bock (1978) identified a protein called synaptyn. It is found in all brain structures; its content in the membrane is ten times greater than in cytoplasm; it is absent in glia; and it is linked with vesicle exocytosis during impulse transmission.

There are at least another half a dozen brain-specific proteins that have been found by immunochemical methods. They are awaiting investigation to assign them specific functions.

The effects of learning on protein metabolism in the brain have been studied in various ways. The most popular method, however, has been with the aid of radioactively labeled amino acids that are injected before, during, or after a learning experience. These amino acids are incorporated in the formation of new RNA, which leads to the formation of new proteins. Estimation of labeled RNA in brain cells is presumed to indicate the influence of new learning when it is found to be different from RNA in the control subjects.

In order to stimulate the synthesis of new proteins, a learning experience must be able to penetrate to the nucleus of brain cells and activate the genetic mechanism which produces messenger RNA (mRNA). Early studies were able to collect only indirect evidence for RNA production in the brain cells of learning animals. Recent studies (Hyden, 1977), however, have demonstrated that hippocampal nerve cells in a learning rat show an increased synthesis, compared with active controls, of mRNA. These findings do not exclude the possibility that the mRNA which is already present in the cell body can be utilized for protein synthesis before the new mRNA has been assembled. The sample studies in this area are summarized below.

*Studies of the Effects of Stimulation on RNA and Protein Turnover.* Bratgaard (1952) reported that with light deprivation, the concentration of RNA in the ganglion cell dropped rapidly to an exceedingly low level. Upon stimulation, the rate of synthesis of RNA in the ganglion cell was proportional to the total light stimulation received by the cell. Rasch *et al.* (1961) also showed that normal light stimulation was a major factor controlling the development of normal ribonucleoprotein levels in the retinal cells of rat, cat, and chimpanzee.

*Effects of Decreased RNA on Learning.* A number of studies have explored the effects of interference with RNA synthesis or destruction of RNA on the storage and retrieval of information (by injection of ribonuclease into the growing medium to destroy RNA synthesis or with the use of RNA inhibitors such as 8-azaguanine). Most of these studies are inconclusive.

*Effects of Increased RNA on Learning.* Studies of the facilitation of RNA synthesis by use of drugs (e.g., strychnine and magnesium pemoline) indicate some improvement in learning.

Matthies *et al.* (1979) investigated the correlates of the acquisition and consolidation of a shock-motivated brightness discrimination in rats. Trained animals showed significantly increased incorporation of radioactively labeled RNA precursors (uridine or uridine nucleotides) into hippocampal cells over passive and active controls. An enhanced labeling was also observed in the visual and cingular cortex. Other cortical as well as thalamic and hypothalamic structures showed no differences between the experimental and control groups. The increased incorporation of amino acids during learning mainly occurred in neurons. In order to prove that the increased incorporation of the labeled amino acids indicated an increased protein synthesis, radiochemical methods were used to measure the specific activity of the precursor pool and to calculate the rate of protein synthesis in the hippocampus. The results indicated that an increase in macromolecular synthesis correlated with learning.

Hyden (1977) and associates have studied protein metabolism quite extensively in relation to various learning situations. They have suggested that when an animal begins to learn a suitable and sufficiently difficult task, short-lasting production of proteins starts within minutes in experimental animals, but is absent in control animals subjected to the same experimental procedure. This production of proteins starts in the hippocampus and spreads to cortical areas after a certain delay. Learning stimuli cause electrical field changes which induce the short-lasting synthesis of at least two brain-specific proteins. One of the proteins is S-100 which is brain specific and is incorporated into the outer membrane of nerve cells during the early part of the animal's life. The protein S-100 in the membrane constitutes about 10% of the total S-100 which is in turn 0.1% of the total brain cell protein. It is produced by glial cells, but is localized to the outer membrane and nuclear membrane of the nerve cell. Characteristically, S-100 binds calcium and during this process undergoes conformation changes that partially open up the protein molecule thus exposing other groups of molecules. This process enables the S-100 protein to react with membranes which then are able to regulate the in- and outflux of ions. Shortly after learning begins, the amount of S-100 in the hippocampus increases by 15–20% and the incorporation of radioactive amino acids into cell protein by 300%. A similar increase is shown by another brain-specific protein that is localized to the neurons and is called 14-3-2. The short-lasting synthesis of S-100 helps the nerve cell attain a metabolic state that favors the process of membrane differentiation.

During learning, calcium also increases in the hippocampus. This is a learning-specific reaction and not due to circulation. Calcium transforms S-100 and perhaps acts as a translator of electrical phenomena to molecular changes.

Several hours after finishing training, when the animals are back in their cages, a protein fraction with a molecular weight of 60,000 is synthesized in the cortex and other parts of the brain. Synthesis begins 8 hr after the finished training, reaches a peak after 24 hr and stops after 48 hr. This protein is presumed to help consolidate new information into LTM.

Shashoua (1976) has found an increased synthesis of three different protein fractions from nerve cells in goldfish trained to acquire new behavior.

According to Hyden (1977) the new synthesis of proteins causes biochemical differentiation of nerve cell membranes and synapses. Thus, in biological terms, learning would mean protein differentiation of brain cells. At retrieval, it is supposed that the same stimuli that induced a growth of brain cell differentiation can activate all brain cells wherever they are located, provided only that they share the same pattern of protein differentiation. It should be emphasized that Hyden does not believe that protein molecules synthesized by a given learning–memory situation act as storage bins for that particular situation and its associated information. Instead, he hypothesizes that the newly synthesized situationally unique protein(s) simply determines whether or not a neuron will fire when stimulated by a particular pattern of incoming neural activity.

*Structural Changes.* Research related to the effects of enriched or impoverished environments on brain structure indicates that the brain grows with use and every part of the neuron, from nucleus to synapse, can increase, decrease, or change depending on whether the environment is stimulating or not. In a preliminary study, Holloway (1966) detected an increased branching of dendrites of stellate neurons in the occipital cortex of rats (25 to 105 days old) exposed to an enriched environment. Greenough and Volkmar (1973) noted that rats raised in enriched environments had more higher-order dendritic branches than their impoverished littermates. Similarly, significant increases in dendritic branching have been found in older enriched rats (Uylings and Smit, 1975).

Changes in synapses have long been considered a mechanism of memory. Many of the synapses in the cerebral cortex are found on dendritic spines. Globus *et al.* (1973) found that basal dendrites from the occipital cortical pyramidal neurons of enriched animals had a greater number of spines when compared with basal dendrites from impoverished animals, implying an increased number of intracortical connections.

Rosenweig *et al.* (1972) examined synapses at the electron microscopic level and provided evidence that synapses respond to environmental changes by either increasing or decreasing their dimensions. Diamond (1976) studied synapses in enriched, impoverished, and standard colony animals from 25 to 55 days of age. They found a significant difference in postsynaptic thickening length in layer 4 of the cortex. This synaptic difference was considered primarily due to impoverishment, as shown by comparison with standard colony littermates.

*Neurotransmitters and Memory.* The idea that facilitation of synaptic function is a crucial phenomenon occurring during the process of learning and memory consolidation has gained increasing acceptance. Understanding the molecular events of synaptic facilitation appears to be a major prerequisite before the mechanisms of such functions of the CNS can be clarified.

Electron microscopic examination of neuronal circuits has revealed several modes of synaptic connectivity. These include reciprocal electronic functions, mixed chemical and electrical functions, and other forms of dendrite to dendrite (D–D) synapses, including triads and serial synapses.

Transmission at most of the synaptic junctions is chemical. At some of the junctions, however, transmission is electrical, and at a few conjoint synapses it is both electrical and chemical. Various chemical agents have been suspected of being transmitters. In fact, the list of these agents found in the CNS has been growing very rapidly. More than a dozen chemical transmitters have been shown to provide transmission in various parts of the CNS.

Although it is agreed that neurotransmitters maintain an STM trace by excitation and inhibition of various synaptic junctions in some areas of the CNS, the role of neurotransmitters in the consolidation of LTM is not clear. Since protein synthesis has been considered a possible mechanism underlying memory consolidation, it has been suggested that neurotransmitters may influence memory consolidation by their effects on protein synthesis or vice versa. There are two ways of visualizing this relationship: first, the neurotransmitters may influence the metabolism of macromolecules directly; second, the proteins may act by modifying the metabolism and function of neurotransmitters. The second possibility is, of course, verified since neurotransmitters are synthesized by enzymes that must be available in the synaptic terminals. Thus an inhibition of protein synthesis from any cause would be expected to produce a decrease in the neurotransmitter pool as soon as the concentration of the synthesizing enzymes falls to a certain value.

The results of the experiments with three of the neurotransmitters in the CNS—serotonin, dopamine and gamma-aminobutyric acid (GABA)—indicate that they may be regulating the rate of protein synthesis at the synaptic level. Gamma–aminobutyric acid stimulates protein synthesis when added *in vitro* to brain ribosomal and mitochondrial systems, to brain cell suspensions, and also to cortex slices. Similarly, inhibition of GABA synthesis (by introducing glutamate decarboxylase) *in vivo* or in brain slices causes decreased synthesis of proteins. It seems that GABA influences protein synthesis in all subcellular fractions, including isolated nerve endings. Gromova (1980) suggested activation of the adrenergic system during learning, which promotes the synthesis of the specific proteins. Similar experiments with dopamine and serotonin, however, indicate that they inhibit the synthesis of proteins in the stimulated neurons.

Learning has also been shown to be associated with the cholinergic system, which promotes the synthesis of definite proteins, fermentative and receptive type. The synthesis of acetylcholine receptors has been found to be activated during learning in the rat (Aleksidze *et al.*, 1975). Deutsch (1973) has summarized the main role of the cholinergic system in memory consolidation.

Thus a modification of the receptor quantity or conformation induced by the synaptic transmitter could result in an increase or decrease in synaptic conductivity with a subsequent modification of its functions.

## Retrieval of Information

Research data seem to indicate that LTM may be divided into at least two categories on the basis of time. Theoreticians have used various labels such as secondary and tertiary (Ervin *et al.*, 1970), intermediate and long-term (McGaugh and Dawson, 1971), long-term working memory and long–term store (Shiffrin, 1973), and recent long-term and remote long-term (Kesner, 1973). The recent LTM refers to memory for events during a period extending from the present to a few weeks back in time. The remote LTM refers to memory of a more permanent kind back to childhood. These terms represent a continuum in depth and organization of information processing within LTM.

The fact that hippocampal dysfunction can induce retrieval failure one day, but not seven days after criterion training, suggests that the hippocampus plays a critical role in retrieval of information from recent LTM, but plays a more limited role in information retrieval from remote LTM. The development of remote LTM is assumed to develop with time when an important and critical item of information is subjected to repeated rehearsal in a variety of cognitive environments. The rehearsal process leads to either the formation of multiple representations of or to the elaboration of multiple interconnections with the specific items within various functional systems in the brain.

In addition to the hippocampus, retrieval of information from remote LTM is assumed to be mediated by a number of independent neural systems (e.g., neocortex) that gain access to the memory functions of patients with hippocampal lesions. However, except for a certain amount of retrograde amnesia for preoperative events, these patients are capable of retrieving information from remote LTM stored prior to the operation (Milner, 1966).

Kesner (1973) has presented the following model of information storage and retrieval. He suggested that mnemonic information is processed in STM and two components of LTM (recent and remote). Data suggest that the midbrain reticular formation constitutes one of the most important neural substrates mediating functions of recent LTM, and the neocortex with the hippocampus may be maximally involved with the development of remote LTM. The data also suggest that the duration of STM ranges from seconds to minutes, for recent LTM seconds to days, and for remote LTM from minutes to a lifetime.

The fundamental operating process for STM is assumed to be the decay of the memory trace, but for recent LTM it is assumed to be the growth or consolidation of the memory trace leading to an increase in its strength and retrievability; for remote LTM it is assumed to be higher-order organization via construction of multiple representations or multiple access routes to the memory trace leading to an increase in resistance to forgetting. Information stored within the recent LTM can be transformed to remote LTM by a number of control processes such as rehearsal, higher-order organization, and perhaps dreaming.

## Influence of Sleep on Memory

There is little doubt that sleep facilitates memory. This effect (called the sleep effect) was first demonstrated in 1924 by Jenkins and Dallenbach and has been replicated many times. To be specific, the sleep effect in behavioral terms refers to the fact that performance is better when sleep occurs during the interval between learning and recall than when there is no sleep during this retention interval. Several psychological theories have been advanced to explain the mechanism of the sleep effect. *Decay theory* says that forgetting is a matter of the decay of the neurobiological traces that underlie learning. Presumably, there is some ongoing, catabolic process that is responsible for the decay of the traces. It is a fact that general body metabolism is slower during sleep than wakefulness. So it is reasonable to assume that any neurological process is taking place at a slower rate during sleep than during wakefulness. If the decay process is slower during sleep, then we would expect to find the sleep effect. *Interference theory* says that during wakefulness there is other learning that is taking place, and it is this new learning that interferes with the recall of the original learning. Going to sleep prevents interfering learning, so there is better recall. *Consolidation theory* says that sleep facilitates memory by promoting the persistence of neurobiological processes that occur during learning. Data supporting this theory indicate that delayed sleep is less effective than immediate sleep after the learning experience.

Although total sleep has been found to be beneficial for improving retention, REM sleep has been found especially beneficial for improving LTM. A number of researchers have suggested that dreaming enhances memory by either reprogramming the brain (Dewan, 1970) through a direct involvement with memory consolidation (Hennevin *et al.*, 1971) via an integration of recently perceived input into existing internal structures (Breger, 1967) or by a recording of recent memories into long-term storage tapes (Greenberg and Liedderman, 1966). Kesner *et al.* (1975) suggested that dreaming may serve as a process associated with transformation of information from recent to remote LTM.

Many data suggest that the processing of new information is not complete for many hours after the initial learning and that the first episode of REM sleep following acquisition of information could be involved in memory consolidation. Greenberg and Pearlman (1974) showed that REM sleep deprivation immediately after learning impaired memory, especially for complex tasks. Also, learning sessions were followed by an increase of time spent in REM sleep. Since REM sleep is associated with reticular and cortical activation, it is speculated that the facilitation of memory by REM sleep may be related to the activation of the reticular activating system (RAS). This hypothesis has been supported by the findings of Denti *et al.* (1970) who showed that the amnesic effect of sleep deprivation was much less in rats whose RAS was electrically stimulated during the consolidation period after learning.

Since the hippocampus has been shown to play a special role in retrieval of information from recent LTM (Kesner *et al.*, 1975), there is a great deal of indirect evidence in support of possible hippocampal involvement with REM sleep. For example, the appearance of theta rhythm during REM sleep indicates hippocampal activation; stimulation of the hippocampus facilitates the manifestation of REM sleep; septal lesions that suppress theta rhythm also produce a reduction in REM sleep. These data suggest that the hippocampus, probably through access to information stored in recent LTM, plays a significant role in determining the nature, structure, and content of dreams, which in turn may be significant for promotion of organizational changes within remote LTM.

Data also suggest that protein synthesis in the brain is intimately related to the physiological processes regulating REM sleep. Bobillier *et al.* (1974) have reported that rats deprived of REM sleep show a decrease in protein synthesis in the brain. Drucker-Colin and Spanis (1975) studied the effects of protein synthesis inhibition on sleep. Administration of anisomycin prevented the appearance of REM sleep, while growth hormone produced a dose-dependent increase in REM compared with controls. Drucker-Colin and Spanis (1975) have proposed a model in which REM sleep is seen as affecting the process of storage of learned information through neurotransmitters. Consolidation of STM, thus leading to LTM, is seen as being influenced by REM sleep through its effect on protein synthesis. Simultaneously, brain excitability induced or associated with REM sleep may be seen as subserving neural reprogramming processes throughout the lifetime of the organism, thus permitting appropriate recall of learned material and appropriate daily behavior. This model also suggests that disorganized pattern of dream content may be produced by the excitability changes in the neural circuitry during REM sleep.

## Theories of Memory

Broadly speaking, theories of memory can be divided into theories focusing on events at the molecular level and theories that emphasize changes in large clusters or ensembles of neurons and are thus of a more molar or holistic nature. The holistic theorists do not dispute the importance of the events and processes occurring at the molecular level, but believe that it is the patterning and sequence of events in large groupings and systems of neurons that constitute the true and essential basis of memory. There is no necessary incompatibility between these two types of theories since each deals with phenomena at a different level of observation and analysis.

At the molecular level, theorists have seized upon every newly discovered structure, structural change (e.g., dendrite branching), endogenous chemicals (especially the neurotransmitters and peptides), protein synthesis, or electrical phenomena (such as reverberating electrical activity), and have proclaimed each to be at least a mediator or modulator of memory. Some of these theories have been described in detail in the previous section.

Holistic theories of memory postulate that the most important factors in memory formation and retrieval are not the changes occurring in one neuron (which simply result in its having an increased or decreased probability/capacity of firing) but the patterning and sequence of firing in large groupings and clusters (systems) of neurons. Memory, from this point of view, is "encoded by changes in the state (i.e., the momentary pattern of organization) of the neural network" and not by the various mechanisms that alter synaptic conductivity. The chief proponents of the holistic viewpoint are E. Roy John and Karl Pribram.

Pribram's holographic theory of memory seizes on the fact that synaptic potentials are accompanied by a wave front which intersects with other wave fronts at a given neuron to produce interference patterns (interfering wave fronts). Memories are hypothesized to be stored or encoded by these interfering wave fronts and to be retrieved whenever the pattern of neural activity in the brain corresponds to the pattern that was present when the given memory was first encoded. The theory is termed holographic because holograms are also the product of interfering wave fronts and because holograms exhibit some of the same properties as memory (any portion of the hologram, however small, contains the entire image; for example, a phenomenon reminiscent of the brain's distributed rather than localized storage of memory). The holographic theory of memory also postulates that the brain operates in accordance with the principles of Fourier analysis, which transforms complex patterns into their component sine waves.

E. Roy John's statistical configuration theory of memory postulates that a particular memory is encoded or represented by "the average behavior of a responsive neural ensemble" and not by a biochemical change in one neuron. Each memory is represented or encoded by a unique pattern of neuronal firing and is retrieved whenever that unique pattern of neuronal firing reoccurs. The same ensemble or network of neurons is thus capable of encoding many different memories. No new physical pathways or connections are assumed to be formed since it is the sequence and patterning of the firing of large numbers of neurons that is presumed to encode memory (this is why the theory is termed configurational).

## Genetic–Evolutionary Theory of Memory (Khan, 1985)

Direct analysis of the evolution of the brain from the data of fossil endocasts indicates that the relative size of the brain increased with the passage of geological time. Evolution of the cortex led to changes in all parts of the brain. The association areas of the cerebral cortex have increased progressively in their size in mammals and especially in man. The increase in the association cortex has occurred in successive stages through evolution. New groups of neurons have developed and specialized in handling the demands and challenges of the environment. Thus, it is presumed that there is a direct relationship between a specific aspect of the environment and a specific group of neurons in the association cortex. This specificity exists at the level of a single cortical neuron that responds, by varying degrees of excitation and inhibition, to a fragment or a trace of environment such as a line, curve, angle, texture, color, sound frequency, odor, and so forth. Because various groups of neurons have developed in direct association with primary sensory and motor cortex, their specificity to respond to a particular aspect of environmental energy is greatly determined by the discriminating or resolving capacity of the sensory receptors. Consequently, there is a great deal of overlapping in the response of individual neurons.

Hubel and Wiesel (1974) demonstrated the presence of specific neurons in visual cortex that responded to specific environmental stimuli. They found at least four types of specific neurons with varying degrees of complexity. The "simple neurons" responded to a narrower segment or trace of a visual stimulus, whereas "complex neurons" responded to a larger segment of the stimulus alone or through collaboration with several simple cells.

The association cortex probably contains thousands of types of neurons with varying degrees of specificity and complexity. Each sensory–motor modality has its own pool of specific neurons and shares other groups of neurons with other sensory–motor modalities. This arrangement leads to a greater amount of plasticity of the cortical areas. Since an environmental stimulus is frequently processed by several sensory and motor modalities simultaneously, it is represented in multiple areas of the cortex. In case of destruction in one area of the cortex, other areas may still retain some memory of the stimulus. Since most neurons respond to only a very narrow aspect of the environmental energy, the system provides for a tremendous amount of plasticity. Destruction of a major part of the association cortex will still leave behind some neurons that may process a stimulus in an appropriate manner.

The basic thesis of this theory is that the memory of a stimulus trace resides in the cells that have specialized through evolution to handle that particular aspect of the environmental energy. Learning of a complex stimulus requires a group of cells to bend together to process the stimulus, each cell in the group responding to a different aspect of the stimulus. The selection of the group of cells for response is directed by the sensory–motor cortex and depends upon the availability of the specific cells from a pool of similar neurons. The practice in learning strengthens the connections among the individual cells in the group. Multiple representations of the stimulus are formed with further practice (or deeper levels of processing) in association with other sensory–motor modalities. Individual neurons of a group are not exclusively tied up in processing any one complex stimulus. In fact, by virtue of their narrow specialization, they participate in processing multiple stimuli forming overlapping groups, networks, or assemblies of neurons.

Neuronal circuits of the RAS are probably involved in the process of recall through focusing attention on specific assemblies of cortical cells.

The role of neurons with a higher order of specialization (complex cells) may be especially important in processing higher intellectual functions such as abstraction. Although experimental evidence for the major tenents of this theory is lacking, this form of theorizing may help future directions of memory research.

## C. SUMMARY

### Psychology of Memory

Memory may be defined as a persistent change in the central nervous system brought about by environmental input and by the activities of the organism such as self-generation of an image, idea, or thought that is retained as memory. Memory processes include sensory memory, STM, encoding, LTM, retrieval, and forgetting.

The first impression that an incoming stimulus makes is called sensory memory. All sensory modalities (visual, auditory, tactile, olfactory, and kinesthetic) are involved in this process. These sensory impressions are either lost with time or processed further for later remembering. It is not yet clear whether the sensory memory is a peripheral phenomenon, a central phenomenon, or some combination of the two. The duration of sensory memory is very short and it varies in time for different sensory modalities: visual sensory memory (iconic memory) may last from 250–500 msec; auditory sensory memory (echoic memory) from 2 to 10 sec; tactual memory about 4 sec; and motor memory (kinesthetic) as long as 80 sec.

Items from sensory memory may be lost or transferred to STM storage. Short-term memory is conceived as a system of limited capacity in which information is maintained by constant attention and rehearsal; it can usually retain 7 items ($\pm$ 2). Short-term memory is considered to be equivalent to "working memory," whose principal function is the active control of thinking and problem solving. Attentional processes select important information for maintenance by rehearsal or transfer it to LTM. Unattended information is lost rapidly from STM. Sensory information from auditory, visual, and other sensory modalities is encoded distinctly in STM and is carried through in a distinct manner to LTM.

The process of encoding implies that information in STM is selectively processed or transferred before it is stored in LTM. The transformation may include addition, subtraction, substitution, and elaboration.

Long-term memory is more or less a permanent record of events. Formation of LTM usually begins 0.5 sec after an item enters STM. However, consolidation of information for permanent retention in LTM may take a much

longer time. The content of LTM is classified into two broad categories: episodic and semantic. The episodic memory consists of the events that have
been given a temporal and spatial coding—where and when something happened. The semantic memory is called retrieval. A distinction is made between
an item that is available in the memory but not accessible at certain times or
under certain conditions. However, appropriate cues are able to enhance
retrieval. There is a growing consensus that similar types of processes may
be involved, in encoding. Thus, effective retrieval cues may resemble the
original events at the time of encoding in its entirety or may represent only
a fraction of the original episode.

In retrieval research, recognition and recall are considered distinct processes. The distinction involves whether or not alternatives are presented to
the subjects. For example, if a person is asked, "What is the capital of X"
recall is being tested. But if the subject is asked, "What is the capital of X,"
and is given several possible answers, then recognition is being tested.

Forgetting is said to occur when a performance loss is observed in some
memorized items after a retention interval. Several theories have been advanced
to explain the process of forgetting. The "trace decay theory" proposes that
forgetting results from spontaneous degeneration of memory with time. The
"interference theory" dictates that events occurring between learning and
recall may induce interference in retention and consequent forgetting. The
"cue-dependent theory" suggests that it may be the loss of retrieval cues with
time that leads to forgetting. The "level of processing theory" would indicate
that events processed superficially are forgotten easily while deeper levels of
processing result in durable memory. However, forgetting appears to be a
complex phenomenon and none of the theories are able to explain it fully.

### Neurobiology of Memory

The nature of biological processes involved in the formation of memory
has eluded investigators despite intensive efforts during the past several decades. However, a great deal of knowledge has been accumulated on the roles
of sensory receptors and primary sensory areas of brain in the formation of
memory. Stimulation of sensory receptors gives rise to specific patterns of
neural activity in the primary sensory areas of the brain. Attention is necessary
to process this neural activity further for retention in memory.

Biological events of memory formation in the central nervous system
are divided into two phases: a labile and a stable phase. The labile phase is
the initial phase, occurring immediately after an experience, during which
memory formation is in a labile phase and is easily disrupted by various types
of interferences and distractions. In the stable phase, the memory is laid down
in a durable and permanent form and is quite resistant to erasure, persisting
through sleep, unconsciousness, head trauma, and seizures.

Exact mechanisms of labile and stable phases are unknown. A large number of theories and hypotheses have been advanced, some of them partially supported by experimental data. The assumption most frequently encountered as an explanation or mechanism of the labile phase of memory is that it depends upon the activity of the specific neural circuits to sustain a reverberatory activity. The spontaneous neural activity, which occurs in thalamic and cortical networks in the absence of an external stimulus, is modified by incoming sensory information. Specific changes in the characteristics of sensory stimuli (such as frequency or intensity) cause specific changes in the pattern of the spontaneous neural activity. The modified patterns of spontaneous neural activity caused by sensory stimulation have been shown to last for several minutes if they are left uninterrupted.

Multiple processes proposed for the stable phase of memory formation include actual growth of new connections between nerve cells, synthesis of substances inside neurons or glial cells, and formation of specific patterns of excitation in groups of neurons selected on random basis.

Structural changes in neurons with learning have been supported by the research relating to the effects of enriched or impoverished environments. An increase in higher-order dendritic branching and in dendritic spines has been demonstrated in animals raised in enriched environment and with learning.

Molecular changes with learning are frequently related to the formation of new proteins (neurotransmitters and receptors). Although the formation of several new proteins specific to the nervous system has been demonstrated during learning, the role of these proteins in memory formation remains unclear. Various neurotransmitters participate in maintaining an STM trace by excitation and inhibition of synaptic functions, but their role in LTM formation is not clear. It has been suggested that neurotransmitters may influence memory consolidation by their effects on protein synthesis or vice versa. It is also possible that an increase in protein synthesis during learning may alter the quantity of neurotransmitter receptors which in turn would result in altered conductivity of neural synapses.

## D. REFERENCES

Akert K, Gruesen R, Woolsey C, et al: Bucy syndrome in monkeys with neocortical ablations of temporal lobe. *Brain* 1961; 84:480–98.

Aleksidze NG, Balavadze MV: The inductive synthesis of cholinesterase in brain during learning and training of rats. *Vopr Biochim Mozza* 1975; 10:97–106.

Arbuckle, T, Katz W: Structure of memory traces following semantic and nonsemantic orientation tasks in incidental learning. *J Exp Psychol Hum Learn Mem* 1976; 2:362–369.

Atkinson RC, Shiffrin RM: Human memory: A proposed system and its control process, in Spence KW, Spence JT (eds): *Advances in the Psychology of Learning and Motivation Research and Theory*. New York, Academic Press, 1968, vol 2, pp. 89–195.

Baldwin B, Soltysik S: Acquisition of classical conditioned defensive responses in goats subjected to cerebral ischemia. *Nature* 1965; 206:1011–1013.

Bauer JH, Cooper RM: Effects of posterior cortical lesions on performance of a brightness-discrimination task. *J Comp Physiol Psychol* 1964; 58:84–92.

Bobillier P, Sakai F, Sequin S, et al: The effect of sleep deprivation upon *in vivo* and *in vitro* incorporation of tritiated amino acids into brain proteins in the rat at three different age levels. *J Neurochem* 1974; 22:23–31.

Bock E: Nervous system specific proteins. *J Neurochem* 1978; 30:7–14.

Bogoch S: *The Biochemistry of Memory*. London-Toronto-Oxford, University Press, 1968.

Bower G: A multicomponent theory of the memory trace in Spence KW, Spence JI (eds): *The Psychology of Learning and Motivation*. New York, Academic Press, 1967, vol 1, p. 381.

Brady J, Nauta W: Subcortical mechanisms in control of behavior. *J Comp Physiol Psychol* 1955; 48:412–20.

Bratgaard SO: RNA increase in ganglion cells of retina after stimulation by light. *Acta Radiol Supp* 1952; 96:80.

Breger L: Functions of dreams. *J Abnorm Psychol* (Monograph No. 641), 1967.

Brown J, Lewis V, Monk A: Memorability, word frequency and negative recognition. *Q J Exp Psychol* 1977; 29:461–473.

Bures J, Buresova O: Plasticity at the single neuron level, in *Proceedings of the 23rd International Physiology Congress*. Tokyo, 1965, pp. 359–364.

Burns BD: *The Mammalian Cerebral Cortex*. London, Arnold, 1958.

Cerf J, Otis L: Heat narcosis and its effect on retention of a learned behavior in goldfish. *Fed Proc* 1957; 16:20–21.

Chow KL, Randall W: Learning and retention in cats with lesions in reticular formation. *Psychosom Sci* 1964; 1:259–60.

Corsi PM: Verbal memory impairment after unilateral hippocampal excisions. Paper presented at the 40th Annual Meeting of the Eastern Psychological Association, Philadelphia, April, 1969.

Craik FI, Lockhart T: Levels of processing: A framework for memory research. *J Verb Learn Verb Behav* 1972; 11:671–684.

Dallett J: Theories of dream function. *Psychol Bull* 1973; 79:408–16.

Dejerine J: Sur un cas de cecite verbal avec agraphie suivi d'autopsie. *Mem Soc Biol* 1891; 3:197–201.

Delgado JM: Free behavior and brain stimulation. *Int Rev Neurobiol* 1964; 6:349–449.

Denti A, McGaugh J, Landfield P, et al.: Effects of post-trial electrical stimulation of the mesencephalic reticular formation on avoidance learning in rats. *Physiol Behav* 1970; 5:659–62.

Deutsch JA: Cholinergic synapse and memory, in Duetsch JA (ed): *Physiological Basis of Memory*. New York, Academic Press, 1973, pp. 59–76.

Dewan EM: The programming "P" hypothesis for REM sleep, in Hartmann E (ed): *Sleep and Dreaming* (International Psychiatry Clinics Series, vol 7). Boston, Little Brown, 1970.

Diamond MC: Anatomical brain changes produced by environment, in McGaugh J and Petrinovich L (eds): *Knowing, Thinking and Believing*. New York, Plenum Press, 1976.

DiLollo V: Temporal characteristics of iconic memory. *Nature* 1977; 267:241–243.

Dooling D, Christiaansen R: Levels of encoding and retention of prose, in: Bower GH (ed): *The Psychology of Learning and Motivation*, vol 11. New York, Academic Press, 1977, pp. 1–39.

Drucker-Colin R, Spanis C: Neurohumoral correlates of sleep: Increase of proteins during REM sleep: *Experientia* 1975; 31:551–52.

Ervin F, Sweet W, Mark V: Amygdala function in man; the problem of violent behavior. *Acta Nerv Supp* 1970; 12:185.

Fedio P, Van Buren J: Memory deficits during electrical stimulation of the speech cortex in conscious man. *Brain Lang* 1974; 1:29–42.

Fernandez-Guardiola A: Bases electrofisiologicas de la epilepsia: Sistema limbico y activadad convulsia. *Gac Med Mex* 1976; 112:13–20.

Flexner A, Tulving E: Retrieval independence in recognition and recall. *Psychol Rev* 1978; 85:153–171.

Frieder B, Allweis C: Memory consolidation: Further evidence for the four-phase model from the time-courses of diethyldithiocarbamate and ethacrynic acid amnesia. *Physiol Behav* 1982a; 1071–1075.

Freider B, Allweis C: Prevention of hypoxia-induced transient amnesia by post-hypoxic hyperoxia. *Physiol Behav* 1982b; 29:1065–69.

Gerstmann J: Syndrome of finger agnosia, disorientation for right and left, agraphia, acalculia: Local diagnostic value. *Arch Neurol Psychiatr* 1940; 44:398–408.

Geschwind N: Disconnexion syndromes in animals and man. *Brain* 1965; 88:237–294.

Glendenning RL: Effects of training between two unilateral lesions of visual cortex upon ultimate retention of black–white discrimination habits by rats. *J Comp Psychol* 1972; 80:216–29.

Globus A, Rosenzweig, Bennett E, *et al*: Effects of differential experience on dendritic spine counts in rat cerebral cortex. *J Comp Physiol Psychol* 1973; 82:175–81.

Goldman S, Pellegrino J: Processing domain, encoding elaboration and memory trace strength. *J Verb Learn Verb Behav* 1977; 16:29–43.

Graesser A, Mandler G: Limited processing capacity constrain the storage of unrelated sets of words and retrieval from natural categories. *J Exp Psychol Hum Learn Mem* 1978; 4:86–100.

Greenberg R, Liedderman PH: Perceptions, the dream process and memory. *Comp Psychiatr* 1966; 7:507.

Greenberg R, Pearlman C: Cutting the REM nerve: An approach to the adaptive role of REM sleep. *Perspect Biol Med* 1974; 17:513–21.

Greenough W, Volkmar F: Pattern of dendritic branching in occipital cortex of rats reared in complex environments. *Exp Neurol* 1973; 40:491–504.

Gromova EA: Emotional memory and its mechanism. *Nauka Moskva* 1980.

Hebb DO: *The Organization of Behavior*. New York, Wiley, 1949.

Hecaen H, Kremin H: Reading disorders resulting from left hemisphere lesions: Aphasic and "pure" alexia, in Whitaker H, Whitaker H (eds): *Studies in Neurolinguistics*. New York, Academic Press, 1977, vol 2.

Hennevin E, LeConte P, Bloch V: La function du sommeil paradoxical: Faits et hypotheses. *L'Annee Psychol* 1971; 2.

Henschen SE: Clinical and anatomical contributions on brain pathology. *Arch Neurol Psychiatr* 1925; 13:226–249.

Hilgard E, Marquis D: *Conditioning and Learning*. New York, Appleton, 1940.

Holloway R: Cranial capacity, neural reorganization and Homonid evaluation: A search for neone suitable parameters. *Am Anthropol* 1966; 68:103–21.

Horel JA, Bettinger LA, Royce GJ, *et al*: Role of neocortex in the learning and relearning of two visual habits by the rat. *J Comp Physiol Psychol* 1966; 61:66–78.

Hubel D, Wiesel T: Sequence of regularity and geometry of orientation columns in the monkey striate cortex. *J Comp Neurol* 1974; 158:267–294.

Hunt R, Elliott J: The role of nonsemantic information in memory: Orthographic distinctiveness effects on retention. *J Exp Psychol Gen* 1980; 109:49–74.

Hyden H: The differentiation of brain cell protein, learning and memory. *Biosystems* 1977; 8:213–18.

James W: *The Principles of Psychology*. New York, Henry Holt, 1890.

John ER: *Mechanism of Memory*. New York, Academic Press, 1967.

Jones G: Fragmentation hypothesis of memory: Cued recall of pictures and of sequential position. *J Exp Psychol Gen* 1976; 105:277–293.

Jouvet M: The role of monoamines and acetylcholine–containing neurons in the regulation of sleep–waking cycle. *Ergebn Physiol* 1972; 64:166–307.

Kaada BR: Stimulation and regional ablation of the amygdaloid complex with reference to functional representations, in Eleftheriou BF (ed): *The Neurobiology of the Amygdala*. New York, Plenum Press, 1972.

Katz J, Halstead W: Protein organization and mental functions. *Comp Physiol Monogr* 1950; 20(103):1–38.

Kelly HP: Memory abilities: A factor analysis. *Psychol Monogr* 1964; Vol. 2.

Kesner RP: A neural system analysis of memory storage and retrieval. *Psychol Bull* 1973; 80:177–203.

Kesner RP, Dixon D, Pickett D, *et al*: Experimental animal model of transient global amnesia: Role of the hippocampus. *Neuropsychologia* 1975; 13:465–80.

Kesner RP, Fiedler P, Thomas G: Function of the midbrain reticular formation in regulating level of activity and learning in rats. *J Comp Physiol Psychol* 1967; 63:452–57.

Khan A: Genetic-evolutionary theory of memory. Paper presented at Neurology Conference, Loyola University Medical Center, Chicago, Illinois, March, 1985.

Kirby RJ, Kimble DP: Avoidance and escape behavior following striatal lesions in the rat. *Exp Neurol* 1969; 20:215–27.

Kluver H, Bucy P: "Psychic blindness" and other symptoms following bilateral temporal lobectomy in Rhesus monkeys. *Am J Physiol* 1937; 119:352–53.

Korsakoff SS: Etude Medico-psychologique sur une forme des maladies de la memoire. *Revue Philosophique* 1889; 28:501.

Lashley KS:P The mechanism of vision XII. Nervous structures concerned in the acquisition and retention of habits based on reaction to light. *Comp Psychol Monogr* 1935; 11:43–79.

Lashley KS: In search of the engram. *Symp Soc Exp Biol* 1950; 4:454–482.

Lorente de No R: Analysis of the activity of the chains of internuncial neurons. *J Neurophysiol* 1938; 1:207–244.

Mandler G: Recognizing: The judgment of previous occurrence. *Psychol Rev* 1980; 87:252–271.

Matthies H, Krug M, Porov V: Biological aspects of learning and memory formation and anatomy of the CNS. *Acad Verlag* 1979.

McGaugh JL, Dawson RG: Modification of memory storage processes. *Behav Sci* 1971; 16:45–63.

Melton A, Irwin J: The influence of degree of interpolated learning on retroactive inhibition and the overt transfer of specific responses. *Am J Psychol* 1940; 53:173–203.

Meyer GE, Maguire WM: Spatial frequency and the mediation of short-term visual storage. *Science* 1977; 198:524–25.

Miller GA: The magical number seven, plus or minus two: Some limits on our capacity for processing information. *Psychol Rev* 1956; 63:81–97.

Milner B: Amnesia following operation on the temporal lobes, in Whitty CW and Zangwill OL (eds): *Amnesia*. London, Butterworths, 1966; pp. 109–120.

Moor BW: Brain specific proteins, in Schenider D (ed): *Proteins of the Nervous System*. New York, Raven Press, 1973, pp. 1–13.

Murdock BB Jr: Item and order information in short-term serial memory. *J Exp Psychol* 1976; 105:191–216.

Myers RE: Visual deficits after lesions of brain stem tegmentum in cats. *Arch Neurol* 1964; 11:73–90.

Nelson T: Repetition and depth of processing. *J Verb Learn Verb Behav* 1977; 16:151–171.

Norman DA (ed): *Models of Human Memory*. New York, Academic Press, 1970.

Norman DA: What have the animal experiments taught us about human memory? in Deutsch GA (ed): *Physiological Basis of Memory*. New York, Academic Press, 1973.

Norman DA: *Memory and Attention: An Introduction to Human Information Processing* (2nd ed). New York, Wiley, 1976.

Olds J: Self-stimulation of the brain. *Science* 1958; 127:315–24.

Penfield W, Rassmussen T: *The Cerebral Cortex of Man*. New York, MacMillan, 1950.

Postman L: Mechanisms of interferences in forgetting, in Talland GA, Waugh NC (eds): *The Pathology of Memory*. New York, Academic Press, 1969, pp. 195–209.

Ransmeier R, Gerard R: Effects of temperature, convulsion and metabolic factor on rodent memory and EEG. *Am J Physiol* 1954; 179:663–64.

Rasch E, Swift H, Riesen A, *et al:* Altered structure and composition of retinal cells in dark-reared mammals. *Exp Cell Res* 1961; 25:348–63.

Rosenweig M, Mollgaard K, Diamond M, *et al:* Negative as well as positive synaptic changes may store memory. *Psychol Rev* 1972; 79:93–96.

Rozin P: Psychobiological approach to human memory, in Rosenzweig MR, Bennett EL (eds): *Natural Mechanisms of Learning and Memory.* Cambridge, Mass, MIT Press, 1976.

Russell W, Nathan P: Traumatic amnesia. *Brain* 1946; 69:280–300.

Sakitt B: Iconic memory. Psychol Rev 1976; 83:257–276.

Scoville WS, Milner B: Loss of recent memory after bilateral hippocampal lesions. *J Neurol Neurosurg Psychiatr* 1957; 20:11–21.

Sem-Jacobsen C: *Depth Electrographic Stimulation of the Human Brain and Behavior.* Springfield, Ill, Thomas, 1968.

Shashoua VE: Brain metabolism and the acquisition of new behavior. *Brain Res* 1976; 111:347.

Shiffrin RM: Information persistence in short-term memory. *J Exp Psychol* 1973; 100:39–49.

Shiffrin RM, Schneider W: Controlled and automatic human information processing: II Perceptual learning, automatic attending and a general theory. *Psychol Rev* 1977; 84:127–90.

Shulman HG: Encoding and retention of semantic and phonemic information in short-term memory. *J Verb Learn Verb Behav* 1970; 9:499–508.

Simons D, Puretz S, Finger S: Effects of serial lesions of somatosensory cortex and further neodecortication on tactile retention in rats. *Exp Brain Res* 1975; 23:353–65.

Sperry RW, Gazzaniga MC: Language following surgical disconnection of hemispheres, in Millikan C, Darley F (eds): *Brain Mechanisms Underlying Speech and Language.* New York, Grune and Stratton, 1967.

Spiliotis PH, Thompson R: The "manipulative response memory system" in the white rat. *Physiol Psychol* 1973; 1:101–14.

Thompson R: Localization of the "maze memory" system in the white rat. *Physiol Psychol* 1974; 1:1–17.

Thompson R: Card displacement response as affected by neocortical, cerebellar and limbic forebrain lesions in the rat. *Bull Psychonom Soc* 1976a; 8:103–104.

Thompson R: Stereotaxic mapping of brain stem areas critical for memory of visual discrimination habits in rat. *Physiol Psychol* 1976b; 4:1–10.

Thompson R: *A Behavior Atlas of the Rat Brain.* London/New York, Oxford University Press, 1978.

Thompson R: Functional organization of the rat brain; in Orbach J (ed): *Neuropsychology after Lashley.* Hillsdale, NJ, Erlbaum, 1982.

Thompson R, Myers R: Brain stem mechanisms underlying visually guided responses in the rhesus monkey. *J Comp Physiol Psychol* 1971; 74:479–512.

Tulving E: Episodic and semantic memory, in Tulving E, Donaldson W (eds): *Organization of Memory.* New York, Academic Press, 1972.

Tulving E: Encoding specificity retrieval processes in episodic memory. *Psychol Rev* 1973; 80:352–373.

Tulving E: Synergistic: Ecphory in recall and recognition. *Can J Psychol* 1982; 36:130–147.

Tulving E, Watkins O: Recognition failure of words with a single meaning. *Mem Cognit* 1977; 5:513–522.

Uylings HB, Smit G: Proceedings: Branching structure of cortical dendrites. *Acta Morphol Neerl-Scand* 1975; 13:110–11.

Underwood BJ, Erlebacher AH: Studies of coding in verbal learning. *Psychol Monogr* 1965; 79:25.

Verzeano M: Pacemakers, synchronization and epilepsy, in Petche H, Brazier M (eds): *Synchronization of EEG Activity in Epilepsies.* New York, Springer-Verlag, 1972.

Verzeano M, Negishi K: Neuronal activity in cortical and thalamic networks. *J Gen Psychiatr* 1960; 43(suppl):177.

Von Forester H: *Das Gedachtnis, Deuticke.* Vienna, Deuticke, 1948.

Watkins MJ: The intricacy of memory span. *Mem Cognit* 1977; 5:529–534.

Watkins M, Gardner J: An appreciation of generate–recognize theory of recall. *J Verb Learn Verb Behav* 1979; 18:687–704.

Woodward A Jr, Bjork R, Jongeward R: Recall and recognition as a function of primary rehearsal. *J Verb Learn Verb Behav* 1973; 12:608–617.

Zangwill OL: Neuropsychological models of memory, in Talland GA, Waugh NC (eds): *The Pathology of Memory*. New York, Academic Press, 1969, pp. 161–165.

Zornetzer SF, Gold M: The locus coeruleus: Its possible role in memory consolidation. *Physiol Behav* 1976; 16:331–36.

CHAPTER 2

# Memory Assessment

An ideal test of memory should estimate deficits in all types of memory processes and should suggest anatomical localization as well as the etiological nature of the pathology. There are no biological tests that indicate memory deficits. The currently available neuropsychological tests are also far from meeting this ideal goal.

Most of the tests used at present may be grouped under the following categories:

1. Single tests of memory:
   a. Verbal tests.
   b. Nonverbal tests.
2. Test batteries for memory.
3. Neuropsychological test batteries including tests for memory.
4. Questionnaires to assess memory.
5. Clinical examinations of memory.
6. Specific rating scales and inventories.

## A. SINGLE TESTS OF MEMORY (VERBAL)

Several books and review articles exist that describe and critically evaluate these tests in detail (Lezak, 1983). The verbal tests require recall of previously learned material and learning of new material such as a series of digits, letters, words, sentences, and paragraphs. The tasks are varied in length, stimulus repetition, timing, and the use of interference techniques. A few examples of these tests are as follows.

### Digit Span Tests

The Wechsler Adult Intelligence Scale includes a digit span subtest in which an increasing number of digits are presented for immediate verbal recall. The digits are recalled both in a forward and a reverse order. The rate of presentation for all digits is 1/sec.

Several variations of this test have been designed. For example, in The Point Digit Span Test (Smith, 1975) the examiner asks his subject to point out the digit series on a numbered card. This form of administration does not require a verbal response. Thus a patient with a speech problem can be tested for digit span on this test.

In the Number Span technique (Barbizer and Cany, 1968), the patient is given increasingly longer number sequences. However, each succeeding sequence differs from the one before it in its last number, e.g., 6–2, 6–2–4, 6–2–4–8, and so forth. Barbizet and Cany reported that young adults could recall an average of 9.06 numbers, whereas older persons (> 65 years) could retain only 5.87 numbers.

In the Digit Sequence Learning Test (Hamsher *et al.*, 1980; Benton *et al.*, 1983), subjects learn varying lengths of digit sequences based on their level of education. The subjects with less than 12th grade education usually learn the 8-digit sequence (Form D8); subjects with 12 or more years of education are given the 9-digit sequence (Form Kq). The task continues until the patient has repeated the digit sequence correctly for two consecutive trials or after the 12th trial. This technique is reported to be quite sensitive to memory changes accompanying normal aging (Benton *et al.*, 1981).

### Letter Span Tests

These tests are similar to the digit span tests except that letters are substituted for digits. The norms for letter span are 6.7 letters for people in their 20s and 6.5 letters for people in their 50s.

### Syllable Span Tests

Syllables, especially nonsense syllables, are used in psychological research on memory. Nobles' Tables (1961) contain 2,100 nonsense syllables of the consonant–vowel–consonant (CVC) type. The use of these syllables is a particularly good choice in memory recall when the examiner wants to minimize the confounding effects of word meaning. Talland (1965) found that normal subjects could recite as many CVC syllables as three-letter words on immediate recall.

### Word Span Tests

The use of words offers a wide variety of formats for assessing learning and recall. However, a test using words is influenced by multiple factors such as familiarity–unfamiliarity, concreteness–abstraction, and low–high association level. Toglia and Battig (1978), in their *Handbook of Semantic Word Nouns*, give ratings for 2,854 English words (and some nonwords) along seven dimensions: concreteness, imagery, categorizability, meaningfulness, familiarity, number of attributes or features, and pleasantness. Several other lists of words have been developed to help examiners choose words on the basis of their research needs (Locascio and Ley, 1972).

## Brief Word Learning Test

This test is frequently used as part of the neuropsychiatric examination. The patient is given three or four familiar but unrelated words. The patient is asked to repeat them to ensure that the words have been clearly registered. The examiner continues to question the patient on other matters for 5 min before the patient is asked to recall the words. Most patients have no difficulty in recalling three or four words 5 min later. A recall of one of three or two of four words usually indicates some impairment of verbal learning.

Several variations of this test are in vogue. In one, the examiner identifies the category after each words such as, "Chicago, a city; blue, a color; rose, a flower; orange, a fruit." If the patient misses any of the words on spontaneous recall, the examiner provides the clue to its category. Other clues such as the initial letter or the phoneme of the forgotten word or multiple choice format may be provided. If the patient is able to recall the words with the help of clues, it usually implies that the patient has a retrieval problem rather than a storage problem. The recall of the words may be delayed for 10 or 30 min or more to assess delayed recall.

Word span may be tested, like "Number Span Technique," beginning with a two-word list and adding a word after each successful repetition. Miller (1973) found that a group of control subjects achieved on the average a word span of five words. The word span remains fairly stable during the early years. There is a tendency for people in their 50s and 60s to do less well than the younger groups.

## Memory for Sentences

An average adult can correctly recall sentences of 24 or 25 syllables in length (Williams, 1965). The Stanford-Binet Scales include a sentence memory test at several age levels, beginning with 12-syllable sentences for 4-year-olds, 16 to 19-syllable sentences for 11-year-olds, and 20-syllable sentences for 13-year-olds. The syntax and vocabulary become more complex at higher age levels.

## Memory for Paragraph and Stories

It is generally not possible to memorize a paragraph or a story word by word. However, most people can recall the ideas presented in the paragraph using some of their own words and some from the actual presentation. Scoring paragraph recall presents a number of problems due to substitutions, omissions, additions, elaborations, and shifts in the story's sequence. Several methods of scoring have been suggested. Rapaport *et al.* (1968) developed a system in which they scored as correct all segments of the story in which "the change does not alter the general meaning of the story or its details." They also included a four-point "distortion score" that reflects the extent to which alterations change the gist of the story. Thus they give credit to all minor alterations as accurate "meaningful memories."

Another scoring method suggested by Talland and Ekdahl (1959) makes a distinction between verbatim and content (semantic) recall of the story. They divided meaningful verbal material into separate scoring units for verbatim recall and for content ideas. The content ideas are scored as correctly recalled if the subject makes substitutions with synonyms or with suitable phrases for the exact wording.

Several of the paragraphs and stories that have been standardized for testing immediate and delayed recall include stories in the Stanford-Binet Test, the Wechsler Memory Scale, the Babcock Story Recall Test, and the Cowboy Story.

### The Babcock Story Recall Test (Babcock, 1930; Babcock and Levy, 1940)

This is a paragraph recall test to assess both immediate and delayed recall. The following paragraph is divided into 21 measuring units for recall:

> December 6./Last week/ a river/ overflowed/ in a small town/ ten miles/ from Albany./ Water covered the streets/ and entered the houses./ Fourteen persons/ were drowned/ and 600 persons/ caught cold/ because of the dampness/ and cold weather./ In saving/ a boy/ who was caught/ under a bridge,/ a man/ cut his hands.

The examiner starts with the instruction, "I am going to read a story to you now. Listen carefully because when I finish I'm going to ask you to tell me as much of the story as you can remember." After the paragraph is read, the subject is asked, "Now tell me everything you can remember of the story." The examiner may encourage the subject by providing some structure for recall with questions such as "what happened," "where did it happen," or "who was involved?"

After the first recall the paragraph is read again to assess delayed recall with the instruction, "In a little while I'm going to ask you to tell me how much of the story you can still remember. I'm going to read the story to you again now so that you have it fresh in your memory for the next time." The examiner continues testing the patient on other material for 20 min before the subject is asked to recall the story for an assessment of delayed recall. Again, the examiner may encourage the subject to recall the story as before.

The number of memory units recalled constitutes the score for immediate and delayed recall. Four points are added to the immediate recall score to equate for the second reading of the paragraph before the delayed recall trials. The total scores for immediate recall usually vary from 13 to 15 and for delayed recall 15 to 17 depending upon the intellectual abilities of the subjects.

*The Cowboy Story*

The following story is used frequently in the mental status examination for the assessment of immediate recall:

> A *cowboy*/ from *Arizona*/ went to *San Francisco*/ with his *dog,*/ which he *left*/ at a *friend's*/ while he *purchased*/ a *new* suit of *clothes.*/ Dressed finely,/ he *went back*/ to the *dog,*/ *whistled* to him,/ *called him* by name/ and *patted* him./ But the dog *would have nothing to do* with him,/ in his new *hat*/ and *coat,*/ but gave a *mournful*/ *howl.*/ *Coaxing* was of no effect/; so the cowboy *went away*/ and donned his *old garments,*/ whereupon the *dog*/ *immediately*/ showed his wild *joy*/ on *seeing his master*/ as he thought he *ought* to be./ (Talland, 1965)

Talland (1965; Talland and Ekdahl, 1959) divided the above story into 17 memory units for quantitative verbatim recall and identified 24 content ideas (italicized words or phrases) which are credited as correctly recalled even if the subject substitutes synonyms or suitable phrases for them. The average score for verbatim recall of the story is 8.32 memory units and for content recall 9.56 units.

## B. SINGLE TESTS OF MEMORY (NONVERBAL)

Immediate and delayed recall may also be tested with stimuli that do not require verbal responses such as copying a figure, matching a design, or responding to specific sounds. Unfortunately, there is a lot of silent verbal labeling of the stimuli during the performance of these tests so that they cannot be considered pure tests of nonverbal memory abilities. To reduce verbal mediation, nonsense figures or shapes are used. However, even the most complex of such figures cannot escape some verbal mediation.

### Visual Memory Tests

*Recurring Figures Test (Kimura, 1963)*

In this test, 20 cards with geometric or irregular nonsense figures are shown to the subjects, one at a time. At the completion, another pack of 140 cards is shown, 3 sec for each card. The second pack of cards contains seven sets of eight of the original 20 designs which are interspersed throughout the rest of the 84 one-of-a-kind-design cards. The subject is asked to indicate the cards that he has seen previously. False positives are subtracted from the right responses to correct for guessing. A perfect performance score is 56 on this test. The average score for young adults is 44 which decreases with increasing age. Newcome (1969) found that the average score was 28.5 ± 6.92 for a group of 28 subjects who were mostly in their forties.

### Visual Retention Test (Warrington and James, 1967)

This test includes 20 5 × 5 inch white cards containing four blackened squares that are positioned in various ways so that no two designs are alike. Each card is presented for 2 sec. After each exposure, subjects are asked to choose the identical figure from a set of four similar figures. During the second administration, the stimulus figures are rotated 180° and the exposure of each figure is extended to 10 sec. This multiple choice recognition task was designed to minimize verbal mediation. Ten control subjects made, on the average, 3.3 errors on the first administration and 2.2 errors on the second administration with combined errors of 5.5 out of a maximum possible error score of 40.

### Object and Picture Memory Span Tests

Real objects or pictures may be used to test visual span. The tests vary in the type of objects, exposure time, and the length of interval before recall. Unfortunately, verbal mediation plays a major role in the recall of familiar objects and this effect cannot be separated from visual retention in these tests.

In the Memory Span for Objects Test (Wells and Ruesch, 1969), the subject is shown pictures of objects which he then names aloud. At the completion, the subject is asked to recall them much like a wordspan test. An adult, on the average, recalls 11 out 20 pictures and 7 ± 1.4 out of 10 pictures.

Squire (1974) tested remote memory with 15 pictures of objects that were presented one at a time for 3 sec each. Thirty minutes later the subject was shown a series of 30 pictures with 15 original and 15 new pictures mixed together. The task was to recognize the original pictures. Each correct answer was given one point with a maximum of 30 points.

### The Nonlanguage Paired-Associate Learning Test (Fowler, 1969)

This test was designed for individuals whose language deficits did not allow them to take verbal learning tests. The test is patterned after the Associate Learning Test of the Wechsler Memory Scale with the exception that real objects are used instead of words. The test material includes six sets of objects that are easily associated in pairs (such as fork and knife) and four sets of objects that make hard-to-associate pairs (such as a cigar and a red rubber ball). The subject is presented all of the pairs of objects for visual association. Then one item of each pair is shown and the subject is expected to pick out the second item of the pair from a set of 22 items. Several trials of ten pairs are given, but the order in which each item is presented varies from trial to trial.

## Design Reproduction Tests

There are several design reproduction tests used for immediate visual recall. Several standardized tests such as the Wechsler Memory Scale and the Binet Test contain designs that are exposed for 10 sec each before the subject is expected to reproduce them on paper. The designs can be used both for immediate and delayed recall. The following are the commonly used single design reproduction tests.

*The Benton Visual Retention Tests (Benton et al., 1974).* This is a widely used visual recall test. It has three forms that are roughly equivalent in difficulty level. Each form has ten cards with designs. Most cards have three figures, two large and one small. The small figure is always placed at one side or the other of the large figures. There are three administration procedures for this test. The figures are exposed for 10 sec during administration A and for 5 sec during administration B with immediate recall of the figures by drawing. In administration procedure C, the subject is encouraged to copy the figures as accurately as possible. Each administration is scored for both the number of correct designs and the number of errors. Six types of errors are recognized: omission, distortion, perserveration, rotation, misplacement, and size. There are separate normative tables for the expected number of correct scores and for the expected error scores by estimated premorbid IQ and age. Taking the subject's age and intellectual endowment into account, one can determine from these tables whether the subject's correct and error scores fall into the impairment category.

## Visual Sequence Recall Tests

Several tests have been designed to test the visual memory for a sequence of blocks, pictures, or numbers.

*Learning a Place in Space.* A square frame or a card is divided into nine $3 \times 3$ sets of squares. Nine pictures of different objects are placed in the squares, one at a time, for 5 sec each then removed. After all of the nine pictures have been placed in their predesignated places and removed, the subject is asked to locate their original place on the board. The examiner confirms the right responses and corrects the errors immediately. This procedure is continued until the subject learns the correct places for all of the nine pictures. If the subject continues to fail by the tenth trial, the examiner modifies the procedure by leaving correctly identified pictures in their squares, thus reducing the probability of making a mistake. This modified procedure is then continued until the subject succeeds on three consecutive trials. The test is discontinued if the subject does not learn by the tenth trial with the modified procedure. The subject is then tested for delayed recall at varying intervals (3 min, 24 hr, and 4 days) in three ways: (1) by pointing to the square and naming the picture that belonged there without the picture being present; (2) by placing the pictures in the correct squares. The pictures are presented in the same order as in the original presentation; and (3) by placing the pictures in the correct squares when they all are handed together to the subject.

A control group of subjects is reported to have learned the test in one to four trials and made six to nine correct identifications on the three types of recall.

*Learning a Code.*   This test requires a subject to learn the principle involved in the sequential arrangement of bead colors. The examiner begins by hiding a bead of a specified color and asking the subject to guess the first color in the bead sequence and then showing the bead. The subject learns several sequences of colors of different lengths. The criteria for learning a sequence are three correct consecutive trials. Most subjects usually learn all code lengths in six or fewer trials.

*The Corsis Block-Tapping Test (Milner, 1971).*   This test consists of nine numbered black 1½ inch cubes fastened in a random order to a black board. The examiner taps the blocks in a prearranged sequence and the subject is asked to copy each tapping pattern. By adding one tap to each succeeding successful sequence, the examiner determines the tapping span for immediate recall. Twenty-four test trials of tapping sequences of increasing length are administered.

*The Knox Cube Imitation Test.*   This test consists of four cube blocks affixed in a row on a strip of wood. The examiner taps the cubes in a prearranged sequence of increasing length and complexity. The subject is asked to copy the pattern after the examiner. This is a simple test and may require only about 5 min for administration.

### Tests of Tactile Memory

Tactile memory is frequently tested by blindfolding the subjects then having them recognize the forms and shapes by moving their fingers over them.

### Senquin Formboard

This test was originally designed for testing visuospatial performance. Halstead (1947) converted it into a tactile memory test by blindfolding the patients and having them recognize the shapes on the board. There are several variations of the use of the Senquin Formboard for testing tactile memory. It has been integrated in the Halstead–Reitan Neuropsychiatric battery.

## Tactile Nonsense Figures (Milner, 1971)

This test consists of four pieces of wire twisted into different nonsense shapes. Subjects are asked to draw the shapes after they have felt the wire figures with their fingers.

## Fuld Object-Memory Evaluation (Fuld, 1977, 1980)

This test consists of a bag containing ten small common objects such as a ball, bottle, button, card, cup, key, matches, nail, ring, and scissors. The subject is asked to name or describe each of the ten objects by feeling them in the bag using the right and left hands alternatively as requested by the examiner. Each item identified by the subject is pulled out of the bag so that the subject can see it and check his guesses until all the items are identified and labeled. Then a distractor task is given by asking as many names as the subject can think of in 1 min. After the distractor task, the subject is asked to recall all the items that he had identified in the bag. This is followed by four learning and recall trials. One distractor task is inserted between each learning trial. The next 15 min are spent on other test material after which the subject is asked again to recall all ten items. The test is terminated if all ten items are recalled correctly. If not, the missed items are presented in a three-item multiple choice format.

Several memory scores are derived from this test: (1) *Total Recall* is the sum of items correctly named in all five trials. (2) *Storage* is the total number of items recalled at least once during the first five recall trials. (3) *Repeated Retrieval* is the sum of items named without reminding. (4) *Ineffective Reminders* is the sum of instances in which a reminder was not followed by correct recall on the next trials.

## Tests for Remote Memory

Tests designed to test remote memory include recognition of faces of famous people and recalling past important public events.

Albert and associates (Albert, 1981; Butters and Albert, 1982) collected 25 photographs of persons who achieved fame in each of the six decades (1920s to 1970s) making a total of 180 pictures that were presented as a recognition test. In a variation of this test, patients are given several names if they are unable to recognize a face to enhance their recall.

Warrington and Silberstein (1970) developed a multiple choice questionnaire for assessing memory of events that had occurred in the previous year. This method was later extended to cover events for the four preceding decades. Sanders (1972) has criticized this examination technique because of the extensive variations of individual interest in local and worldwide events.

## C. TEST BATTERIES FOR MEMORY

### The Wechsler Memory Scale (WMS)

Wechsler published his "rapid, simple and practical memory examination" in 1945. It consists of the following seven subtests:

1. Personal and Current Information: The subject is asked for age, date of birth, and identification of current and recent public officials.
2. Orientation: is assessed by questions about the time and place.
3. Mental Control: This subcategory is designed to test automatism such as repeating the alphabet and simple conceptual tracking as in counting by fours from 1 to 53.
4. Logical Memory: This subtest includes immediate recall of verbal ideas from two paragraphs. The examiner first reads the two paragraphs but stops after each paragraph to get the subject's immediate free recall. Paragraph A contains 24 memory units or ideas and paragraph B contains 33. The subject is given one point of credit for each correct idea recalled. The total score is the average recalled. The total score is 23.
5. Digit Span: This subject differs from the Digit Span Subtest of the Wechsler Adult Intelligence Scale by omitting the three-digit trial of digit forward and the two-digit trial of digit backward and not giving score credits for performance of nine or eight backward.
6. Visual Reproduction: Each of three cards with a printed design is shown for 5 sec. Following each exposure, the patient draws what he remembers of the design. This is an immediate recall test but some examiners also recommend a delayed trial.
7. Associate Learning Test: consists of ten word pairs, six forming "easy" common associations such as "baby–cries" and the other four pairs are uncommon or "hard" associations such as "cabbage–pen." The list of the word pairs is read three times. The subject tries to recall as many pair associates as he can remember after each reading. The total score is one half the sum of all correct associations to the easy pairs plus the sum of all correct associations to the hard pairs. The highest possible score is 21.

Erickson and Scott (1977) criticized the WMS on the basis of the relatively small normative population, the lack of normative data for all ages, and its poor record in differentiating between organically impaired and normal individuals. This test combines the scores of various subtests to estimate Memory Quotient. This concept is overly inclusive and tends to ignore the multidimensional aspects of memory functions. Dissatisfaction with the WMS led Russell (1975) to revise it. He identified two subtests of the WMS, logical memory and visual reproduction, as measures of immediate recall which together provide an assessment of verbal and configurational memory. Half an hour after the administration of each subtest, a second recall trial is given which produces a score for delayed recall.

### Cronholm and Molander Memory Test Battery

Cronholm and Molander (1957) developed a memory test battery which they employed to study the efect of electroconvulsive treatment, brain injury, and cerebral palsy. The battery consists of the following three sets of material (each with two forms, A and B).

1. Fifteen Word Pair Test: The word pairs used in this test have a low association value (less than 1%).
2. Fifteen Figure Test: This test has 15 drawings of familiar objects which are first shown to a subject for visual retention. They are then mixed with 15 other drawings and the subject is required to identify the original drawings.
3. The Nine Personal Data Test: In this test the subject is required to associate three fictitious facts with each of the three photographs of persons.

Both word pairs and personal data tests require a recall response, while the figure test requires a recognition of the learned material when it appears in a larger picture with drawings of 15 other objects. The test is used for both immediate and delayed recall. The battery has been useful in demonstrating how levels of immediate and delayed recall may vary in depression and as a consequence of different disorders of the central nervous system (Cronholm and Ottoson, 1963).

### Randt Memory Test Battery (Randt *et al.*, 1980)

This test is brief and contains seven subtests referred to as modules: general information, recall of five words, digit forward, digit backward, recall of paragraph, and incidental learning. The test takes approximately 20 min for administration and was designed for the longitudinal follow-up of drug effects, especially the memory-enhancing drugs in the older population. The test has five different forms for repeated examinations. The first and the last modules of each form are identical in all forms. An interesting feature of this test is the use of telephone interviews to obtain 24-hr recall data.

## D. NEUROPSYCHOLOGICAL TEST BATTERIES

Several neuropsychological batteries have been constructed to meet clinical and research needs. Most of these batteries were designed to assess brain damage. They include, however, tests of memory functions. Since brain damage is frequently associated with impairment of memory functions, these batteries have been popular in assessing both brain damage and memory impairment. The Halstead–Reitan Neuropsychological Battery, neuropsychiatric batteries derived from Luria's work, (Christensen, 1979) and the Michigan Neuropsychological Battery (Smith, 1980) are the commonly used test batteries.

## The Halstead–Reitan Neuropsychological Battery

Ward Halstead, through his observation of brain-damaged individuals, attempted to measure behavioral characteristics of brain-damaged individuals more formally through modification and development of various psychological tests. Factor analytic techniques were applied to the data derived from these tests to obtain the optimum set of procedures for exploring further the psychology of brain functions and damage. Halstead's interpretation of these analyses led to the inclusion of ten measures in his battery and the adoption of a four-factor theory of human performance. Ralph M. Reitan, a student of Halstead, included several additional procedures in the battery. These additional measures included age, the appropriate Wechsler Intelligence Scale, an aphasia and sensory perceptual battery, the Trail Making Test, and a measure of grip strength.

The tests that make up the complete set of the neuropsychological examination vary somewhat according to the patient's age. The Halstead Neuropsychological Test Battery and Allied Procedures are used for persons 15 years of age and older. For children ages 9 to 15, the Halstead Neuropsychological Test Battery for Children and Allied Procedures are used. The Reitan Indiana Neuropsychological Test Battery for Children is used for children ages 5 to 9. The Halstead Neuropsychological Test Battery for adults has been modified considerably from its original form. Two of the tests have been eliminated. The Critical Flicker Fusion Test was eliminated because of a failure of statistical validation. The second test, the Time Sense Test, was eliminated because it was not helpful in evaluating the performance of patients considered individually. This leaves five tests and seven variables in the Halstead Battery from which the Impairment Index is computed. The five tests in the Halstead Battery are the following:

1. Category Test: This consists of 208 items divided into seven subtests. The items on slides are presented one at a time by a self-contained projection apparatus on a screen that is placed in front of the subject. In the front of this apparatus there is a panel with four lights numbered one to four and beneath each light is a lever. The patient is told that the stimulus on the screen will suggest a number between one and four. The patient then must press the lever under the number thought to be correct. Only one response is allowed for each item. The patient is provided immediate feedback via a pleasant doorbell for a correct answer or a buzzer for an incorrect answer. The patient is told that in each subtest responses are based on a single principle.

The responses to the first few items in each subtest are usually made randomly until the principle is found through feedback. The patient is never told the principle either during or after the test. However, the patient is told at the end of each subtest that a new subtest is about to begin in which the principle may be the same or may be different from that of the last subtest. There is no time limit for this test. The score is the total number of errors on the seven subtests. The category test is considered to be a learning experiment and supposedly taps current learning skills, abstract concept formation, and mental efficiency. Patients who do poorly on these tests are often characterized as having poor judgment and memory problems.

2. Tactual Performance Test: This test is a modified Senquin-Goddard Formboard. This board contains ten spaces for blocks of various shapes. The board is placed vertically in a stand in front of the patient. The blocks are placed in between the patient and the board. The patient is blindfolded before the start of this test and is not allowed to see the board or the blocks before, during, or after the test. The patient is instructed to place the blocks with the preferred hand into the proper spaces of the board as quickly as possible. At the end of the first trials all the blocks are removed from the board and are placed in front of the patient. The patient is asked to perform the same task with the nonpreferred hand. A third trial is carried out in a similar manner with the use of both hands. The total time for all three trials is the score that contributes to the impairment index. Time for each trial is also noted separately. The time score allows for evaluation of the data in terms of the level of performance and comparative efficiency of the two sides of the body working alone and together.

After the board and the blocks are placed out of sight, the blindfold is removed and the patient is asked to draw the board on a piece of paper with all the spaces or blocks in their proper places. If an exact place for a block is forgotten, it can be drawn anywhere on the board. A score for memory (number of blocks remembered) and localization (number of correctly placed blocks) is obtained. Credit is given if a shape is drawn that does not look like any of the blocks but is correctly identified verbally.

This test is supposed to assess several abilities including motor speed, use of tactile and kinesthetic cues to enhance psychomotor coordination, learning, response to the information, and the ability to remember things when not explicitly directed to do so (incidental memory).

3. Rhythm Test: This is a subtest of Seashore's Test of Musical Talent. In this test 30 pairs of rhythmic beats are presented by a tape recorder. The patient is asked to identify the pairs as either the same or different. The score is a scaled score based on the number of correct identifications, with one being the best and ten the worst possible scaled score. This task is supposed to measure nonverbal auditory perception, attention, and sustained concentration.

4. Speech-Sounds Perception Test: Sixty nonsense words are presented on a tape recorder. The patient is given a paper containing six subtests with

ten rows of four words in each subtest. After a word is spoken, the patient is asked to identify it from the four words on the appropriate line. The score is the total number of misidentifications. This test is supposed to assess auditory–verbal perception, auditory–visual coordination of language processing, and sustained attention and concentration throughout a relatively complex and rapid task.

5. Finger Oscillation Test: This is a test of motor speed. The patient is asked to depress a lever with the index finger of each hand. The lever is connected to a manual counter. The patient is given several consecutive trials (usually five) with each hand and is encouraged to tap as rapidly as possible. Each trial lasts ten seconds. The score for each hand is the average of five trials. The test assesses motor speed. The preferred hand speed is expected to exceed the nonpreferred hand speed by 10%.

### Allied Procedures

These tests are generally included in a comprehensive neuropsychological examination. They include the following:

1. Trail-making Test: The test is divided into two parts; A and B. Part A consists of 25 circles drawn over an 8½ × 11 inch sheet of white paper. The circles are numbered from 1 to 25. The patient is required to connect the circles with a pencil in numerical order from 1 to 25 as rapidly as possible. Before the main task is carried out, practice is provided on a brief example on a separate sheet. During the task, if a circle is connected out of order the patient is stopped, corrected, and begun again from that point. The score is the total time spent due to errors.

Part B of the test also contains 25 circles drawn on a paper. The circles are either numbered from 1 to 13 or lettered A to L. The patient is required to connect the circles in order by alternating between numbers and letters, that is 1-A, 2-B, 3-C, and so on. The score is the total time spent in completion. Part B is roughly two and a half times more difficult than part A.

The test is supposed to assess motor speed, visual scanning, and the ability to progress in sequence.

2. Strength of Grip Test: A plunger-type dynamometer, with an adjustable hand grip, is used to measure hand strength. Two trials alternating between preferred and nonpreferred hand are given. The score is the average of two trials for each hand. The test measures grip strength in the upper extremities and also provides left–right comparison.

3. Sensory-Perceptual Examination: In this test, tactile, auditory, and visual stimuli are first presented unilaterally to one side of the body, then they are presented bilaterally in a simultaneous manner.

a. Tactile: The back of each hand and each side of the face are touched lightly when the patient's eyes are closed. The patient is asked to identify the side touched. The patient is then touched bilaterally simultaneously to determine whether the patient perceives both stimuli or whether the stimuli on one side of the body are ignored. The score is the number of times only one side is reported on bilateral simultaneous stimulation. The patient is never told that the stimuli are applied to both sides of the body.

b. Visual: Stimuli are presented in the peripheral field of vision unilaterally and bilaterally. The examiner sits facing the patient who focuses on the examiner's nose. The examiner stretches his arms out at an equidistance between himself and the patient. The examiner wiggles his finger in all quadrants of the peripheral vision, first unilaterally then bilaterally in a simultaneous manner.

c. Auditory: The examiner first presents a slight noise (such as pressing of fingers and separating them) to each ear separately. If the patient can hear unilateral stimulation, he is presented bilateral stimuli simultaneously. The score is equal to the number of suppressions on bilateral simultaneous trials.

4. Tactile Perception:

a. Beginning with the preferred hand, all the fingers of both hands are touched lightly one by one. A system allowing the patient to identify which finger is touched is established before the test begins. The fingers are identified by numbers from one to five starting with the thumb. The order of finger touch is predetermined and stimuli are presented with the patient's eyes closed. Each finger is touched four times. The score is the number of errors out of twenty trials for each hand.

b. Fingertip Number-Writing Perception: The numbers are written with an empty ballpoint pen on the balls of the patient's fingertips, the patient's eyes being closed. The numbers 3, 4, 5, and 6 are written four times on each hand in a predetermined order. The numbers are first written larger on the palm of the hands to identify the way the numbers will be written. The score is the number of errors out of 20 trials for each hand.

c. Tactile Form Recognition: The patient places one hand through a hole in a board. One of four forms (square, cross, circle, and triangle) of plastic chips is placed in the fingers of that hand. The patient is asked to point to the corresponding chip displayed on the board facing the patient. No verbal response needs to be made. Each of the four forms are placed twice in each hand. The score is the number of errors for each hand and the total response time for each hand from the time the form is placed on the fingers until the identification is made with the other hand.

## Modified Halstead–Wepman Aphasia Screening Test

This test is designed to assess various aspects of language ability. The patient is asked to name objects, read, spell, identify letters and numbers, write, calculate and identify body parts, pantomime simple actions, understand the meaning of spoken language, differentiate right and left, and follow verbal directions.

## Criticism

This battery was devised in the 1930s and has undergone few alterations. The diagnostic data derived from the tests relate to older disease classifications, making interpretation difficult. Efforts to use the Halstead–Reitan Battery to localize lesions in the brain have produced equivocal results. The battery does elicit differential performance patterns between right and left hemisphere lesions (Klove, 1974; Reitan, 1955). However, without the sensory examination added to the battery by Reitan (1966), the remaining tests do not identify right–left hemispheric differences with sufficient consistency (Schreiber *et al.*, 1976). It should be noted that the battery's greatest strength in making left–right discrimination in lesion localization comes from several brief sensory and motor tests that neurologists have relied on for decades to make the same diagnostic distinctions. A few other studies (Dodrill and Troupin, 1975; Matarazzo *et al.*, 1974) also suggest that neither the Impairment Index nor several of the subtests are highly stable measures in some specific populations.

## Luria's Neuropsychological Battery

Christensen (1979) brought together Luria's neuropsychological exmaination techniques in a single set of materials. This collection is organized into ten sections: motor functions, acousticomotor organization, higher cutaneous and kinesthetic functions, higher visual functions, impressive (i.e., receptive) speech, expressive speech, writing and reading, arithmetic skills, mnestic processes, and investigation of intellectual processes. This battery is not comprehensive and does not satisfy all the requirements of a neuropsychological examination. For example, few techniques are included to assess nonverbal memory or nonverbal concept formation. The subtests of verbal memory and learning are not of sufficient difficulty to pick up subtle learning deficits.

Golden and associates (1981) have developed a neuropsychological battery (the Luria-Nebraska Neuropsychological Battery) which incorporates items drawn from Luria's work in a standardized test format. This battery has limitations for predicting the site of lesion. Crossen and Warren (1982) reported that the battery misidentified the site of lesion in an aphasic patient with a posterior lesion and another patient with two right-sided cerebral vascular attacks had significant scale elevation indicating both left- and right-sided lesions.

## E. QUESTIONNAIRES TO ASSESS MEMORY

Several investigators have independently developed questionnaires to assess people's beliefs about their memory performance in natural circumstances. These questionnaires describe prototypical memory situations and ask respondents multiple choice questions about how their memory performs in the situations specified. The content of these questionnaires vary to fit the specific needs of the clinical or research situations, such as:

1. Questionnaires that test memory for historical facts (Squire and Slater, 1975).
2. Questionnaires about salient life events (Jenkins *et al.*, 1979).
3. Clinical interviews about memory (Talland, 1968).
4. Experimental memory tasks used in clinical assessment of memory aptitude (Erickson and Scott, 1977).
5. Questionnaires asking the respondent to evaluate their memory performance in specified situations on the basis of repeated experience with everyday memory tasks.

People's beliefs about their memory result from their subjective experiences in performing memory tasks and from feedback from friends and relatives about their memory performance. As a consequence, the beliefs themselves influence memory performance. A person falsely believing he is good in remembering directions is less likely to pay attention when specific directions are given. Similarly, a person is less likely to do well in remembering names if he falsely believes he is poor at remembering names. Thus people's beliefs may facilitate as well as impair memory performance.

Many questionnaires in their present form correlate only moderately with performance of laboratory and everyday memory tasks. People's beliefs about their memory performances tend to be stable but not very accurate. Research reports indicate that responses to many questionnaires vary with several variables, such as the kind of memory failure, susceptibility to cognitive failure under stress (Broadbent *et al.*, 1982), confidence in memory performance (Schulster, 1981), and the age of the subject. In order to obtain more accurate assessment of memory, all present-day questionnaires should be supplemented with objective measures of memory.

## F. CLINICAL EXAMINATION OF MEMORY

Most neuropsychiatric examinations include a mental status examination to determine the patient's neurological and psychiatric status. Memory assessment is an important part of a comprehensive mental status examination. However, in order to reach some conclusion about memory deficits, it is necessary to assess other mental functions such as the patient's level of awareness, verbal functions, attention and concentration, emotional status, and intellectual potential. A deficit in any one of these areas is likely to affect functions in other areas as well as memory. In fact, most mental functions overlap with each other and a separation of such functions is artificial.

Many tests assess immediate, recent, and remote memory. The confusion created by the use of different terms should be kept in mind. For example, the term "short-term memory" is used by psychologists for what neurologists call immediate memory. Similarly, psychological "long-term memory" is similar to the neurological term "recent memory."

Immediate memory is tested by asking patients to recall a series of numbers, words, or events immediately after they are uttered by the examiner. The Digit Span Test (discussed earlier in this chapter) is usually a good test to assess immediate recall. Normal persons can recall seven digits forward and five digits backward. Some authors suggest that this is not a memory function since material handled in immediate recall is not necessarily retained for later recall. This is, however, an important initial process in learning retention.

Recent memory is tested by asking about events of the day that may have occurred several hours earlier. The examiner may use words, names or a sentence for the patient to memorize for later recall, making sure that the patient has repeated the material correctly. Recall of the material 5 to 10 min later would be a test of recent memory. Most persons can recall four names after 10 min. Recent memory reflects the ability to learn new material. Nonverbal tests may also be used to test recent memory. The patient may be asked to point to three objects in the room and recall them a few minutes later.

Remote or long-term memory is tested by asking the patient the events of the past that may be corroborated by close relatives. Similarly, recall of political figures and major social world events will serve the same purpose.

A failure to recall recent or remote events requires a discrimination between impairment in the initial process of registration and inability to retrieve already-learned material. The latter process is designated as forgetting. Everybody has a tendency to forget and it is exaggerated with advancing age. To demonstrate forgetting, three stages in the testing process must be undertaken. First, there is the memorization task. Second, a test must be given to show that the material presented was actually present in the memory storage. Third, a later test is given to demonstrate that there has been a loss between the first and second testing. In the clinical setting, the examiner may provide clues for the recall of remote events. Severe retrieval problems do not respond to memory cues.

## G. SPECIFIC RATING SCALES AND INVENTORIES

The specific rating scales and inventories discussed here have been designed for specific populations that have memory deficits as an essential or prominent aspect of their disorder such as Alzheimer's disease, multi-infarct dementia, and brain damage. Only a few of the scales are mentioned here.

## Sandoz Clinical Assessment—Geriatric (Shader *et al.*, 1974)

The 19 items in the scale rate behavior disorder, mood states, and cognitive functions. Behavioral items focus on activities such as self-care, eating, unsociability, and emotional lability. Each item is scored on a seven-point scale that ranges from one (= not present) to seven (= severe). The scale is reported to discriminate between groups of normal volunteers and elderly patients with mild and severe dementia. (See appendix for the scale.)

## Dementia Score Scale (Hachinsky *et al.*, 1975)

This scale measures how well the patient gets along in his usual environment. It contains 22 items that rate changes in the performance of everyday activities and changes in habits such as eating, dressing, sphincter control, and emotional control. The patients suffering from primary degenerative disease (i.e., Alzheimer's and related diseases) or multi-infarct dementia score from 4 to 25 with group averages of 11.6 (SD = 5.4) and 12.0 (SD = 5.1), respectively. Another scale, Ischemic Score (Hachinski *et al.*, 1975), distinguishes well multi-infarct dementia from degenerative diseases.

## The Alzheimer's Disease Assessment Scale (Rosen *et al.*, 1984)

The authors of the scale claim that the scale is a valid indicator of the increasing severity of dysfunction occurring over time in Alzheimer's disease. The scale rates cognitive and noncognitive behavior on 21 items. Each item is rated one (= not present) to five (= severe). The cognitive behavior is rated on nine items which include spoken language ability, comprehension of spoken language, recall of instructions, word finding difficulty, following commands, naming objects and fingers, constructional praxis, ideational praxis, and orientation with a maximum score of 48 points. There are two memory items: (1) a word-recall task in which the patient reads ten high-imagery words exposed for 2 sec each. The patient then recalls the words aloud. Three trials of reading and recall are given. The score equals the mean number of words not recalled on three trials (maximum = 10); (2) a word-recognition task in which the patient reads aloud 12 high-imagery words. These words are then randomly mixed with 12 words the patient has not seen. The patient indicates whether the words were shown previously. Then two more trials of reading the original words and recognition are given. The score equals the mean number of incorrect responses for three trials (maximum = 12). The noncognitive subscale has ten items such as depression, distractibility, delusions, and hallucinations with a maximum score of 50 points. Subjects with Alzheimer's disease have significantly more cognitive and noncognitive dysfunctions than normal elderly subjects.

## Brief Psychiatric Rating Scale (Overall and Gorham, 1962)

This scale has been used by psychiatrists and psychologists in evaluating primarily psychiatric patients. The scale, however, contains items that rate prominent features of some organic conditions (e.g., motor retardation, conceptual disorganization, blunted affect). The scale consists of 19 items. Each item represents a relatively discrete symptom area. Ratings are made on a seven-point scale (1 = not present; 7 = extremely severe).

## Brief Cognitive Rating Scale (BCRS) (Reisberg *et al.*, 1983)

Patients with Alzheimer's disease show a fairly uniform decline on BCRS which utilizes seven rating categories for each of the five axes. Several other diagnostic categories such as mania and acute anxiety will cause some deficits on the concentration axis. The five axes include the following: concentration and calculating ability, recent memory, past memory, orientation, and functioning and self-care. Items in each axis are scored from information obtained during a clinical interview with the patient in the presence of spouse or the caretaker. (See appendix for the scale.)

## Global Deterioration Scale (GDS) (Reisberg *et al.*, 1982)

The Global Deterioration Scale is a clinical scale that describes clinical characteristics of Alzheimer's disease in seven stages that correspond to seven clinical phases as follows:

| GDS Stages | Clinical Phases |
|---|---|
| 1. No cognitive decline | Normal |
| 2. Very mild cognitive decline | Forgetfulness |
| 3. Mild cognitive decline | Early confusion |
| 4. Moderate cognitive decline | Late confusion |
| 5. Moderately severe decline | Early dementia |
| 6. Severe cognitive decline | Middle dementia |
| 7. Very severe cognitive decline | Late dementia |

Clinical characteristics of each stage and phase are described in a fairly clear-cut manner.

## H. SUMMARY

Assessment of memory functions is generally included in a comprehensive mental status examination. Clinical tests of memory frequently test immediate, recent, and remote memory. The confusion created by the use of different terms should be kept in mind. For example, the term "short-term memory" is used by psychologists for what neurologists call "immediate memory" and the psychological term "long-term memory" is similar to the neurological term "recent memory."

Among the large number of tests designed to test various memory processes, it is at times difficult to select an appropriate test for a particular type of memory problem. It is, however, helpful to become familiar with a few selected tests for routine clinical screening. For example, immediate memory may be tested by asking patients to recall a series of numbers or words immediately after they are uttered by the examiner. The Digit Span Test is usually a good test to assess immediate recall. A normal person can recall seven digits forward and five digits backward.

Recent memory may be tested by asking about events of the day that may have occurred several hours earlier. Patients may be given words, names, or a sentence for later recall, making sure that the patient comprehends it well by asking him to repeat after the examiner. Recall of the material 5 to 10 min later would be a test of recent memory. Most persons can recall four names after 10 min. Recent memory reflects the ability to learn new material. Nonverbal tests may also be used to test recent memory. The patient is asked to point to three objects in the room and recall them a few minutes later.

Remote or long-term memory is tested by asking the patient some events from his past. They should be corroborated by close relatives. Recall of political figures and major social world events will serve the same purpose. It is, however, important to demonstrate that the events tested were actually present in the memory storage before an impairment of memory is declared.

Complex memory problems are assessed with neuropsychological test batteries. The Wechsler Memory Scale and the Halstead–Reitan Neuropsychological Batteries are more popular among the psychologists. Most of these batteries were designed to assess brain damage. Since brain damage is frequently associated with impairment of memory functions, the neuropsychological batteries have been popular in assessing both brain damage and memory impairment. None of the batteries, however, are specific to memory problems.

Burgeoning interest in Alzheimer's disease has led to the development of several rating scales and inventories such as the Sandoz Clinical Assessment—Geriatric, Alzheimer's Disease Assessment Scale, and Brief Cognitive Rating Scale. These scales are particularly useful in the follow-up of the changes in the memory and cognitive functions of patients with degenerative diseases.

## APPENDIX A

### The Brief Cognitive Rating Scale (BCRS)

*Axis I: Concentration and Calculating Ability*

1. No objective or subjective evidence of deficit in concentration.
2. Subjective decrement in concentration ability.

3. Minor objective signs of poor concentration (e.g., on subtraction of serial 7s from 100).
4. Definite concentration deficit for persons of their background (e.g., marked deficit on serial 7s; frequent deficit in subtraction of serial 4s from 40).
5. Marked concentration deficit (e.g., giving months backward or serial 2s from 20).
6. Forgets the concentration task. Frequently begins to count forward when asked to count backward from 10 by 1s.
7. Marked difficulty counting.

### Axis II: Recent Memory

1. No objective or subjective evidence of deficit in recent memory.
2. Subjective impairment only (e.g., forgetting names more than formerly).
3. Deficit in recall of specific events evident upon detailed questioning. No deficit in the recall of major recent events.
4. Cannot recall major events of previous weekend or week. Scanty knowledge (not detailed) of current events, favorite TV shows, etc.
5. Unsure of weather; may not know current president or current address.
6. Occasional knowledge of some recent events. Little or no idea of current address, weather, etc.
7. No knowledge of any recent events.

### Axis III: Past Memory

1. No subjective or objective impairment in past memory.
2. Subjective impairment only. Can recall two or more primary school teachers.
3. Some gaps in past memory upon detailed questioning. Able to recall at least one childhood teacher and/or one childhood friend.
4. Clear-cut deficit. The spouse recalls more of the patient's past than the patient. Cannot recall childhood friends and/or teachers but knows the names of most schools attended. Confuses chronology in reciting personal history.
5. Major past events sometimes not recalled (e.g., names of school attended).
6. Some residual memory of past (e.g., may recall country of birth or former occupation).
7. No memory of past.

### Axis IV: Orientation

1. No deficit in memory for time, place, identity of self or others.
2. Subjective impairment only. Knows time to nearest hour, location.

3. Any mistake in time, by 2 hrs; day of week, by 1 day; date, by 3 days.
4. Mistakes in month, by 10 days, or year, by one month.
5. Unsure of month and/or year and/or season; unsure of locale.
6. No idea of date. Identifies spouse but may not recall name. Knows own name.
7. Cannot identify spouse. May be unsure of personal identity.

## Axis V: Functioning and Self-Care

1. No difficulty, either subjectively or objectively.
2. Complains of forgetting location of objects.
3. Decreased job functioning evident to co-workers. Difficulty in traveling to new locations.
4. Decreased ability to perform complex tasks (e.g., planning dinner for guests, handling finances, marketing, etc.).
5. Requires assistance in choosing proper clothing.
6. Requires assistance in feeding, and/or toileting, and/or bathing, and/or dressing.
7. Requires constant assistance in all activities of daily life.

## SCAG Variables

1. Mood depression
2. Confusion
3. Mental alertness
4. Motivation initiative
5. Irritability
6. Hostility
7. Bothersome
8. Indifference to surroundings
9. Unsociability
10. Uncooperativeness
11. Emotional lability
12. Fatigue
13. Self-care
14. Appetite
15. Dizziness
16. Anxiety
17. Impairment of recent memory
18. Disorientation
19. Overall impression of patient

# I. REFERENCES

Albert MS: Geriatric neuropsychology. *J Consult Clin Psychol* 1981; 49:835–850.

Babcock H: An experiment in the measurement of mental deterioration. *Arch Psychol* 1930; 117:105.

Babcock H, Levy L: *The Measurement of Efficiency of Mental Functioning* (revised examination). *Test and Manual of Directions*. Chicago, CH Stoelting, 1940.

Barbizet J, Cany E: Clinical and psychometrical study of a patient with memory disturbances. *Int J Neurol* 1968; 7:44–54.

Benton A, Eslinger P, Damasio A: Normative observations on neuropsychological test performances in old age. *Clin Neuropsychol* 1981; 3:33–42.

Benton A, Hamsher K, Varney N, *et al*: *Contributions to Neuropsychological Assessment*. New York, Oxford University Press, 1983.

Benton A, Levine H, Van Allen M. Geographic orientation in patients with unilateral cerebral disease. *Neuropsychologia* 1974; 12:183–191.

Broadbent D, Cooper P, Fitzgerald P, *et al*: The cognitive Failures Questionnaire (CFQ) and its correlates. *Br J Clin Psychol* 1982; 21:1–16.

Butters N, Albert M: Process underlying failures to recall remote events, in Cermak LS (ed): *Human Memory and Amnesia*. Hillsdale, NJ, Lawrence Erlbaum Associates, 1982.

Christensen A: Luria's neuropsychological investigation (text), ed 2. Copenhagen, Munksgaard, 1979.

Cronholm B, Molander L: Memory disturbances after electroconvulsive therapy. *Acta Psychiatr Neurol Scand* 1957; 32:280–306.

Cronholm B, Ottoson J: Reliability and validity of a memory test battery. *Acta Psychiatr Scand* 1963; 39:218–234.

Crossen B, Warren R: Use of the Luria-Nebraska Neuropsychological Battery in aphasia: A conceptual critique. *J Consult Clin Psychol* 1982; 50:22–31.

Dodrill C, Troupin A: Effects of repeated administrations of a comprehensive neuropsychological battery among chronic epileptics. *J Nerv Ment Dis* 1975; 161:185–190.

Erickson R, Scott M: Clinical memory testing: A review. *Psychol Bull* 1977; 84:1130–1149.

Fowler RS Jr: A simple non-language test of new learning. *Percept Mot Skills* 1969; 29:895–901.

Fuld P: *Fuld Object-Memory Evaluation*. Chicago, CH, Stoelting, 1977.

Fuld P: Guaranteed stimulus-processing in the evaluation of memory and learning. *Cortex* 1980; 16:255–272.

Golden CJ: A standardized version of Luria's neuropsychological tests, in Filskov S, Boll TJ (eds): *Handbook of Clinical Neuropsychology*. New York, Wiley-Interscience, 1981.

Hachinski V, Iliff L, Zilhka E, *et al*: Cerebral blood flow in dementia. *Arch Neurol* 1975; 32:632–637.

Halstead W: *Brain and Intelligence*. Chicago, University of Chicago Press, 1947.

Hamsher K deS, Benton A, Digre K: Serial digit learning: Normative and clinical aspects. *Clin Psychol* 1980; 2:39–50.

Jenkins C, Hurst M, Rose R: Life changes: Do people really remember. *Arch Gen Psychiatr* 36:379–384, 1979;

Kimura D: Right temporal lobe damage. *Arch Neurol* 1963; 8:264–271.

Klove H: Validation studies in adult clinical neuropsychology, in Reitan RM, Davison LA (eds): *Clinical Neuropsychology*. Washington, DC: Hemisphere, 1974.

Lezak M: *Neuropsychological Assessment*. New York, Oxford University Press, 1983.

Locascio D, Ley R: Scaled-rated meaningfulness of 319 CVCVC words and paralogs previously assessed for associative reaction time. *J Verb Learn Verb Behav* 1972: 11:243–250.

Matarazzo J, Wrens A, Matarazzo R, *et al*: Psychometric and clinical test–retest reliability of the Halstead Impairment Index in a sample of healthy, young, normal men. *J Nerv Ment Dis* 1974; 158:37–49.

Miller E: Short- and long-term memory in patients with presenile dementia (Alzheimer disease). *Psychol Med* 1973; 3:221–224.

Milner B: Interhemispheric differences in the localization of psychological processes in man. *Br Med Bull* 1971; 27:272–277.

Newcome F: *Missile Wounds of the Brain*. London, Oxford University Press, 1969.

Nobles CE: Measurement of association value (a), rated associations (a¹), and scaled meaning-fulness (m¹) for 2100 CVC combinations of the English alphabet. *Psychol Rep* 1961; 8:487–521.

Overall J, Gorham D: The Brief Psychiatric Rating Scale. *Psychol Rep* 1962; 10:799–812.

Randt D, Brown E, Osborne D: A memory test for longitudinal measurement of mild to moderate deficits (rev). Unpublished manuscript, Dept. of Neurology, New York University Medical Center, 1980.

Rapaport D, Gill M, Schafer R: *Diagnostic Psychological Testing*, rev ed, Holt RR (ed). New York, International University Press, 1968.

Reisberg B, Ferris S, de Leon M, *et al.*: The global deterioration scale (GDS): An instrument for the assessment of primary degenerative dementia (PDD). *Am J Psychiatry* 1982; 139:1136–1139.

Reisberg B, Schneck M, Ferris S, *et al.*: The brief cognitive rating scale (BCRS): Findings in primary degenerative dementia (PDD). *Psychopharmacol Bull* 1983; 19:47–50.

Reitan RM: Certain differential effects of left and right cerebral lesions in human adults. *J Comp Physiol Psychol* 1955; 48:474–477.

Reitan RM: A research program on the psychological effects of brain lesions in human beings, in Ellis NR (ed): *International Review of Research in Mental Retardation.* New York, Academic Press, 1966, vol 1.

Rosen W, Mohs R, Davis K: A new rating scale for Alzheimer's disease. *Am J Psychiatry* 1984; 141:1356–1364.

Russell EW: A multiple scoring method for the assessment of complex memory functions. *J Consult Clin Psychol* 1975; 43:800–809.

Sanders H: Problems of measuring very long-term memory. *Int J Ment Health* 1972; 1:98–102.

Schreiber D, Goldman H, Kleinman K *et al*: The relationship between independent neuropsychological and neurological detection and localization of cerebral impairment. *J Nerv Ment Dis* 1976; 162:360–365.

Schulster J: Structure and pragmatics of a self-theory of memory. *Mem Cognit* 1981; 9:263–276.

Shader R, Harmatz J, Salzman C: A new scale for clinical assessment in geriatric populations: Sandoz Clinical Assessment-Geriatric (SCAG). *J Am Geriatr Soc* 1974; 22:107–113.

Smith A: Neuropsychological testing in neurological disorders, in Friedlander WJ (ed): *Advances in Neurology.* New York, Raven Press, 1975, vol 7.

Smith A: Principles underlying human brain functions in neuropsychological sequelae of different neuropsychological processes, in Filskovet SB, Boll TJ (ed): *Handbook of Clinical Neuropsychology.* New York, Wiley-Interscience, 1980.

Squire LR: Remote memory as affected by aging. *Neuropsychologia* 1974; 12:429–435.

Squire L, Slater P: Forgetting in very long-term memory as assessed by an improved questionnaire taxonomy. *J Exp Psychol Hum Lang Mem* 1975; 104:50–54.

Talland GA: *Deranged Memory.* New York, Academic Press, 1965.

Talland GA: *Disorder of Memory and Learning.* Middlesex, England, Penguin Books, 1968.

Talland GA, Ekdahl M: Psychological studies of Korsakoff's Psychosis: IV. The rate and mode of forgetting narrative material. *J Nerv Ment Dis* 1959; 129:391–404.

Toglia MP, Battig W: *Handbook of Semantic Word Nouns.* Hillsdale, NJ, Lawrence Erlbaum Associates, 1978.

Warrington E, James M: Disorders of visual perception in patients with localized cerebral lesions. *Neuropsychologia* 1967; 5:253–266.

Warrington E, Silberstein M: A questionnaire technique for investigating very long-term memory. *Q J Exp Psychol* 1970; 22:508–512.

Wechsler, D: A standardized memory scale for clinical use. *J Psychol* 1945; 19:87–95.

Wells FL, Ruesch J: *Mental Examiner's Handbook* (rev ed). New York, Psychological Corporation, 1969.

Williams M. *Mental Testing in Clinical Practice.* Oxford, England, Pergamon, 1965.

CHAPTER 3

# Drugs Influencing Learning and Memory

## A. INTRODUCTION AND HISTORICAL OVERVIEW

Prior to the 20th century, there were no true scientific studies of the effects of drugs on human memory, only anecdotal information such as De Quincey's treatise on opium and some scattered clinical observations on the various mental effects of such substances as alcohol, coffee, and anesthetics. The term "psychopharmacology" was coined in 1920 to denote the study of the effects of drugs in experimental psychiatry, but the literature on psychopharmacology remained sparse until the discovery and introduction of the major tranquilizers in the 1950s beginning with chlorpromazine and reserpine. As the psychopharmacology literature began to increase at exponential rates during the 1950s, a subliterature devoted to the effects of drugs on learning and memory processes began to accumulate. Prior to the mid 1960s, most of the subliterature dealt with the effects of drugs on learning processes rather than memory processes since the drug was usually administered prior to a learning task. In addition, much of the literature published prior to 1965 on the effects of drugs on learning and memory processes (animal as well as human) was badly flawed methodologically by the absence of adequate control groups and the lack of double-blind procedures.

With widespread adoption and use of the posttraining drug administration procedure in the mid 1960s, a literature on the effects of drugs on memory processes rather than on learning processes came into existence.

At present, the literature on the effects of drugs on memory processes is dominated by studies employing animals as subjects, such studies probably composing 75% to 85% of the total literature. The rest of the studies published since 1950, employing human subjects, aimed to determine whether a given drug had a facilitating or impairing effect on human memory processes. No attempt will be made in this section to discuss every drug studied for memory-altering properties. Rather, only those drugs that have aroused enough interest or controversy to be tested in at least several studies will be discussed.

## B. DRUGS IMPAIRING MEMORY

To demonstrate that a drug impairs human memory, the drug should be administered *after* a given task has been learned to a specified criterion. If the drug is administered before learning/training, any inferiority in measures of retention shown by subjects receiving the drug over control subjects receiving a placebo or no drug at all can be as easily attributed to an impairing of learning effect as to an impairing of memory effect, thus making it impossible to draw any conclusions about the drug's impairment of only the memory processes.

There are relatively few studies in the literature that have used human subjects to demonstrate a given drug's impairing effect on memory. Researchers have always been more interested in finding drugs that could facilitate learning and memory and have been understandably reluctant to expose themselves to the lawsuits that might ensue in this type of research.

When one turns to studies using animals, one finds relatively few experiments using the posttraining drug administration format so that a number of drugs with a reputation for impairing learning in animals have as yet not been convincingly shown to impair memory.

### Protein Synthesis Inhibitors

The drugs for which there is the best evidence of an impairing effect on memory (but animal rather than human memory) are the protein synthesis inhibitors, puromycin (an antibiotic and an aminonucleotide) and cycloheximide [an antibiotic and a glutarimide which can suppress protein synthesis in the mouse brain by 95% to 97% for several hours (Squire, 1976)]. Research on the effects of these drugs on memory processes began in the early 1960s and was originally designed to test the hypothesis that macromolecules such as proteins, RNA, and DNA were the substrata of memory or the much sought after "engram." Many of the now widely adopted tasks, experimental paradigms, and experimental controls used in research today were first originated in the course of testing this macromolecular theory of memory and it is largely to the testing of this theory that we owe our current concepts of short-term and long-term memory.

Both drugs produce a partial or total amnesia for a previously learned task when injected into the brains of fish and mice, although puromycin produces amnesia whether injected in a range between 5 hr before training to 24 hr after training, whereas cycloheximide usually does not produce amnesia unless injected either before training or no more than 30 min after training (Burrell *et al.*, 1978).

Both drugs selectively impair only long-term memory and do not block acquisition (learning) or short-term memory as evidenced by the ability of animals trained under these drugs to demonstrate the same behaviors as uninjected controls when tested immediately after training. Well-learned tasks are resistant to the amnesic effects of both drugs and are usually retained. Since the amnesia produced by both drugs can be reduced or eliminated by various physiological treatments (such as the bitemporal injection of isotonic saline in the case of puromycin and the injection of dextroamphetamine or the use of corticosteroids in the case of cycloheximide), the amnesia produced by both drugs probably results from their effects on memory retrieval processes rather than memory storage processes. Both of these drugs inhibit protein synthesis via different mechanisms: puromycin, by substituting for aminoacyl, transfers RNA in newly forming polypeptide chains causing the release of these incomplete peptide chains (called peptidyl-puromycin fragments) from the polyribosomes; cycloheximide by inhibiting polysome aggregation and inactivating aminoacyl transferase. There is considerable debate as to whether their amnesic effects may be attributed solely or even partially to their protein-suppressing action. In the case of cycloheximide, persuasive arguments have been made that its amnesic effect results from its ability to reduce the level of norepinephrine in the brain (perhaps by depleting an enzyme required for the production of norepinephrine) or from its ability to inhibit the secretion of adrenocortical steroid hormone (the adrenal gland mediation hypothesis). In the case of puromycin, an alternative explanation for its amnesic effect is that the amnesia is the result of the peptidyl-puromycin fragments binding to norepinephrine receptor sites at the synapse, thus displacing normal peptides from neuronal membranes.

Other protein synthesis-inhibiting drugs that produce amnesia in animals are anisomycin, hydroxycycloheximide (Streptovitacin A), and acetoxycycloheximide.

There do not seem to be any reports of memory disturbance in humans resulting from the use of various antibiotics currently used to treat infection, perhaps because antibiotics do not as a rule penetrate the blood–brain barrier. There is, however, a suggestive study in which cancer patients deprived of the two amino acids, tyrosine and phenylalanine, in order to retard the growth of their rapidly growing tumors developed an inability to remember new information coupled with delusions characteristic of delirium (Agranoff et al., 1976).

Retention of memories may require synthesis of brain proteins, for example, to make small structural changes at dendritic synapses more durable. Antibiotics that are protein synthesis inhibitors interfere with retention in animals. Sleep aids long-term retention in humans. Sleep also provides conditions favorable to protein synthesis. The tetracycline antibiotics at clinical dosages are protein synthesis inhibitors not only in bacteria but also in humans.

Allen (1974) reported that a combination of selective REM sleep deprivation with doxycycline administration impaired the memory retention of sentences. In a subsequent study (Idzikowski and Oswald, 1983), 32 volunteers learned a sentence after awakening from the third REM period under experimental conditions that controlled for state dependency. Doxycycline (200 mg), taken at bedtime, impaired recall possibly through a putative inhibitory mechanism on brain protein synthesis.

Some important recent findings bearing on the protein synthesis-inhibiting drugs are:

1. The interval between training and the administration of puromycin which will produce amnesia can be lengthened in both fish and mice by keeping them in their training apparatus following training. This has been interpreted to mean that heightened arousal delays the onset of the memory consolidation process perhaps by delaying the onset of a hypothetical endogenous memory fixation signal (reduction in arousal) necessary to initiate the conversion of short-term memories into long-term memories (to put short-term memories into long-term storage). It suggests that experiments in which amnesia-producing agents fail to produce retention deficits should be examined for variables that might heighten or prolong arousal.

2. Cycloheximide impairs memory formation when bilaterally injected following training into the hippocampus, the striatum, or the amygdala of mice, but does not impair memory when injected into the cortex, the midbrain, the reticular formation, or the thalamus. This suggests that impairment of memory does not require inhibition of protein synthesis throughout the entire brain but only regional inhibition of protein synthesis (Agranoff, 1975).

3. Injections of various peptides will prevent the amnesia induced by antibiotics. The mechanism by which they prevent the amnesia is not yet known.

4. Since puromycin-induced amnesia can be reversed in mice by such adrenergic stimulants as dextroamphetamine and imipramine and since the amnesia produced by cycloheximide can also be reversed by dextroamphetamine or monoamine oxidase inhibitors, there is increasing interest in the hypothesis that the mechanism by which puromycin and cycloheximide produce their amnesic effect is that of interfering with enzymes necessary for the synthesis of catecholamines (especially norepinephrine).

### RNA Synthesis Inhibitors

A second group of drugs for which there is convincing evidence of an impairing effect on memory are drugs that inhibit RNA synthesis including 8-azaguanine, actinomycin D, camptothecin, and 2,6-diaminopurine. Research with drugs inhibiting RNA synthesis grew out of the attempt to test and refine the macromolecular theory of memory, beginning with a study by Hyden published in 1943. Like protein synthesis inhibitors, drugs inhibiting RNA synthesis do not impair acquisition (or learning) or short-term memory but do impair the formation of a permanent or long-term memory. Ribonucleic acid synthesis-inhibiting drugs are usually more toxic than protein synthesis-inhibiting drugs and have not therefore been used on humans. They block the synthesis of RNA by various mechanisms: actinomycin D, for example, by binding to guanosine residues in DNA thus blocking RNA polymerase activity (which is DNA dependent); alpha-amanitin by blocking the enzyme RNA polymerase II which is involved in the synthesis of messenger RNA.

Ribonucleic acid synthesis-inhibiting drugs eventually inhibit protein synthesis as well. Studies with RNA synthesis-inhibiting drugs suggest that messenger RNA synthesis must occur in addition to normally ongoing protein synthesis for short-term memory to be placed in long-term storage. There is no evidence as yet to suggest that brain DNA is involved in memory processes since drugs inhibiting the synthesis of DNA do not impair learning or memory in organisms such as the goldfish (Arganoff, 1976).

## Anticholinergic Agents

Unlike the drugs inhibiting protein and RNA synthesis, drugs interfering with the production of the neurotransmitter acetylcholine have been studied using human as well as animal subjects. The most intensively studied of the anticholinergic agents are atropine and scopolamine with the study and use of scopolamine dating back to the early 1900s when it was used in obstetrical procedures to produce (in combination with other medications) a state of twilight sleep/amnesia. Both atropine and scopolamine block muscarinic acetylcholine receptors and both cross the blood–brain barrier. Although the posttraining administration of scopolamine (which has more profound CNS effects than atropine) has not impaired memory in some experiments, there is substantial and convincing documentation that it impairs both retrieval from long-term memory and the ability to store new information in humans. A series of experiments by David Drachman indicate that scopolamine impairs memory processes and not attentional or arousal processes. Drachman has also pointed out the striking similarities between the memory impairment produced by scopolamine and that found in normal aged subjects and has suggested that chemicals increasing the level of acetylcholine in the brain might reverse these memory deficits. Interestingly, there is some evidence that low doses of atropine (and presumably low doses of other anticholinergic agents) may facilitate retention (Zornetzer, 1978).

Sadeh *et al.* (1982) examined 41 parkinsonian patients for the effect of anticholinergic drugs on memory functions. Nineteen of the patients were tested while both receiving and not receiving treatment. The results pointed toward a possible deleterious effect on memory of standard anticholinergic therapy in Parkinson's disease patients.

## Barbiturates

The barbiturates, phenobarbital, pentobarbital, amobarbital, and secobarbital, all seem capable of imipairing memory in animals when administered after training. The barbiturates tend to impair acquisition and retention of learned behavior. The performance of learned responses, which depend upon a motor component, appears to be facilitated, whereas a verbal or associative component of acquired behavior is impaired.

A single dose of pentobarbital (100 mg/68 kg body weight, IV) reduces memory span (Quarton and Talland, 1962). Thiopental (an ultra short-acting agent) produces an amnesic effect upon the recognitive memory for pictures and the recall memory for words and letter association.

Secobarbital has been shown to exert an anterograde amnesic effect. In one study (Bixler *et al.*, 1979), subjects were given 100 mg of secobarbital at bedtime. They were later awakened to complete four tasks (sharpen a pencil, describe a familiar topic, write a check, and describe an important event) and then were allowed to return to sleep. Next morning most subjects showed a significant decrement in the recall of those tasks.

Biochemical studies indicate that sedative doses of barbiturates produce a generalized reduction of serotonin turnover. Pentobarbital produces an increase in monoamine oxidase activity in the diencephalon. Monoamine oxidase type A activity (for which serotonin is a substrate) was inhibited in the diencephalon, the telencephalon, and the brain stem by phenobarbital (Tagliente, 1979).

An injection of sodium amytal into the carotid artery on the side opposite to the one in which humans had previously undergone a temporal lobectomy produces a temporary but massive memory deficit that is quite similar to the memory deficits produced by bilateral medial temporal lobectomy.

## Anesthetics

Non-hydrogen-bonding anesthetics, carbon dioxide, ether (diethyl ether), and nitrous oxide normally produce retrograde amnesia in animals and impair memory processes in humans, with higher doses producing increasing retrograde amnesia and an increasing interval between training and anesthetic administration reducing the retrograde amnesia in animals or memory impairment. In some studies, however, particularly those using human subjects, these agents have facilitated memory processes. This facilitation may result from the low doses employed and is in accordance with the theory that the increased CNS excitation produced by all non-hydrogen-bonding anesthetics upon introduction will at first facilitate memory consolidation until increasing dose or concentration produces either very high levels of CNS excitation (as is the case with nitrous oxide and carbon dioxide) or CNS depression (as is the case with halothane and the barbiturates) whereupon memory consolidation will be impaired (Porter, 1972). In addition, anesthetics should facilitate learning and possibly memory processes whenever the arousal or anxiety produced by the given task or experiment is too high.

Since many anesthetics, barbiturates, and sedatives produce state-dependent learning, it is necessary to confirm that published studies have controlled for this effect before accepting their conclusions. The most widely accepted way to control for state-dependent learning effects is to use a factorial design in which half the subjects are given the drug before training and half are given a placebo before training following which half of each group is given either the drug or the placebo and then tested. The existence of state-dependent learning has interesting implications for the psychotherapeutic treatment of alcoholism, suggesting that therapy might be more effective if the patient were under the influence of alcohol. It also implies that persons receiving both drug therapy and psychotherapy at the same time should gradually reduce their drug dose so that new learning will transfer to the nondrug state.

The anesthetic thiopental produces an amnesia in humans for material discussed under sedation which is not state dependent since reinstatement of the anesthetic does not facilitate recall.

The use of premedication with a general anesthetic also may influence memory. The use of a narcotic as a premedication in obstretic patients within 6 hr of general anesthesia reduced the frequency of unpleasant stimuli recalled during a cesarean section by 18% (Wilson and Turner, 1969).

## Benzodiazepines

Benzodiazepines, used as a preanesthetic medication or as a hypnotic, produce a potent anterograde memory impairment. In a study (Pandit and Dundee, 1970), 144 patients were given diazepam (10 mg IM) as premedication 60–90 min before anesthesia. Memory was tested 6 and 24 hr after the surgery. Two of the patients showed hazy memory of the trip to the operating room, one had no recollection of the intravenous injection, and four had only a hazy memory of this event. In another study (Gregg et al., 1974), patients were given intravenous injections of diazepam (1 mg/7 lb, 1 mg/14 lb, or 1 mg/21 lb body weight) or a placebo. They were then exposed to various visual, auditory, and painful stimuli either immediately or 10, 20, and 30 min following the injection. The memory for the stimuli was tested 24 hr after the exposure. A dose-related amnesia for all the sensory stimuli was apparent. For the highest dose of diazepam (1 mg/7 lb of body weight), less than 30% of the stimuli were recalled.

Diazepam-induced anterograde amnesia has also been shown in normal young volunteers (Clarke et al., 1970) usually with a peak effect within the first 10 min after diazepam administration. Diazepam has also been shown to impair driving skills (Linnoila, 1973).

The effects of intravenous injection of diazepam appears to show a consistently rapid onset (2 to 3 min) and brief anterograde amnesia (29 to 30 min). The duration of amnesia is increased as a function of increase in dosage. Intravenous administration of lorazepam has a delayed onset of effect (30 to 40 min) and produces a prolonged amnesia, lasting up to 270 min.

## Antipsychotic Drugs

The effects of these drugs on memory processes is complicated by their sedative and motor effects. In general, clinically effective doses of chlorpromazine lead to a reduced activity level associated with increased unresponsiveness, passivity, and motivational decrement.

Kornetsky *et al.* (1959) found that individuals given 200 mg of chlorpromazine performed at a reduced level on various intellectual and motor tasks such as digit copying, digit symbol substitution, addition speed, pursuit rotor performance, visual discrimination, and tactual performance. However, vigilance tasks such as pursuit rotor performance, tapping speed, and continuously maintained performance were impaired by chlorpromazine to a greater degree than was a digit symbol substitution.

In a series of double-blind studies normal subjects were given single doses of four different phenothiazines, chlorpromazine, promethazine, perphenazine and trifluoperazine. They were tested 2, 4, and 7 hr after the ingestion of the drug. Chlorpromazine and promethazine produced psychomotor retardation, impairment of intellectual functions, and drowziness. Perphenazine and trifluoperazine produced an elevation of mood. In other studies, the effects of chlorpromazine (50 mg) showed reduced verbal and numerical performance on the Morrisby Differential Test Battery, accompanied by drowziness and other side effects. The tests that involved judgment of conceptual relationships were also affected by this drug.

Prolonged use of chlorpromazine (5 weeks) reduces performance on the critical flicker fusion test, but the performance is normalized with continued drug use (Hoehn-Saric *et al.*, 1964).

It appears that neuroleptics have little or no effect on short-term or long-term memory processes. Most of the effects reported on intellectual functions appear to result from sedation and motor effects induced by neuroleptics.

### Marijuana

The emerging consensus is that marijuana impairs acquisition rather than retrieval of previously stored information in humans. There is evidence for state-dependent learning effects in that material learned under the influence of marijuana is better recalled under marijuana than under a placebo. One hypothesis for marijuana's impairing effect on acquisition is that subjects under its influence do not rehearse the information they have been asked to learn. This lack of rehearsal, in turn, is attributed to marijuana's disrupting influence on attentional processes which has been reported anecdotally and demonstrated experimentally.

## C. DRUGS FACILITATING MEMORY

To demonstrate a facilitating effect on memory rather than acquisition (or learning), arousal, attention, motor behavior, or perception, it is necessary to administer the drug *after* a given task or body of information has been learned to a specified criterion. It must then be shown that subjects receiving the drug are superior in measures of retention than a matched group of subjects receiving a placebo. Where human subjects are used, the experiment should be of the double-blind type in which neither the subjects nor the experimenter know which drug is the experimental agent and which placebo. In addition, there should be controls for the state-dependent learning effects that some of these drugs can produce. Drugs that have been used to improve memory include:

1. Central nervous system stimulants
2. Convulsant stimulants
3. Cholinergic drugs
4. Vasodilators
5. Anabolic agents
6. Pyrrolidinone derivatives
7. GABA-ergic drugs

## Central Nervous System Stimulants

This group of drugs includes several subcategories such as amphetamines and xanthines. Stimulants such as caffeine and amphetamines were among the first chemical agents to be tested on human subjects with the aim of determining whether they facilitated memory, learning, and performance. They have generated the largest literature of all the agents reputed to facilitate memory and have been tested on the largest number of human subjects.

### Amphetamine

Amphetamine is a sympathomimetic amine, a derivative of phenylethylamine. When administered peripherally, amphetamine crosses the blood–barrier and produces marked stimulant effects on the central nervous system, especially the reticular activating system, the respiratory and vasomotor centers, and the cerebral cortex. Although some of the earliest experiments conducted in the late 1930s showed an impairing effect on learning and performance in the rat, the majority of experiments since then have found amphetamine to have a facilitating effect on animal learning and performance when given in small, subconvulsive doses prior to training (McGaugh, 1973). And there is a growing number of animal studies in which the posttraining administration of low, subconvulsive doses of amphetamine have facilitated both learning and retention (although repeated posttraining administration of amphetamine impairs retention as do high doses of posttraining amphetamine). In addition, amphetamine has been found capable of blocking or preventing the amnesia resulting from the administration of the protein synthesis inhibitors puromycin and cycloheximide.

Studies employing human subjects tend to demonstrate that in tasks and learning situations in which fatigue, persistence, and speed of performance are important factors, amphetamine can facilitate performance.

Amphetamines have been observed to facilitate learning in children with attention deficit disorders (Conners *et al.*, 1964). Proteus maze performance was improved by amphetamines in normal as well as in hyperactive children. Methamphetamine (15 mg/68 kg IV) improved recall of strings of digits from 8 to 20 times (Talland and Quarton, 1982).

Crow and Bursill (1970) investigated the effects of amphetamines on short-term memory. Subjects were asked to reproduce lists of digits after various delay times following their presentation. Error rates for drug-treated subjects exceeded those of the controls at all delay intervals. However, the results were not significant. Hurst *et al.* (1969) reported completely negative findings, showing no facilitating effects of amphetamines on the recall of paired-associate verbal stimuli of low association.

The mechanism of action of amphetamine in humans has not yet been determined, but it is presumed to be similar to the mechanism of action found in studies of the rat. These studies at first pointed to the inhibition of mono-amine oxidase as being the primary mechanism of amphetamine's action. Currently, however, the central stimulant effects of amphetamine are believed to be the result of its ability to trigger the release of newly synthesized dopamine and norepinephrine from nerve terminals and its ability to block or inhibit the neuronal reuptake of dopamine and norepinephrine. The increase in norepinephrine levels may explain why amphetamine reverses or blocks the amnesia caused by the protein synthesis inhibitors puromycin and cyclo-heximide since it has been demonstrated that norepinephrine, when administered intracranially, reduced the inhibition of protein synthesis produced by electroconvulsive shock.

In normal dosages, amphetamine does not seem to trigger the release of serotonin, but in doses larger than 5 mg/kg amphetamine can trigger the release of extragranular stores of serotonin into extraneural space, but depletion of serotonin does not occur. In addition, there appears to be an antagonistic pattern of interaction between the acetylcholinergic neuronal system and the dopaminergic neuronal system in the brain as evidenced by the ability of cholinergic agonists like physostigmine to reduce the central stimulant actions of amphetamine and the ability of cholinergic antagonists like sco-polamine to enhance the central stimulant actions of amphetamine.

## Magnesium Pemoline

Although pemoline, the active ingredient of Cylert and an oxazolidine derivative, was first chemically synthesized in 1913, its central stimulant effects were not recognized until 1956. Interest in pemoline remained subdued until 1966 when two articles appeared in *Science,* one claiming that magnesium pemoline stimulated RNA polymerase activity in the rat brain both *in vitro* and *in vivo* (RNA polymerase catalyzing the synthesis of messenger RNA); the second claiming that magnesium pemoline enhanced the learning and retention of an active avoidance response in rats. A flurry of studies followed focused on the learning and memory-facilitating properties of magnesium pemoline, but by 1973 it was clear that magnesium pemoline did not, as initially reported, stimulate RNA polymerase activity, and that any reported enhancement of learning and retention, especially in humans, was most likely due to an increase in general alertness, arousal, interest, and motivation. Since 1960, pemoline has been clinically studied in and administered to large numbers of adult patients in the United States, primarily as an antidepressant and antifatigue agent. In 1975, the Food and Drug Administration approved the use of Cylert for the treatment of hyperkinetic children. Although the precise mechanism of its action is not yet known, the evidence to date points to its ability to increase the rate of dopamine synthesis and dopamine levels in certain areas of the brain such as (in young rats) the basal ganglia and brain stem as being at least one if not the primary mechanism of pemoline action.

## Caffeine

Caffeine was independently discovered by German and French scientists in the early 1820s. A small number of posttraining administration experiments using animals point to a possible facilitating effect on memory. There are considerable interindividual differences in the effects of caffeine in coffee upon simple learning functions in man. Gililand and Nelson (1939) noticed that coffee given 20, 100, and 140 min prior to memory span tests increased the accuracy of performance of most individuals. The central effects of coffee, however, appear to depend upon the activation and behavioral baselines upon which the drug is superimposed.

It appears that caffeine reduces drowziness and increases alertness through stimulation of reticular activating system. Tasks requiring sustained alertness and attention such as automobile driving (Regina et al., 1974) and sequential memory tasks (Mitchel et al., 1974) show significant improvement in performance after caffeine ingestion.

The use of caffeine in hyperactive children has not shown any beneficial effects (Gross, 1975). Most of the children were, in fact, worsened by caffeine as compared with other stimulants such as amphetamines. These findings may be parallel to the effects of caffeine in animals. Caffeine given to mice during the nadir of their activity cycle significantly increased subsequent locomotor activity, but the same dose given during the activity peak depressed locomotor activity levels (Essman, 1971).

## Convulsant Stimulants

These drugs include strychnine, pentylenetetrazol, and bemegride. They act on the brain stem selectively to augment its descending influences and are often called medullary stimulants. In small doses, they cause stimulation of respiratory, vasomotor, and vagal centers of the medulla. Slightly larger doses cause convulsions comparable to a grand mal seizure.

### Strychnine

Strychnine's effects on learning and memory processes in animals (but not humans) have been studied more intensively and for a longer period of time than have the effects of other convulsants. The earliest study to show a facilitating effect was conducted by Lashley who found that pretraining administration of strychnine sulfate facilitated maze acquisition in rats. Lashley published this study in 1917, but his finding did not stimulate additional research until 1959 when a published study reported that strychnine had a facilitating effect on the acquisition of a discrimination response in rats.

Between 1960 and 1974, 19 published studies have examined strychnine's effect on learning and memory processes in the rat and mouse. Eleven of these studies (of which five used the posttraining administration procedure) found strychnine to be a facilitator of both learning and memory processes whereas eight studies (including five using the posttraining administration procedure) found either no effect or an impairing effect. Given these conflicting results and the lack of any hypothesis accounting for them, it would be premature to conclude that strychnine is a facilitator of memory consolidation although there is evidence to support such a conclusion.

### Other Convulsants: Bemegride, Pentylenetetrazol, and Picrotoxin

Posttraining subconvulsive injections of bemegride, pentylenetetrazol (Metrazol), and picrotoxin have been found to facilitate retention in animals in some studies, usually only when the drug was administered within the first 30 min after training. Pentylenetetrazol has been extensively used in the treatment of chronic organic brain syndrome patients and has been the subject of over 50 published studies, all but 12 reporting a favorable therapeutic effect. Of the 16 best-controlled studies, pentylenetetrazol produced favorable clinical results in only five (Ban, 1978).

Given the sparse number of studies on bemegride and picrotoxin and the conflicting results of geropsychiatric studies using pentylenetetrazol, it is again necessary, as in the case of strychnine, to reserve judgment on the question of whether these convulsants enhance memory process when administered in subconvulsive doses.

## Cholinergic Drugs

Some of the cholinergic drugs tested for memory-enhancing effects include choline esters such as arecoline and choline-sterase inhibitors such as physostigmine. The choline esters act directly on postganglionic neurons and on the effector tissues. The cholinesterase inhibitors act indirectly through delaying hydrolysis of liberated acetylcholine by cholinesterase. The cholinesterase occurs in neurons known to be cholinergic and is concentrated in nerve terminals and also in a postsynaptic site if it is part of a cholinergic neuron. It is distributed throughout the central nervous system in a pattern presumed to identify cholinergic neurons.

Arecholine and physostigmine appear to enhance learning and memory in normal young volunteers. In one study (Davis et al., 1978), 19 normal male volunteers were given 1.0 mg of physostigmine or 1 mg of saline by a slow intravenous infusion on two consecutive days. The short-term memory was tested with the digit span and memory scanning tasks. The long-term memory was assessed by two verbal learning tasks. Physostigmine significantly enhanced storage of information into long-term memory. Retrieval of information from long-term memory was also improved. Short-term memory processes were not significantly altered by physostigmine. Sitaram and Weingartner (1978) found that arecholine (4 mg) and choline (a precursor of acetylcholine) significantly enhanced serial learning in normal young volunteers. The serial learning task consisted of learning a fixed sequence of ten words belonging to a familiar category.

Davis et al. (1980) did not find any beneficial effect of choline chloride in young and nondemented elderly volunteers on their ability to learn new information. However, physostigmine improved the learning ability of elderly individuals (including some demented persons). The physostigmine was given in doses of 0.125 mg, 0.25 mg, or 0.5 mg by a constant infusion for 30 min.

Several studies have pointed out that there is a narrow dosage range within which memory is potentiated by these drugs. Most individuals show a U-shaped effect—no effect at low doses, some improvement at a restricted range of doses, and deficits at the highest dose. The effects of physostigmine and arecholine in demented individuals appears similar to those in normal subjects, although the optimal dosage seems more variable. It is desirable to try a range of doses. There are some patients who respond to physostigmine in a wider dosage range. These patients are not clinically distinguishable by any particular pattern of deficits.

The improvement with either physostigmine or arecholine is in no way dramatic and memory functions remain grossly impaired as compared with normal subjects. In fact, several recent studies failed to find any beneficial effects of these drugs in demented patients. Caltagirone et al. (1983) administered physostigmine in individual optimal dose orally or subcutaneously to eight patients affected by Alzheimer's disease. Memory was tested with Rey's 15 Words Test and the Digit Span Test. All patients showed a slight behavioral activation, but no significant change occurred in performance. Similarly, no significant difference was found after chronic oral administration of physostigmine (1 mg four times a day for one month) to a group of Alzheimer's patients (Caltagirone et al., 1982).

## Vasodilators

Cerebral arterioslerosis and a consequent decrease in blood perfusion of the brain are considered partially responsible for the memory impairment in old age. A great deal of research has centered around testing vasodilator drugs in improving blood flow to the brain. The intracranial blood vessels do not respond to the same neural and humoral influences that control other vascular beds. The vascular tone is regulated by the intrinsic contractibility of the vessels which is modified by the pressure perfusing them and by changes in $CO_2$ tension. They do not respond to drugs that mimic or block autonomic nervous system effects. There is no reason to believe that the occlusion caused by arteriosclerosis can be modified by vasodilator drugs any more than in the vessels of the heart or the extremities. However, the drugs may relieve vasospasm that may be present in these vessels.

The most extensively clinically studied cerebrovasodilator is Hydergine, a mixture of three dihydroergot alkaloids. It has proved superior to placebo in the treatment of senile behavior in at least 12 double-blind studies, although not all these studies have noted improvements in memory processes (Ban, 1978). There appears to be a renewed interest in this drug. A nationwide trial of Hydergine is being conducted for the treatment of senile dementia. A recent review of 38 clinical studies conducted between 1969 and 1981 and using 3 or 4.5 mg/day concluded: "Hydergine is influential in alleviating or inhibiting certain target symptoms associated with senile dementia as detected by clinicians using behavioral rating scales" (McDonald, 1982).

The exact mechanism of action of Hydergine is unknown. The original inference that it modified dementia by vasodilation in the brain has been abandoned in favor of its effects on noradrenergic, dopaminergic, and serotonergic functions. Hydergine is an ergot and has several well-documented pharmacologic effects such as dopamine agonist, phosphodiesterase inhibitor, stimulator of cerebral metabolism, and a mild vasodilator.

Another extensively studied and widely used drug in the treatment of arteriosclerotic dementia is papaverine, an alkaloid derivative of opium. Three uncontrolled and three placebo-controlled studies have shown papaverine to be therapeutically helpful to geropsychiatric patients although improvements in memory and intellectual functioning were often absent. Although there is evidence that papaverine increases cerebral circulation in both normal and arteriosclerotic brains, it is possible that its therapeutic effect is a result of dopamine receptor blockage or phosphodiesterase inhibition rather than cerebral vasodilation.

Cyclandelate, a drug with structural similarities to papaverine, has also been found to benefit patients with cerebral arteriosclerosis and impaired mental abilties by at least five double-blind clinical studies, although memory processes were not always improved. As with Hydergine, the therapeutic effect of cyclandelate may result from its effect on cerebral metabolism rather than increased cerebral blood flow since improvement in mental function tests is not always accompanied by significant cerebral blood flow increases.

Other cerebral vasodilators that have been reported to improve mental symptoms of senility are nicotinic acid (which may, unlike Hydergine, papaverine, and cyclandelate, increase blood flow only in persons with cerebral arteriosclerosis but not in normal persons), isoxsuprine [which has proved therapeutically helpful in three uncontrolled and two placebo-controlled clinical studies (Ban, 1978)], and the anticoagulant dicumarol.

None of the cerebral vasodilators has yet been shown to facilitate memory processes per se and none has yet been shown to reverse intellectual impairment. In addition, there is the possibility that cerebral vasodilators may actually divert blood away from ischemic areas (since arteriosclerosis impairs the dilation ability of affected cerebral blood vessels) so that the presumed increase of blood and oxygen in ischemic areas never really occurs. Thus any clinical improvements noted with the use of cerebral vasodilators may be due to mechanisms other than increased oxygenation of hypoxic brain tissues.

## Anabolic Agents

Anabolic agents, which are hypothesized to correct disturbances of protein synthesis, have not been as frequently or widely used as either cerebral vasodilators or CNS stimulants in the treatment of senile dementias. Two of these agents, pyritinol (a bisdisulfide hydrochloride) and naftidrofuryl (an acid oxalate) have been shown to either normalize or increase cerebral glucose consumption (which is often more reduced in aged psychiatric patients with organic brain syndrome than is cerebral oxygen consumption) and to improve intellectual performance in aged psychiatric patients. No studies pertaining solely to memory processes have yet been conducted using these two drugs, but the possibility that reduced cerebral glucose consumption may be an important factor in the onset of senile dementias warrants and will no doubt receive further clinical study.

## Pyrrolidinone Derivatives

These are a new class of drugs which Giuryea has designated as "nootropic," meaning drugs that selectively influence only the higher integrative mechanisms of the mind. Piracetam, an original structure chemically related to GABA, is the first member of this group studied for its memory-enhancing effects. Research with piracetam began in 1963 and has shown it to be nontoxic (even at extremely high doses), to be devoid of behavioral, sedative, or stimulant effects, to be devoid of state-dependency effects, and to be capable of crossing the blood–brain barrier. Piracetam is alleged to facilitate learning and memory processes in animals and is supposed to be equally capable of facilitating these processes in normal humans, patients recovering from head injuries, geriatric patients, and alcoholics.

Aniracetam, another member of the group, has been tested in rodents on various forms of learning and memory tasks (Cumin *et al.*, 1982). The results show (1) almost complete prevention of incapacity to learn a discrete response in rats exposed to sublethal hypercapnia immediately before acquisition session; (2) partial or complete prevention of scopolamine-induced short-term amnesia for a passive avoidance task; and (3) complete protection against amnesia for a passive avoidance task in rats submitted to electric shock immediately after avoidance acquisition. These improvements of impaired functions were observed at oral doses of 10–100 mg/kg. The mechanism of action remains unknown.

## GABA-ergic Drugs

There is an increasing interest in the participation of gamma-aminobutyric acid (GABA) in the behavior of animals and man. Gamma-aminobutyric acid was found to have a modulating effect on the activity of the nigrostriatal and the mesolimbic dopaminergic system, providing the subcortical control of locomotor functions and higher nervous activity. High levels of GABA and glutamic acid decarboxylase (GAD) activity, the enzyme responsible for GABA synthesis, were found in the substantia nigra, the caudate nucleus, the globus pallidus, and the nucleus accumbens. Therefore, GABA-ergic agents capable of changing brain GABA levels, imitating or enhancing the inhibitory effects of GABA on its receptors, or finally, blocking the latter, may affect in a variety of ways locomotor activity, exploratory behavior, and conditioning. The influence of GABA-ergic compounds on behavior remains poorly studied in spite of the available reports on the favorable effects of GABA itself and some of its derivatives on mental development and memory in humans.

General GABA-mimetic and GABA-blocking drugs have been tested for their effects on conditioned avoidance response (CAR) in rats. Sodium valproate slowed the acquisition of CAR and failed to affect the latency of a well-learned CAR, but interestingly, showed a marked anticonflict effect similar to that of benzodiazepine. The similarity of effects of drugs such as benzodiazepines and sodium valproate in potentiating possible GABA-ergic transmission suggests that GABA may play a role in conditioning, learning, and memory processes (Rayevsky *et al.*, 1983).

## Other Drugs

### Yeast RNA

A number of studies in the early 1960s in which yeast RNA was given either orally or intravenously to geriatric patients diagnosed as having chronic brain syndrome found significant improvement in memory and retention. Later studies, however, failed to replicate these findings and there is currently no clinical interest in yeast RNA. Ribaminol, a combination of yeast RNA and diethylaminoethanol, was reported to enhance memory processes in humans in the late 1960s, but this finding does not seem to have been replicated in a controlled study.

## Tricyanoaminopropene

Tricyanoaminopropene (TCAP), an alleged elevator of RNA levels in the mouse brain, facilitator of protein synthesis, and reducer of the amnesia effects of electroconvulsive shock in mice, has not been found to facilitate learning and memory processes in senile patients (Essman, 1971). Chronic administration of TCAP does seem, however, to facilitate some types of learning in rats.

## Nicotine

Nicotine is a central nervous system stimulant and cholinergic agonist that has been experimentally studied since the early 1920s. Daily administration of nicotine over long periods of time has usually impaired performance in rats while small doses have often, but not always, facilitated learning in rats (McGaugh *et al.*, 1965). Posttraining administration of nicotine given in the lower dosage has been shown to facilitate memory processes in animals. Whether nicotine impairs or facilitates learning and memory processes is probably partially determined by the level of arousal induced in the animal by the given task. The performance of the tasks that induce high arousal levels is impaired by nicotine. In man nicotine appears to reduce performance, but this effect may be related to a number of factors other than the central action of the drug per se. Heimstra (1962) showed that cigarette smoking increased the onset of fatigue and did not affect vigilance or tracking behavior. The tracking performance was, however, decreased by inhalation of four cigarettes over a brief period. There are wide interindividual variations in the amount of absorption and elimination of nicotine from cigarette smoking.

The mechanism of nicotine action on learning and memory is not known. Nicotine appears to influence the cholinergic, the adrenergic, and the serotonergic systems of the brain. The cholinergic mechanism of action was suggested by the finding that the facilitation of memory consolidation could be achieved by posttraining administration of atropine. When atropine was given to rats in shuttle avoidance task, its stimulant effect upon performance added to the stimulant effect of nicotine. The adrenergic mechanism was proposed from the observation that nicotine facilitated conditioned response in rats and this facilitative effect was reduced if the animal was pretreated with a-methyl-p-tyrosine, which causes reduced brain levels of catecholamines.

*Hyperbaric Oxygenation*

Although three studies conducted between 1969 and 1972 found that hyperbaric oxygenation (100% oxygen under 2.5 atm of pressure for 90 min, twice each day for 15 days) improved performance on three tests of cognitive functions (including the Wechsler Memory Scale) in elderly male subjects diagnosed as having chronic organic brain syndrome, these three studies were severely flawed by incorrect diagnoses, scoring techniques, and tests of questionable validity, failure to maintain a true double-blind status, practice effects, and experimenter effect. Studies attempting to replicate these studies but employing true double-blind placebo controls have not found any appreciable improvement in cognitive functioning following hyperbaric oxygenation. As a result, there is no convincing evidence as yet that hyperbaric oxygenation facilitates human memory processes.

*Naloxone*

Naloxone, an opiate antagonist, when given up to 20 mg (0.3 mg/kg) intravenously, showed no consistent alterations in cognitive test performance. Cohen *et al.* (1983) agreed that this dose of naloxone may not be sufficient to overcome the activity of the endogenous opioid system. They administered increasing intravenous doses of naloxone (0.3 mg/kg, 1 mg/kg, and 2 mg/kg). Naloxone at 2 mg/kg, but not at lower doses, impaired aspects of memory as measured by a verbal learning task that assessed direct free recall and recognition. At the same time working memory was left unaffected. These results suggest that the endogneous opioid system may play a role in the acquisition and retention of environmental events.

## D. SUMMARY

To demonstrate that a drug impairs human memory, it should be administered after a given task has been learned to a specified criterion. If the drug is administered before learning or training, any improvement or retardation in learning may be attributed to an impairment of learning rather than to an impairment of memory. Much of the literature published prior to 1965 on the effects of drugs on learning and memory was methodologically flawed because the experimental drugs were given before learning. With widespread adoption and use of the posttraining administration of drugs in the mid 1960s, data on the effects of drugs on memory processes rather than on learning processes were gathered. At present the literature on the effects of drugs on memory processes is dominated by studies employing animals as subjects. Such studies probably compose 75 to 85% of the total literature.

Drugs influencing memory may be divided into two broad categories: drugs that have an impairing effect on memory and drugs that facilitate memory. The first category includes several groups of drugs such as (1) protein synthesis inhibitors, (2) RNA synthesis inhibitors, (3) anticholingergic agents, (4) barbiturates, (5) anesthetics, (6) benzodiazepines, (7) antipsychotic drugs or neuroleptics, and (8) marijuana. Drugs facilitating memory include (1) CNS stimulants, (2) convulsants, (3) cholinergic drugs, (4) vasodilators (5) anabolic agents, (6) pyrrolidinone derivatives, and (7) GABA-ergic drugs.

Increasing use of sedatives and hypnotics makes it necessary for clinicians to become aware of the memory-impairing effects of these drugs. Barbiturates in general tend to impair acquisition of new information. Secobarbital has been shown to exert an anterograde amnesic effect. In a study (Bixler *et al.*, 1979), subjects were given 100 mg of secobarbital at bedtime. They were later awakened to complete four tasks (sharpen a pencil, describe a familiar topic, write a check, and describe an important event) and then were allowed to return to sleep. The next morning most subjects showed a significantly decreased recall of those tasks. Diazepam-induced anterograde amnesia has also been shown in normal young volunteers, usually with a peak effect within the first 10 min after diazepam administration. Diazepam has also been shown to impair driving skills.

In spite of a large number of drugs studied so far for facilitation of memory, none has been shown to produce a dramatic effect. However, there are several groups of drugs that facilitate learning and memory to sufficient degree to make them useful in individuals with severe memory problems. Stimulants such as amphetamines improve learning and memory through decreasing fatigue and enhancing attention.

Cholinergic drugs, including choline esters (arecholine), cholinesterase inhibitors (physostigmine), and choline precursors (lecithin), have been studied extensively both in normal volunteers and in patients with degenerative disease. The findings are inconclusive and even the beneficial effects reported with these drugs are in no way dramatic and the memory functions of these patients remain grossly impaired.

Vasodilator drugs have not been helpful in improving blood flow to the brain since intracranial blood vessels do not respond to the same neural and hormonal influences that control other vascular beds. Their vascular tone is modified by the pressure of the blood perfusing them and by changes in carbon dioxide tension. They do not respond to drugs that mimic or block autonomic nervous system effects. There is no reason to believe that occlusion caused by arteriosclerosis can be modified by vasodilator drugs any more than in the vessels of the heart or the extremities. However, the drugs may relieve vasospasm that may be present in the blood vessels. Hydergine has proved superior to placebo in the treatment of senile behavior. The original hypothesis that Hydergine improved dementia by vasodilation in the brain has been abandoned in favor of its effects on noradrenergic, dopaminergic, and serotonergic functions.

Several pyrrolidinone derivatives (also called nootropics), such as piracetam and aniracetam, appear to have facilitating effects on learning and memory in patients recovering from head injury, senile dementia, and chronic alcoholism. These drugs have few behavioral, sedative, or stimulant side effects. Although the mechanism of action of nootropics is unknown, they seem to influence metabolic processes in the nervous system.

## E.  REFERENCES

Agranoff BW: Biochemical strategies in the study of memory formation, in *The Nervous System*. New York, Raven Press, 1975, vol 1: *The Basic Neurosciences*, pp. 585–589.

Agranoff BW: Learning and memory: Approaches to correlating behavioral and biochemical events, in Seigal G, Albers R, Agranoff B (eds): *Basic Neurochemistry*, ed 2. Little Brown & Co., 1976, pp. 765–784.

Agranoff BW, Springer AD, Quarton GC: Biochemistry of memory and learning, in Vinken PJ, Bruyn GW (eds): *Handbook of Clinical Neurology*. Amsterdam, North Holland Publishing Co, 1976, vol 27, pp. 459–476.

Allen SR: REM sleep deprivation and protein synthesis inhibition effects on human memory, in Levine P, Koella W (eds): *Sleep*. New York, Karger, 1974, pp. 373–376.

Ban TA: Vasodilators, stimulants and anabolic agents in the treatment of geropsychiatric patients, in Lipton MA, Demascio A, Killam K (eds): *Psychopharmacology: A Generation of Progress*. New York, Raven Press, 1978, pp. 1525–1533.

Bixler EO, Scharf MB, Soldatos CR, *et al*: Effects of hypnotic drugs on memory. *Life Sci* 1979; 25:1379–88.

Burrell HR, Dokas LA, Springer AD: Progress in biochemical approaches to learning and memory, in Lipton MA, Demascio A, Killam K (eds): *Psychopharmacology: A Generation of Progress*. New York, Raven Press, 1978, pp. 623–635.

Caltagirone C, Albanese A, Gainotti G: Acute administration of individual optimal dose of physostigmine fails to improve amnesic performances in Alzheimer's presenile dementia. *Int J Neurosci* 1983; 18:143–147.

Caltagirone C, Albanese A, Gainotti G, *et al*: Oral administration of chronic physostigmine does not improve cognitive or amnesic performances in Alzheimer's presenile dementia. *Int J Neurosci* 1982; 16:247–249.

Clarke PR, Eccersley PS, Frisby JP, *et al*: Amnesic effect of diazepam (Valium). *Br J Anaesth* 1970; 42:690–697.

Cohen RM, Cohen MR, Weingartner H, *et al*: High-dose naloxone affects task performance in normal subjects. *Psychiatr Res* 1983; 8:127–135.

Conners CK, Eisenberg L, Sharpe L: Effects of methylphenidate (Ritalin) on paired-associate learning and proteus maze performance in emotionally disturbed children. *J Consul Psychol* 1964; 28:14–22.

Crow, RJ, Bursill AE: An investigation into the effects of methamphetamine on short-term memory in man, in Costa E, Garattini S (eds): *Amphetamine and Related Compounds*. New York, Raven Press, 1970, pp. 889–895.

Cumin R, Bandle E, Gamzu E, *et al*: Effects of novel compound aniracetam (R0-13-5057) upon impaired learning and memory in rodents. *Psychopharmacology* 1982; 78:104–111.

Davis KL, Mohs RC, Tinklenberg J, *et al*: Physostigmine: Improvement of long-term memory processes in humans. *Science* 1978; 201:272–274.

Davis KL, Mohs RC, Davis BM, *et al*: Human memory and the effects of physostigmine and choline chloride. *Psychopharmacol Bull* 1980; 16:27–28.

Essman WB: Drug effects and learning and memory process. *Adv Pharmacol Chemother* 1971; 9:241–330.

Gililand AR, Nelson D: The effects of coffee on certain mental and physiological functions. *J Gen Psychol* 1939; 21:339–348.

Gregg JM, Ryan DE, Levin KH: Amnesic actions of diazepam. *J Oral Surg* 1974; 32:651–664.

Gross MD: Caffeine in the treatment of children with minimal brain dysfunction or hyperactive syndrome. *Psychosomatics* 1975; 16:26–27.

Heimstra NW: Social influence on the response to drugs. *Psychopharmacology* 1962; 3:72–78.

Hoehn-Saric R, Bacon E, Gross M: Effects of chlorpromazine on flicker-fusion. *J Nerv Ment Dis* 1964; 128:287–292.

Hurst PM, Radlow R, Chubb NC, *et al:* Effects of D. amphetamine on acquisition, persistence and recall. *Am J Psychol* 1969; 82:307–319.

Hyden H, Egyhazi E: Nuclear RNA changes in nerve cells during a learning experiment in rats. *Proc Natl Acad Sci USA* 1962; 48:1366–1373.

Idzikowski C, Oswald I: Interference with human memory by an antibiotic. *Psychopharmacology* 1983; 79:108–110.

Kornetsky C, Pettit M, Wynne R, *et al:* A comparison of psychological effects of acute and chronic administration of chlorpromazine and secobarbital in schizophrenic patients. *J Ment Sci* 1959; 105:190–198.

Linnoila M, Mattila M: Interaction of alcohol and drugs on psychomotor skills as demonstrated by a driving simulator. *Br J Pharmacol* 1973; 47:671P–672P.

McDonald RT: Drug treatment of senile dementia, in Wheatley D (ed): *Psychopharmacology of Old Age.* New York, Oxford University Press, 1982, pp. 113–138.

McGaugh JL: Drug facilitation of learning and memory. *Annu Rev Pharmacol* 1973; 13:229–241.

McGaugh JL, Petkinovich LF: Effects of drugs on learning and memory. *Int Rev Neurobiol* 1965; 3:139–196.

Mitchel VE, Ross S, Hurst PM: Drugs and placebos: Effects of caffeine on cognitive performance. *Psychol Rep* 1974; 35:875–883.

Pandit SK, Dundee J: Preoperative amnesia. *Anesthesia* 1970; 24:493–499.

Porter AL: An analytic review of the effects of non-hydrogen bonding anesthetics on memory processes. *Behav Biol* 1972; 7:291–309.

Quarton GC, Talland GA: The effects of methamphetamine and pentobarbital on two measures of attention. *Psychopharmacologia* 1962; 3:66–71.

Rayevsky KS, Kharlamov AN: GABA-ergic drugs: Effects on conditioning, memory and learning. *Pharmacol Res Commun* 1983; 15:85–96.

Regina EG, Smith GM, Keiper CG: Effects of caffeine on alertness in simulated automobile driving. *J Appl Psychol* 1974; 59:483–489.

Sadeh M, Braham J, Modan M: Effects of anticholinergic drugs on memory in Parkinson's disease. *Arch Neurol* 1982; 39:666–667.

Sitaram N, Weingartner H: Human serial learning: Enhancement with arecoline and choline and impairment with scopolamine. *Science* 1978; 201:274–276.

Squire LR: Pharamacology of learning and memory; in Glick SD, Goldfarb F (eds): *Behavioral Pharmacology.* Mosby, 1976, pp. 258–282.

Tagliente T: *Regional Effects of Barbiturates on Monoamine Oxidase Type A and Type B Activity in the Mouse Brain,* PhD dissertation. City University of New York, 1979.

Talland GA, Quarton GC: The effects of methamphetamine and pentobarbital on the running memory span. *Psychopharmacologia* 1982; 7:379–382.

Wilson J, Turner D: Awareness during caesarean section under general anesthesia. *Br Med J* 1969; 1:280–283.

Zornetzer SF: Neurotransmitter modulation and memory: A new neuropharmacological phrenology? in Lipton MA, Demascio A, Killam K (eds): *Psychopharmacology: A Generation of Progress.* New York, Raven Press, 1978, pp. 637–649.

CHAPTER 4

# Alcohol and Memory Impairment

The effects of ethanol on the human body appear to be accumulative. Almost all the physiological systems of the body are affected by alcohol. Chronic consumption of alcohol causes diseases of the liver, pancreas, brain, gastrointestinal tract, and cardiovascular system. Organ sensitivity to alcohol varies widely. A few drinks a day, without producing acute intoxication, may cause liver disease in some persons while others may show no apparent effect. The nervous system, however, appears to be very sensitive to the toxic effects of alcohol.

Even moderate amounts of alcohol, taken in social gatherings, produce definite impairment of mental and motor functions. There appears to be a continuum in the effects of alcohol from social drinking to chronic heavy consumption. Although the effects of a few drinks in a social drinker may disappear by the next day, the effects of chronic consumption of alcohol accumulate to cause brain dysfunction and brain damage with associated intellectual and memory impairments.

## A. SOCIAL DRINKING

Early laboratory studies demonstrated a positive relationship between moderate blood alcohol concentrations (BACs = 0.06–0.10 mg/100 ml) and the impairment of various psychomotor functions (Drew et al., 1958). Subsequent studies have explored the effects of low BACs (< 0.05 mg/100 ml) on complex cognitive functions (Evans et al., 1974; Sidell and Pless, 1971). The results of these studies were not conclusive. Moskowitz et al. (1968, 1976) demonstrated in a series of experiments that low BACs impaired a divided-attention task that measured cognitive decision making rather than simple performance. Mills and Bisgrove (1983) tested the degree of cognitive impairment in 40 men on a complex discrimination task. The men were selected to fit four research subgroups: young/light drinkers; young/heavy drinkers; old/light drinkers; old/heavy drinkers. The mean age of the young drinkers was 28.55 years. The light and heavy drinkers were defined on the basis of their history of past drinking. All the subjects were given a placebo and two doses of alcohol in a random order across sessions. The results indicated a progressive impairment of performance on a discrimination task given at 20, 40, 60, and 80 min after the drinking stopped. The test was relatively insensitive to age and past drinking history. However, young/heavy drinkers showed a tendency to be less impaired at their peak BACs.

MacVane *et al.* (1982) studied the effects of social drinking in 106 men between the ages of 30 and 60 on several memory and cognitive tasks: the Wisconsin Card Sorting Test (a five-word short-term memory test), the Digit-Symbol Substitution, and the Vocabulary Subtests of the Wechsler Adult Intelligence Scale. The results indicated a significant decrease in performance on these tests with light to moderate alcohol consumption.

Jones and Jones (1980) investigated whether cognitive performance is adversely affected in sober women social drinkers. Thirty-two women between the ages of 21 and 55 were tested on a verbal memory task before and after a dose of 0.52 g/kg of body weight of alcohol. Neither immediate nor short-term memory differed for light versus moderate drinkers prior to alcohol consumption. However, moderate drinkers had significantly lower ratios of short-term memory to immediate memory than the light drinkers before the consumption of alcohol. The authors concluded that women, like men, may experience negative cognitive consequences as a function of social drinking.

Hannon *et al.* (1983) tested 92 college students, 52 women and 40 men with a mean age of 20.3 years, on a number of memory and cognitive tasks: the Wisconsin Card Sorting Test, the Shipley-Hartford Institute of Living Scale, the Digit-Symbol Test, the Trail-making Test, and the Textual Performance Test. The subjects were also administered a health questionnaire, a drinking history questionnaire, and a drug-history survey. The results indicated significantly decreased cognitive performance with increased consumption of alcohol per occasion and with total lifetime consumption in both men and women college students tested while sober. In men, however, increased performance on some tasks was also significantly correlated with increased frequency of drinking.

Johnson (1981–1982) administered a drinking survey and a cognitive functioning test to 1365 men and women workers to study the effects of light and moderate social drinking on intellectual abilities. The men reported drinking an average of 1.3 oz of absolute alcohol per drinking occasion, with occasions occurring 2.9 times per week. The women reported drinking an average of 1 oz about 1.6 times per week. As reported drinking per occasion increased, the men exhibited a steady decline in abstraction ability. Women who drank more than once a week followed the same general pattern as men, yet those who drank less than once a week experienced no effect.

In summary, a review of the recent literature indicates that social drinking of light to moderate amounts of alcohol impairs cognitive and memory functions not only during drinking but even in the sober state.

## B. ACUTE ALCOHOLIC INTOXICATION

Several types of cognitive and memory disorders have been investigated during acute intoxication. Memory for events occurring during acute intoxication is generally fuzzy or a total blackout may occur. Three types of memory disturbances are attributed to alcohol intoxication: state-dependent learning, memory storage and retrieval deficits, and blackout.

### Alcohol State-dependent Learning

State-dependent learning (SDL) is a phenomenon in which information learned during a particular drug or psychological state is more completely retrieved in a simlar state than in a dissimilar state. Thus certain types of information acquired during alcohol intoxication may be recalled better during subsequent intoxication than during a sober period.

State-dependent learning has been demonstrated in animals and humans using moderate doses of a variety of drugs, including alcohol, marijuana, and barbiturates. Alcohol has been shown to produce SDL on verbal learning tasks (Young, 1979) and motor and physiological responses (Madill, 1967). Several investigators have tried to define the presence of the specific conditions that lead to SDL. For example, Eich (1977) suggested that SDL is most likely to occur if the following two conditions were present: (1) moderate consumption of alcohol (BACs near 100 mg%), and (2) tasks requiring sequential processing retrieval of information. A low dose of alcohol may not be sufficient for SDL to occur whereas high doses are likely to cause a complete obliteration of memory. It has been further suggested that providing external cues during the acquisition of information may decrease SDL and enhance the recall of the information during the sober state. The question of the specific nature of the information learned during SDL is not settled. There are indications that SDL may include less meaningful, verbal and episodic information.

### Memory Storage and Retrieval Problems

The dual-process model of memory divides normal memory processes into sensory memory, short-term memory (STM), and long-term memory (LTM). Sensory memory is the first impression that incoming information makes on the organism. The information from the sensory memory is transferred to STM. An item can be recalled from STM if tested immediately after its presentation, but it is lost within a few seconds unless it is constantly rehearsed or repeated in some manner. Some of the information from STM is transferred to LTM where it remains unstable for some time before it is sorted for long-term recall. Retrieval problems from LTM storage are common in old age and under toxic conditions.

Alcohol appears to dull sensory processes and impedes acquisition of information or its retrieval from the sensory memory (Moskowitz and Murray, 1976). Riege et al. (1976) suggested that retention also varies with the sensory modality. They found that alcoholics, relative to controls, were deficient in verbal recall and in visual and tactual recognition but showed no deficit in recognition of nonverbal auditory stimuli.

The effects of alcohol in the impairment of STM have been controversial. Parker et al. (1974) and Rosen and Lee (1976) found that alcohol (moderate levels) disrupted STM as tested by digit span tests. In their subjects, performance on digit span tests was significantly impaired as compared with the sober condition. Further analysis of the data indicated that although the difference between the sober and intoxicated conditions was statistically significant, it was quite small in the absolute numbers recalled.

In free recall items of a list, the items from near the end of the list reflect STM function (recency effect) while the items from the beginning of the list reflect LTM function (primacy effect). Jones and Jones (1976) found that in free recall moderate BACs (100 mg%) exerted a depressive effect on "primacy effect" but had no effect on "recency effect," indicating some disruption of LTM but no impairment of STM.

It has been suggested that the formation of LTM may be impaired during alcohol intoxication because of the disruption in the transfer of information from STM to LTM. Although the immediate recall on digit span is minimally affected, the information is not retained long enough in STM, through rehearsal and encoding processes, to be transferred to LTM storage. This hypothesis has not been confirmed.

Alternatively, perhaps the information does enter LTM, but retrieval process may be at fault. Temporary retrieval deficits are caused by other nervous system depressants. Saucedo (1980) reported retrieval failure under alcohol intoxication, as a significant number of subjects, tested 24 hr later, spontaneously recalled the previously inaccessible material.

Birnbaum and Parker (1977) tested subjects on paired associate and free recall tasks. The subjects first performed while sober, then retrieved information in an intoxicated or sober state one week later. It was found that retention losses were equal for both the sober to intoxicated and sober to sober groups. The authors concluded that the information originally learned in a nondrug state is quite resistant to later retrieval deficits.

A few studies suggest that alcohol impairs storage more than retrieval. Parker et al. (1976) found that alcohol disrupted initial learning but had no effect on the later retention of the same material.

In addition, performance is also influenced by several other factors such as history of drinking, age, sex, and expectancy. A long history of drinking leads to more impairment in performance under acute intoxication. Short-term memory is disrupted more in older individuals than in younger persons under alcohol. Women have been found to be more affected by alcohol during the premenstrual phase and in comparison to men show greater memory loss under delayed recall conditions (Jones and Jones, 1976).

An expectancy effect has been shown by observation of subjects expecting alcohol but receiving tonic or subjects expecting tonic but receiving alcohol. They made more errors on cognitive tasks than did the subjects in expectancy-congruent groups (Williams *et al.*, 1978).

In summary, a moderate amount of alcohol dulls the sensory channels and impedes acquisition and recall from sensory storage. Short-term memory is minimally affected by alcohol, but the transfer of information to LTM appears to be disrupted, leading to impairment of retention in LTM. Retrieval of previously learned material may be somewhat impaired during acute intoxication.

## Alcohol Blackouts

This phenomenon is an inability of the person to recall, while sober, events that occurred and the information that was learned during the intoxicated state. Although the blackouts are common in alcoholics, they may also occur in nonalcoholics. The blackouts usually occur at high BACs (200 mg%). This is not an all-or-none phenomenon since there is always some memory for the bits and pieces of the situation. Although soon after recovery from the intoxication there may be a complete blackout for some of the events, some recovery does occur with the passage of time and with the help of associated cues.

The mechanism of the loss of memory during blackouts is not clear. Disruption of consolidation process in LTM appears to be the most likely mechanism involved. Mello and Mendelson (1978), using a simple matching task and short retention intervals (0–6 min), have shown that STM is not impaired even at high BACs (200 mg%). Lisman (1974), on the other hand, found an impairment in STM on a picture recall task at 20 min intervals. However, a 20-min interval of recall in Lisman's study may not qualify as a STM deficit.

Several studies show that when learning parameters are maximized by providing contextual cues during intoxication, the loss of memory for the learned material is minimal. Goodwin *et al.* (1975) compared two groups for recall of material learned during intoxication. The group that was provided contextual cues was better able to recall the learned material 24 hr later than the noncued group, even at a very high BACs (300 mg%). The authors concluded that cuing during initial learning enhanced storage and retrieval even at a very high alcohol level.

There are wide individual variations for the occurrence of blackouts, depending upon the age, sex, past history of drinking, and perhaps expectations of the heavy-drinking person. There are indications that the critical threshold for blackouts may drop with progressive heavy drinking.

## C. CHRONIC ALCOHOLISM

Chronic alcoholism is difficult to define especially with respect to its consequences on the person. However, there are several population surveys indicating that chronic drinking is a major health problem in most western countries. Calahan (1970), in a random survey of the United States population, suggested that approximately 9% of the adult population (15% of the men and 4% of the women) were problem drinkers. Whalley (1980) reported demographic data on hospitalized alcoholics in Scotland. He noted a progressive increase in the rate of admissions between 1965 and 1974. There was an 88% increase in admissions for women and a 49% increase for men; a greater increase for young people than old. Although all social classes were represented, social class IV and V (semiskilled and unskilled workers) (Hollingshead and Redlich, 1958) contributed disproportionately large numbers of men and women to the hospitalized group.

Although all bodily organs are affected by the chronic consumption of alcohol, the nervous system appears to be the most sensitive to its damaging effects. The cognitive and memory deficits that occur in social drinkers and in acute intoxication become progressively worse with continued consumption until all aspects of cognitive functioning are impaired. The worsening in cognitive functions parallels the progressive damage to the nervous system. The Wernicke-Korsakoff syndrome, indicative of severe brain damage, may become clinically apparent after 10 to 15 years of chronic drinking in moderate to heavy amounts.

### Cognitive Changes

A fairly large number of studies show that chronic alcoholics perform poorly on various measures of intelligence and on neuropsychological batteries. Miller and Saucedo (1983) summarized the results of 17 controlled studies contrasting the performance of alcoholics on the Wechsler Adult Intelligence Scale (WAIS) to that of various comparison groups. Alcoholics showed impaired performance on all subtests of the WAIS as compared with a control group. The degree of impairment, however, varied for different subtests. Performance subtests were impaired much more than verbal subtest. The Block Design subtest appeared to be the most severely affected test among the performance subtests. Among the verbal subtests, arithmetic scores were quite low for most alcoholics. Vocabulary seemed to be least affected by chronic drinking.

Lishman *et al*. (1980) reported findings on 93 alcoholics, matched with 36 controls, who were examined with a full battery of psychometric tests. In addition to the New Adult Reading Test, the following tests were employed: a shortened version of the WAIS [vocabulary, similarities and digit span subtests for verbal IQ and digit symbol, picture completion and block design subtests for performance (IQ)]; several tests of new learning ability (such as the Wechsler Logical Memory Test and the Williams Object Memory Test); the Trail-making test; the modified Wisconsin Card-sorting Test; and tests of verbal fluency.

The results indicated that both the verbal and performance IQs of alcoholics were lower than those of the controls. This finding persisted after the data were controlled for age and premorbid IQ differences between the groups. Similar differences were seen on several tests of new learning ability on subtests measuring perceptual motor skills and on abstracting tasks.

Neuropsychological assessment on the Halstead-Reitan Tests reveals that chronic alcoholics are impaired on most of the subtests. These findings indicate that alcoholics are clearly impaired in many areas of cognitive functioning despite being selected on the basis of having no obvious indication of brain damage and despite being tested after a period (6–12 months) of total abstinence.

## Memory Deficits

Ryback (1971) proposed that STM disruption by alcohol was the underlying defect common to a continuum of memory effects seen in social drinkers, chronic alcoholics, and Korsakoff's syndrome. This suggestion highlights the progressive deteriorating influence of alcohol on the memory and the cognitive functions. It is impossible to precisely specify the degree of deficit resulting from a specific duration of chronic heavy drinking because of individual variation in the response to alcohol. Studies testing chronic alcoholics at various intervals invariably find memory deficits, with the majority of the chronic alcoholics placed closer to the deficits found in Korsakoff's syndrome.

Riege *et al*. (1981) tested chronic alcoholics, 54 men (15–63 years of drinking, average alcoholism duration 15.9 years) and 18 matched controls, on visual, auditory, tactual, verbal, and facial recognition tests. In recognition memory for visual patterns, short-term alcoholics (<12 years of heavy drinking) differed significantly from long-term alcoholics (13 to 22 years) and extended long-term alcoholics (>23 years). On visual, auditory, and facial recognition tests, both long-term and extended long-term alcoholics were deficient. Tactual recognition appeared to be unaffected by long-term alcoholism. The number of memory deficits seemed to increase linearly with increased age and length of alcoholism.

Guthrie *et al*. (1980) tested 521 chronic alcoholics (402 males and 119 females), ten days after they were hospitalized for treatment, on the Benton Visual Retention Test for Memory. The mean IQ of the group on the Raven's

Progressive Matrices Test was 110, SD $\pm$ 13.41, and a mean age of 39.6 years, SD $\pm$ 10.6. More than half of the group (57.8%) showed moderate to severe impairment on the memory test.

Although the core of the selective dysfunction in chronic alcoholics is memory impairment, other deficits frequently occur: rigidity of thought processes, impaired abstract thinking, difficulty in learning new material, decrease in visuospatial and visuoreceptive skill, and emotive behavioral changes.

## Neuropathology

Although no direct relationship has been established between memory impairment and specific brain pathology, it is generally assumed that the memory disturbances in chronic alcoholics result from brain damage caused by alcohol.

Central nervous system disturbances resulting from chronic consumption of alcohol were traditionally attributed to malnutrition, especially thiamine deficiency.

However, it has been shown that neurophysiologic deficits are present in individuals without any nutritional deficiency—a direct toxic effect on the CNS. Alcohol is a CNS depressant, having properties in common with general anesthetics.

In nutritionally controlled studies of rodents (Walker *et al.*, 1980) chronic ethanol exposure results in impaired learning in a variety of behavioral tasks including shuttle-box shock avoidance, temporal discrimination, temporal alteration, and complex maze learning. The ethanol-induced impairments appeared to be permanent since the deficit was present even after the ethanol-free period of 18 weeks. Histological examination of the brains of these rodents reveals altered dendritic morphology and a decrease in the number of hippocampal and cerebellar neurons. The number of dendritic spines on pyramidal and granular cells was drastically reduced by 50% to 60% in the alcohol group relative to the controls.

Alcohol has been shown to slow conduction along both sensory and motor pathways. At least two mechanisms for this inhibition of conduction have been identified: demyelination and action on the neuronal membrane. Demyelination in peripheral nerves, pyramidal tracts, the cerebellum, the pons, and the corpus callosum has been demonstrated in chronic alcoholism (D'Amour *et al.*, 1979). Alcohol has a depolarizing effect on the neuronal membrane. The depolarization, however, is dose related and reverses itself after the alcohol is washed away. The effect of alcohol on action potential generation is biphasic. Low concentrations tend to cause increases in excitability (i.e., lower threshold) whereas high concentrations tend to cause a transient increase but then a progressive reduction of excitability finally leading to complete blockage of impulse conduction.

## Neurochemistry

A long-standing and controversial question is whether alcohol exerts its effects mainly by depressing synaptic transmission or mainly by reducing axonal excitability and conduction. Both positions have been supported by a number of studies but neither of the positions have been conclusively proven. There are a variety of mechanisms by which alcohol could alter synaptic transmission. Possible synaptic effects include modification of transmitter synthesis, storage, release, or degradation; postsynaptic effects include changes in the sensitivity of the postsynaptic receptors for the neurotransmitter.

The effects of acute and chronic alcohol administration on neurotransmitter systems are often contradictory and no definite conclusion can be drawn. Alcohol has been shown to enhance the accumulation of labeled catecholamines after administration of labeled tyrosine in both mice and rats. It has not been clear whether this increased accumulation is due to increased synthesis or to more efficient reuptake and/or binding mechanisms at the presynaptic terminal. Borg et al. (1981) measured the levels of the major norepinephrine metabolite, 3-methoxy-4-hydroxy, phenylethylene-glycol (MHPG), in the lumbar cerebrospinal fluid of 45 intoxicated alcoholics after one week (N = 18) and three weeks (N = 27) of abstinence. The MHPG level, which was markedly elevated during intoxication compared with that of 27 healthy controls, declined successively after one and three weeks of abstinence.

Valchar (1980) measured dopamine and its metabolites in acute and chronic administration of ethanol in the rat brain. Dopamine increases in the corpus striatum and continues to increase in chronic administration. Similarly, homovanillic acid and 3,4-dihydroxyphenyl-acetic acid increased progressively, but returned to control levels when ethanol was discontinued. Dopamine and serotonin went up conspicuously 1 hr after the interruption, but returned to control levels 12 hr later.

Earlier studies have shown variable effects of ethanol on brain acetylcholine, some showing an increase (Reisberg, 1974) and others a decrease (Rawat, 1974). Owasoyo and Iramain (1981) measured the activities of acetylcholinesterase (AChE) and choline acetyltransferase (ChAT) in the cerebral cortex cerebellum, the hypothalamus, the hippocampus, the midbrain, and the pons of adult male mice by spectrophotometric methods 30 min after intraperitoneal injection of ethanol 2g/kg of body weight or saline. Ethanol significantly decreased AChE activity only in the cerebral cortex whereas ChAT activity was reduced in the cerebral cortex, the hypothalamus, and the hippocampus. Thus the effect of ethanol on the cholinergic system of the mouse was presumed to be mediated by its effect on AChE and ChAt in specific regions.

A single dose of ethanol has been reported to increase, decrease, and have no effect on brain serotonin levels (Kuriyama et al., 1971). Borisov (1981) showed that rats with less than the normal amounts of brain serotonin prefer alcohol to water. When serotonin level was increased to a normal level, rats completely rejected alcohol. The author concluded that alcoholism may be related to disturbed metabolism of serotonin.

Sytinski *et al.* (1975) reported that GABA levels were slightly increased in the cerebellum and the cerebrum with low doses of alcohol, but large doses of ethanol caused a decrease and lethal doses produced a sharp increase. Such multiphasic effects may explain some of the apparent contradictions in the literature. Edmonds *et al.* (1980) showed that chronic ethanol consumption in rats increases enzyme activities related to GABA metabolism without changing brain GABA levels.

Hiller *et al.* (1981) reported that the addition of ethanol to rat brain membranes strongly inhibits binding of enkephalins at concentrations at which little inhibition of opiate alkaloids is seen. The inhibition is reversible and the potency increases with the chain length of the alcohol.

Several compounds, formed as a result of ethanol metabolism, have been suspected of producing some of ethanol's behavioral effects. Acetaldehyde was once thought responsible, but the administration of pyrazole (which inhibits alcohol dehydrogenase) disproved acetaldehyde's responsibility for the acute effects of ethanol. However, the theories on the long-term effects of alcohol maintain that acetaldehyde and endogenous biogenic aldehydes utilize the same oxidative pathways in the brain. Also, the condensation of aldehydes with the amines can lead to a number of compounds: beta-carbolines, sarsolinal, and tetrahydropapaveroline. These compounds have attracted the most research attention in recent years as possibly being responsible for some of ethanol's action.

## Brain Atrophy

Several studies using computerized tomography have confirmed progressive brain atrophy in chronic alcoholics. Lishman *et al.* (1980) compared CT scans of a group of alcoholics with a control group. The brain of the alcoholics showed both cortical shrinkage and ventricular enlargement. A slight improvement was noted after a year or more of abstinence. In another study, Carlen *et al.* (1981) studied 97 alcoholics with at least a ten-year history of drinking more than 80 g of ethanol daily. Most of the nonimpaired alcoholics had measurable atrophy. Alcoholics of all ages, including the young and clinically unimpaired, demonstrated cerebral atrophy on CT scan.

Brain weight studies of alcoholics show a significant reduction in brain weight compared with controls. Torvik (1982) found that the brains of chronic alcoholics (545 males) weighed significantly less than the brains of 586 controls. The study also revealed generalized brain atrophy in alcoholics.

Deficits on the performance subscales of the WAIS in chronic alcoholics led psychologists to hypothesize greater damage to the right cerebral hemisphere. However, this hypothesis has not been proved by pathological studies. In fact, some of the studies have shown more left- than right-hemispheric damage. Quijo (1981) reported reduced densities in the left brain hemisphere of 11 long-term alcoholics subjected to CT scan.

## Reversibility of Deficits

Victor *et al.* (1971) indicated that Korsakoff's syndrome can reverse over a period of two years with abstinence. This optimism has not been shared by subsequent studies. There is, however, a general agreement among studies that some recovery occurs in the first week of abstinence with conflicting reports on changes during the next nine weeks of abstinence. Guthrie *et al.* (1980) reported that alcoholics tested after 2, 4, 8, 26, and 52 weeks of abstinence showed changes occurring from the first to the last week of testing, with maximal improvement during the period between 4 to 8 weeks, but the overall improvement did not reach statistical significance until 52 weeks. The pattern of improvement was somewhat different in a nutritionally deficient group. This group showed maximal changes between two to four weeks of abstinence with intensive vitamin therapy.

Two other studies of long-term follow-up indicate significant improvement in cognitive functions after one year (O'Leary *et al.*, 1977) and three years of abstinence (White, 1965).

## Alcoholic Dementia

The term alcoholic dementia is usually used when other causes of dementia have been ruled out including Korsakoff's syndrome. The diagnosis of alcohol dementia fell into disrepute after the more specific Korsakoff's syndrome was identified. However, clinical evidence suggests that chronic alcoholics may suffer from intellectual and memory deficits with are distinct from Korsakoff's syndrome. As discussed earlier, the presence of moderate brain atrophy can be demonstrated in many chronic alcoholics, especially in older alcoholics. These individuals may not develop the clinical manifestations of Korsakoff's syndrome. They do, however, suffer from intellectual and memory deficits. Studies indicate the presence of forgetfulness, psychomotor retardation, poor attention, and disorientation. They also show poor abstraction abilities, impaired STM, and disturbed verbal fluency (Blusewicz *et al.*, 1977).

## D. SUMMARY

Alcohol (ethanol) affects all the physiological systems of the body including the liver, pancreas, brain, gastrointestinal tract, and cardiovascular system. Organ sensitivity to alcohol varies widely. The central nervous system appears to be the most sensitive to toxic effects of alcohol. Effects of chronic consumption of alcohol, even in small amounts, seem to accumulate to cause brain dysfunction with associated intellectual and memory impairments. Several studies have shown that social drinking of light to moderate amounts of alcohol impairs cognitive and memory functions not only during drinking but even in the sober state.

Acute alcoholic intoxication has been related to three types of memory disturbances: state-dependent learning (SDL), memory storage and retrieval deficits, and blackouts. State-dependent learning is a phenomenon in which information learned during a particular drug or psychological state is more completely retrieved in a similar state than in a dissimilar state. Thus certain types of information acquired during alcohol intoxication may be recalled better during a subsequent intoxication than during a sober state. It has been suggested that SDL is likely to occur if the following two conditions are present: (1) moderate consumption of alcohol (BACs near 100 mg%), and (2) tasks requiring sequential retrieval of information. A low dose of alcohol may not be sufficient for SDL to occur whereas high doses are likely to cause a complete obliteration of memory. Although the type of information learned during SDL is variable, there are indications that SDL may include less meaningful verbal and episodic information.

Moderate amounts of alcohol dull the sensory channels and impede acquisition and recall from sensory storage. Short-term memory is minimally affected by alcohol, but the transfer of information to LTM appears to be disrupted, leading to impairment of retention in LTM.

Alcohol blackout is referred to as an inability of the person to recall while sober events that occurred and the information that was learned during the intoxicated state. The blackouts usually occur at high blood concentrations of alcohol (200 mg%). This is not an all-or-none phenomenon since there is always some memory for the bits and pieces of the situation. Although soon after recovery from the intoxication there may be a complete blackout for the events, some recovery does occur with the passage of time with the help of associated cues. The mechanism of these blackouts is not clear. A disruption of consolidation process in LTM appears to be the most likely mechanism involved.

The cognition and memory deficits that occur in social drinkers and in acute intoxication become progressively worse with chronic alcoholism until all aspects of cognitive functions are impaired. The worsening in cognitive functions parallels the progressive damage to the nervous system. The Wernicke-Korsakoff's syndrome, indicative of severe brain damage, may become clinically apparent after 10 to 15 years of chronic drinking in moderate to heavy amounts.

It is impossible to precisely specify the degree of deficits resulting from a specific duration of chronic heavy drinking due to individual variation in the response to alcohol. Studies testing chronic alcoholics at various intervals invariably find memory deficits, with the majority of the chronic alcoholics placed closer to the deficits found in Korsakoff's syndrome. Degree of memory deficit seems to increase linearly with increased age and length of alcoholism.

Central nervous system disturbances resulting from chronic consumption of alcohol were traditionally attributed to malnutrition, especially thiamine deficiency. However, it has been shown that neurophysiological deficits are present in individuals without any nutritional deficiency. Alcohol is a CNS depressant, having properties in common with general anesthetics. It slows down conduction along both sensory and motor pathways. Alcohol has also been shown to depress synaptic transmission by influencing metabolism of neurotransmitters. Alcohol consumption enhances accumulation of catecholamines, acetylcholine, serotonin, and GABA in the brain. Several toxic compounds may be formed as a result of ethanol metabolism. They include acetaldehyde, beta-carbolines, satsolinal, and tetrahydropapaveroline.

Computerized tomographic studies of chronic alcoholics frequently show progressive brain atrophy with cortical shrinkage and ventricular enlargement. Similarly, autopsies of chronic alcoholics show a significant reduction in brain weight.

Recovery of cognitive functions with treatment depends greatly upon the degree and duration of chronic alcoholism. In severe cases brain damage is permanent. Some recovery occurs in the first week of abstinence, with maximal improvement during the period between four to eight weeks.

## E.  REFERENCES

Birnbaum I, Parker E: Acute effects of alcohol on storage and retrieval, in Birnbaum IM, Parker E (eds): *Alcohol and Human Memory*. Hillsdale, NJ, Laurence Erlbaum, 1977.

Blusewicz M, Dustman R, Schenkenberg T, *et al*: Neuropsychological correlates of chronic alcoholism and aging. *J Nerv Ment Dis* 1977; 165:348–355.

Borg S, Kvande H, Sedvalle G: Central norepinephrine metabolism during alcohol intoxication in addicts and healthy volunteers. *Science* 1981; 213:1135–1137.

Borisov MM: The role of serotonergic brain structures in alcohol addiction (English translation). *Zh Nevropatol* 1981; 81:1094–1099.

Calahan D: *Problem Drinkers: A National Survey*. San Francisco, Jossey-Bass, 1970.

Carlen P, Wilkenson D, Wortzman G, *et al*: Cerebral atrophy and functional deficits in alcoholics without clinically apparent liver disease. *Neurology* 1981; 31:377–385.

D'Amour M, Shahani B, Young R, *et al*: The importance of studying sural nerve conduction and late responses in the evaluation of alcoholic subjects. *Neurology* 1979; 29:1600–1604.

Drew G, Colquohoun W, Long H: Effects of small doses of alcohol on a skill resembling driving. *Br Med J* 1958; 2:993–999.

Edmonds H Jr, Sylvester D, Bellin S, *et al*: Gamma-aminobutyric acid system and bioelectric activity of the brain in rats during alcohol intoxication. *Fiziol Zh SSSR* 1980; 16:1298–1306.

Eich JE: State-dependent retrieval of information in human episodic memory, in Birnbaum IM, Parker ES (eds): *Alcohol and Human Memory*. Hillsdale, NJ, Lawrence Erlbaum, 1977.

Evans M, Martz R, Rodda B, *et al*: Quantitative relationship between blood alcohol concentration and psychomotor performance. *Clin Pharmacol Ther* 1974; 15:253–260.

Goodwin D, Hill S, Hopper S, *et al*: Alcoholic blackouts and Korsakoff syndrome, in Gross M (ed): *Alcohol Intoxication and Withdrawal: Experimental Studies II*. New York, Plenum Press, 1975.

Guthrie A, Presley A, Greekie C, *et al*: The effects of alcohol on memory, in Sandler M (ed): *Psychopharmacology of Alcohol*. New York; Grune and Stratton, 1980, pp. 79–88.

Hannon R, Day C, Butler A, *et al*: Alcohol consumption and cognitive functioning in college students. *J Stud Alcohol* 1983; 44:283–298.

Hiller J, Angel L, Simon E: Multiple opiate receptors: Alcohol selectively inhibits binding to deltan receptors. *Science* 1981; 214:468–469.

Hollingshead A, Redlich F: *Social Class and Mental Illness: A Community Survey*. New York; John Wiley and Sons, 1958.

Johnson N; Moderate drinkers suffer intellectual impairment. *Alcohol Health Res World* 1981–1982; 6:40.

Jones B, Jones M: Women and alcohol: Intoxication, metabolism and the menstrual cycle, in Greenblatt M, Schuckit M (eds): *Alcoholism Problems in Women and Children*. New York, Grune and Stratton, 1976.

Jones M, Jones B: Relationship of age and drinking history to the effects of alcohol on memory in women. *J Stud Alcohol* 1980; 41:179–186.

Kuriyama K, Rauscher G, Sze P: Effect of acute and chronic administration of ethanol on the 5-hydroxytryptamine turnover and tryptophan hydroxylase activity of the mouse brain. *Brain Res* 1971; 26:450–454.

Lishman W, Ron M, Acker W: Computed tomography of the brain and psychomoter assessment of alcoholic patient—A British study, in Sandler M (ed): *Psychopharmacology of Alcohol*. New York, Grune and Stratton, 1980, pp. 33–41.

Lisman SA: Alcoholic "blackout": state-dependent learning? *Arch Gen Psychiatry* 1974; 30:46–53.

MacVane J, Butters N, Montgomery K, *et al*: Cognitive functioning in new social drinkers. *J Stud Alcohol* 1982; 43:81–95.

Madill M: *Alcohol Induced Dissociation in Humans: A Possible Treatment Technique for Alcoholism*, PhD dissertation. Queens University (Kingston, Ontario, Canada), 1967.

Mello N, Mendelson J: Alcohol and human behavior, in Iverson LL, Iverson S, Snyder S (eds): *Handbook of Psychopharmacology*. New York, Plenum Press, 1978, vol 12.

Miller WR, Saucedo C: Assessment of neuropsychological impairment and brain damage in problem drinkers, in Golden C, Moses J Jr, Coffman J, *et al* (eds): *Clinical Neuropsychology*. New York, Grune and Stratton, 1983, pp. 141–195.

Mills K, Bisgrove E: Cognitive impairment and perceived risk from alcohol. *J Stud Alcohol* 1983; 44:26–46.

Moskowitz H, Depry D: Differential effect of alcohol on auditory vigilance and divided attention tasks. *Q J Stud Alcohol* 1968; 19:54–63.

Moskowitz H, Murray J: Alcohol and backward masking of visual information. *J Stud Alcohol* 1976; 37:40–45.

Naus M, Cermak L, De Luca D: Retrieval processes in alcoholic Korsakoff patients. *Neuropsychologia* 1977; 15:737–742.

O'Leary M, Radford L, Chaney E, *et al*: Assessment of cognitive recovery in alcoholics by use of Trail-Making Test. *J Clin Psychol* 1977; 33:579–582.

Owasoyo J, Iramain C: Effects of acute ethanol intoxication on the enzymes of the cholinergic system in mouse brain. *Toxicol Lett* 1981; 9:267–270.

Parker E, Alkana R, Birnbaum I, *et al*: Alcohol and the disruption of cognitive processes. *Arch Gen Psychiatry* 1974; 31:824–828.

Parker ES, Birnbaum I, Noble E: Alcohol and memory: Storage and state-dependency. *J Verb Learn Verb Behav* 1976; 15:691–702.

Quijo J: Chronic alcoholics may suffer tissue damage in left brain. *Alcoholism/Natl Mag* 1981; I:45.

Rawat AK: Brain levels and turnover rates of presumptive neurotransmitters as influenced by administration and withdrawal of ethanol in mice. *J Neurochem* 1974; 22:915–922.

Reisberg RB: Stimulation of choline acetyltransferase activity by ethanol in in vitro preparations of rat cerebrum. *Life Sci* 1974; 14:1965–1973.

Riege W, Holloway J, Kaplan D: Specific memory deficits associated with prolonged alcohol abuse. *Alcohol Clin Exp Res* 1981; 5:378–385.

Riege W, Miklusak C, Buchhalter J: Material-specific memory impairments in chronic alcoholics. *Biol Psychiatry* 1976; 11:109–113.

Rosen L, Lee C: Acute and chronic effects of alcohol use on organizational processes in memory. *J Abnorm Psychol* 1976; 85:309–317.

Ryback RS: The continuum and specificity of the effects of alcohol on memory: A review. *Q J Stud Alcohol* 1971; 32:995–1016.

Saucedo C: *The Effects of Alcohol State-dependent Learning on an Encoding Variability Task: Clinical and Neuropsychological Implications,* PhD dissertation. University of New Mexico, 1980.

Sidell F, Pless J: Ethyl alcohol blood levels and performance decrements after oral administration to man. *Psychopharmacologia* 1971; 19:246–261.

Sytinski I, Guzikov B, Gomanko M, *et al*: Gamma-aminobutyric acid system in brain during acute and chronic ethanol intoxication. *J Neurochem* 1975; 25:43–48.

Talland GA: *Deranged Memory.* New York, Academic Press, 1965.

Torvik A, Lindboe C, Rogde S: Brain lesions in alcoholics: A neuropathological study with clinical correlations. *J Neurol Sci* 1982; 56:233–248.

Valchar M: Ucast dopaminergniho Systemu V Mechanismu Ucinku Psychofarmak Csl. *Fysiol* 1980; 29:1–32.

Victor M, Adams R, Collins G: *The Wernicke-Korsakoff Syndrome.* Blackwell, Oxford, 1971.

Walker DW, Barnes D, Riley J, *et al*: Neurotoxicity of chronic alcohol consumption: An animal model, in Sandler M (ed): *Psychopharmacology of Alcohol.* New York, Grune and Stratton, 1980, pp. 17–31.

Whalley LJ: Social and biological variables in alcoholism: A selective review, in Sandler M (ed): *Psychopharmacology of Alcohol* New York, Raven Press, 1980, pp 1–15.

White W: Personality and cognitive learning among alcoholics with different intervals of sobriety. *Psychol Rep* 1965; 16:1125–1140.

Williams R, Goldman M, Williams D: Alcohol due and expectancy effects on cognitive and motor performance. Paper presented at the annual meeting of the American Psychological Association,, Toronto, 1978.

Young LD: Alcohol state-dependent effects in humans: A review and study of different task responses. *Br J Alcohol Alcoholism* 1979; 14:100–105.

# Role of Neuropeptides in Memory

Neurotransmitters, neuromodulators, and hormones are being studied extensively to determine their role in memory processes. The research in this area has become complicated with the increasing number of neuropeptides found in the brain. In addition to the classic neurotransmitters (acetylcholine, dopamine, serotonin, etc.), at least 30 to 40 new neuropeptides have been discovered in the last two decades. It is expected that 200 to 400 neuropeptides ultimately will be identified. Most of the neuropeptides so far studied appear to influence memory processes in some manner. Thus a single system of neuropeptides does not control memory processes. A brief review of the research is presented for each of the systems studied so far.

## A. NORADRENALINE AND DOPAMINE SYSTEM

Neurochemical mapping of the brain has revealed the presence of noradrenaline in widespread regions of the brain. The highest concentrations are in the hypothalamus and in the locus coeruleus. The cerebral cortex contains relatively small amounts. The noradrenergic cells in the locus coeruleus send processes widely throughout the brain and spinal cord. This system appears to be important for regulating sleep/wakefulness and attention. Noradrenaline causes hyperpolarization of the postsynaptic neuron.

Dopaminergic neuronal tracts have been demonstrated in the limbic system and in the basal ganglia. They have been of great interest because of their role in the pathology of Parkinson's disease. The primary action of dopamine is inhibition. Neurophysiological data suggest that dopamine hyperpolarizes the postsynaptic neurons by decreasing sodium conductance.

This effect appears to be mediated by an increased synthesis of cyclic adenosine monophosphate (cAMP).

Numerous animal studies have shown that learning and memory are influenced by treatments that affect catecholamines (Oei and King, 1980). Drugs such as amphetamine enhance learning and retention (McGaugh, 1973) whereas diethyldithiocarbamate (DDC) and reserpine, drugs that decrease levels of catecholamines, impair performance. The impairment caused by DDC can be blocked by posttraining administration of noradrenaline and dopamine into the cerebral ventricles. Jensen *et al.* (1977) found that intra-cerebroventricular administration of DDC impaired rats' retention of an inhibitory avoidance response if administered either shortly before or shortly after training. In the doses used, DDC reduced noradrenaline levels to approximately 50% in various brain regions.

Destruction of the noradrenergic system by lesions of the locus coeruleus or lesions of the dorsal noradrenergic bundle severely deplete forebrain norepinephrine, but have yielded mixed results for learning. Some studies report impaired learning while others show no effects.

Injection of DDC in localized areas of the brain such as the amygdala, the hippocampus, and the brain stem have also produced amnesic effects (Flood *et al.*, 1980). Retention of the inhibitory avoidance response in mice is enhanced by posttraining administration of low doses of norepinephrine into the cerebral ventricles and is decreased by posttraining administration of adrenergic antagonists into the amygdala.

The impairing effect of DDC was also achieved by subcutaneous administration of noradrenaline or adrenaline. Since noradrenaline and adrenaline do not readily pass the blood–brain barrier, their central effect was assumed to result from their peripheral influence. Martinez *et al.* (1980a) supported this assumption by showing that retention in rats was enhanced by posttraining peripheral administration of 4-*OH*-amphetamine, a metabolite of amphetamine that does not readily pass the blood–brain barrier. It was further hypothesized that the peripheral effect of noradrenaline was mediated by the adrenal medulla because the effect of noradrenaline was attenuated after the adrenal medulla was surgically removed prior to training. Similarly, the effect of amphetamine and 4-*OH*-amphetamine, given peripherally, were attenuated by adrenal demedullation on active avoidance and inhibitory avoidance tasks (Martinez *et al.*, 1980b).

The effect of posttraining peripheral administration of noradrenaline is dose related in an inverted U-shaped response. A moderate dose of noradrenaline (0.01–0.1 mg/kg) produced the greatest enhancement. A large dose (0.5 mg/kg) appeared to impair retention (Gold *et al.*, 1982). This dose-related response can also be shifted by adrenergic receptor blockers. The adrenaline-induced enhancement of retention is blocked by the β-adrenergic receptor blocker (i.e., propanolol) and adrenaline-induced impairment (from high doses) is blocked by the α-adrenergic receptor blocker phenoxybenzamine hydrochloride (Gold and Van Buskirk, 1978). These results suggest that the effect of peripherally administered adrenaline interact with those produced endogenously during and following training.

The results of intracerebroventricular dopamine administration show that dopamine also facilitates retrieval in a dose-dependent fashion. Relatively high concentrations are necessary to enhance retrieval, but these doses are without behavioral effects in noncontingently trained animals. The significant facilitation of retention by intraventricularly administered lisuride, a dopamine agonist, and its blockade by the dopamine antagonist haloperidol provide additional support for the roles of dopamine in learning and memory.

In summary, a variety of evidence suggest that central and peripheral adrenergic systems can modulate memory storage processes. For example, peripheral posttraining injections of adrenaline or noradrenaline can enhance or impair retention in an inverted-U dose-related manner. Furthermore, under many conditions, retention appears to be well correlated with the posttraining release of peripheral adrenaline and noradrenaline and central noradrenaline. Thus the central mechanisms underlying memory storage seem to be particularly sensitive to adrenergic influences.

## B. SEROTONERGIC SYSTEM

Serotonin is widely distributed in all regions of the brain, but most densely in the hypothalmus. Serotonergic neurons of the raphe nuclei participate in the regulation of sleep and wakefulness. Insomnia is produced by the destruction of the raphe nuclei or by the inhibition of serotonin synthesis. Serotonergic axons descend in the lateral columns of the spinal cord and these pathways appear to mediate the central control of the spinal transmission of pain impulses. The ionic mechanisms for serotonin transmission are not known. Serotonin binds to postsynaptic as well as to presynaptic membranes, suggesting a direct autofeedback that might regulate the release of the transmitter.

Animal studies show that learning and performance are impaired by elevated levels of brain serotonin and are enhanced by decreased levels. Elevated levels of serotonin produced by a combination of 5-hydroxytryptophan (60 mg/kg) and benzylmethoxytryptamine (15 mg/kg) caused a 13% reduction in the average number of correct maze responses by mice. Decreased brain serotonin, produced by either reserpine or oral DL-phenylalanine combined with L-tyrosine, increased correct maze responses by 7% and 9%, respectively (Woolley, 1965). The tryptophan hydroxylase inhibitor p-chlorophenylalanine (pCPA) has been an effective depletor of brain serotonin—up to 90% depletion in rats and 39% in mice. This agent facilitates several types of learning in rats such as the conditioned avoidance response and brightness discrimination.

Mice show diurnal differences in the serotonin depleting effect of pCPA. For the cerebral and the cerebellar cortices, a greater reduction in serotonin content resulted with morning administration of pCPA, although basal serotonin levels were down after noon.

Intracranial injection of serotonin elevates tissue serotonin, causes inhibition of regional protein synthesis, and produces temporary retrograde amnesia in mice. Pretreatment with norepinephrine blocks the retrograde amnesia of serotonin, but other catecholamines (dopamine, epinephrine) had no antiamnesic effect.

There is usually a rise in the serotonin level 15 min after electroconvulsive shock (ECS) which may be related to post-ECS amnesia. Norepinephrine and normetanephrine given intraventricularly 10 min prior to ECS block the rise of serotonin.

Common serotonin receptor antagonists such a methysergide and cyproheptadine have not found good use in the studies of learning and memory. There are several other substances such as nicotine and uric acid that have been shown to affect learning and memory by virtue of alteration in serotonin metabolism. In mice, nicotine reduces the forebrain turnover rate of serotonin by about 20% 45 min following nicotine injection. These changes are related to behavioral effects on mice. Essman (1973) treated mice with nicotine, then trained them for a single-trial passive avoidance response either 15 or 45 min later, followed by a single ECS. Mice trained and shocked 45 min after nicotine showed a 60% reduced incidence of ECS-induced amnesia. Similarly, uric acid has been shown to alternate retrograde amnesia induced by posttraining ECS, presumably through reducing serotonin turnover (Essman, 1970).

In man, disturbances of recent memory have been noticed in certain disease conditions (such as carcinoid syndrome and medullary carcinoma of the thyroid) in which high levels of circulating serotonin lead to some rise in brain serotonin and 5-hydroxyindoleacetic acid in the cerebrospinal fluid. Forgetting of dream content is presumed to be related to the rise of brain serotonin that occurs after a REM sleep episode. The recall of dream content is better if the person is awakened shortly after a REM sleep episode before the rise in brain serotonin occurs.

In summary, serotonin appears to exert a negative influence upon learning and memory. The effects are, however, small and not very dramatic. A variety of agents such as nicotine and uric acid alter learning and retention through changes in serotonin metabolism.

## C. CHOLINERGIC SYSTEM

A great deal of attention has been focused on the cholinergic system of neurotransmission because of its presumed involvement in Alzheimer's disease, Huntington's chorea, and tardive dyskinesia. There are, however, various technical difficulties that have hindered a clear understanding of the relationship between the cholinergic system and these diseases. Acetylcholine turnover cannot be measured in humans with presently available techniques. Acetylcholine levels and choline uptake are too vulnerable to postmortem changes for use. Activity of choline acetyltransferase has been used on postmortem tissue as an index of cholinergic neurons. Assays of the specific binding of [$^3$H]3-quinuclindinylbenzilate are also possible on postmortem tissue and are regarded as an index of muscarinic receptor activity of cholinergic neurons. Human studies are further complicated by the enormous variability in factors such as age, diet, drug exposure, and mode of death.

Several researchers (Carlton, 1961; Deutsch, 1971) had postulated two reciprocal systems of excitation and inhibition in the brain. The system of excitation was assumed to be mediated by noradrenergic functions whereas the system of inhibition was regulated by cholinergic functions. These assumptions were supported by a large amount of data derived from animal studies. Anticholinergic drugs such as scopolamine, given to animals, impaired their performance on various laboratory tasks such as avoidance procedures (Mollenauer et al., 1976), complex maze learning (Van der Poel, 1974), and discrimination tasks (Warburton and Brown, 1976). Similar effects were also noted following localized administration of anticholinergic drugs. For example, intrahippocampal injection of anticholinergic drugs impaired extinction performance (Singh et al., 1974), intracisternal administration impaired reversal learning, and intrahypothalamic injections decreased performance on a variety of operant tasks (Miczek and Grossman, 1972).

Cholinergic agonists, such as arecholine, choline, and pilocarpine, and anticholinesterases (physostigmine, DFP, phosdine) enhance discrimination performance (Warburton and Brown, 1972), habituation (Overstreet, 1975), and passive avoidance tasks in animals (Baratti et al., 1979).

Brain lesions causing the destruction of the cholinergic system also show impaired learning and memory performance parallel to that produced by anticholinergic drugs. For example, lesion of the septohippocampal pathways affects performance of various learned tasks (Morley and Russin, 1978).

Human studies show somewhat inconsistent results. Administration of scopolamine to normal subjects produces amnesic effects that are much greater than can be explained by the presence of the drowziness produced by the drug (Petersen, 1977). Cholinomimetics (arecholine, choline, physostigmine) have been found to improve some aspects of learning in normal human subjects (Sitaram et al., 1978; Davis et al., 1978). Extensive trials of acetylcholine precursors, such as 2-dimethylaminoethanol (deanol acetamidobenzoate), lecithin, or choline have produced significant improvement in learning and memory in only a small percentage of cases (Smith and Swash, 1978; Boyd et al., 1977). This lack of improvement is explained on the following basis: the precursors rarely increase acetylcholine levels in the brain; the action of the precursors depends on the continued integrity of neurons and may be absent in degenerative disease such as Alzheimer's disease. David and Yamamura (1978) found a dose-dependent effect of physostigmine in human subjects in relation to memory storage processes. Although physostigmine by itself did not affect cognitive functions, it antagonized the cognitive impairment induced by scopolamine. Liljequist and Mattila (1979) found that physostigmine (20 mg/kg iv) impaired the performance of good chess players. However, the chess players with low performance level showed improved solutions to chess problems. On the other hand, scopolamine impaired the performance of all players. When the two drugs were combined, they canceled out the effects of each other.

It has been suggested (Glen and Whalley, 1979) that cholinergic agents may produce some improvement in the memory of Alzheimer's disease patients only at the onset of the disease. They may have little effect once the disease has progressed beyond the initial stage. The latter point has been confirmed by two recent studies. In one study (Caltagirone *et al.*, 1982), physostigmine was administered orally 1 mg q.i.d., for one month to eight patients with a clinical diagnosis of Alzheimer's disease. The possible beneficial effects of the drug were evaluated by means of a neurophysiological battery administered to all patients before and after treatment. The drug did not produce any improvement in performance after one month of treatment. In the second study (Caltagirone *et al.*, 1983), eight Alzheimer's disease patients received individual optimal doses of physostigmine orally or subcutaneously. Individual dose was calculated by monitoring serum cholinesterase activity. Possible beneficial effects were evaluated with two memory tests: Rey's 15 Words and the Digit Span Test from the Wechsler Memory Scale. Although a slight behavioral activation was noted in all patients after treatment, no significant improvement occurred on these memory tests.

It has been pointed out that the cholinergic system may not be the sole mediator of inhibitory functions. Remington and Anisman (1976) found that scopolamine differentially affected spontaneous alternations and locomotor activity in mice as a function of age and strain. Furthermore, this relationship was nonlinear. In addition, much of the original data on which the cholinergic inhibitory model is based has been questioned by more recent findings. Ross *et al.* (1975) reported that interference of the cholinergic system at different foci in the brain did not produce a uniform effect. In Mollenauer and co-workers' study (1976), 95% of the errors of scopolamine-treated animals were due to their failure to initiate any response within the time limit. During the second half of each session, their discrimination performance was perfect. These observations suggested that the scopolamine-induced discrimination deficit was not due to a lack of inhibition, but to some delay of initial responding.

The cholinergic system is differentiated into muscarinic and nicotinic effects. The studies of the differential effects of muscarinic (i.e., scopolamine) and nicotinic (i.e., mecamylamine) blocking agents show that both scopolamine and mecamylamine produce a dissociation of learning. However, only scopolamine suppresses habituation by blocking the muscarinic activity of the cholinergic system. It appears that muscarinic receptor involvement in learning and memory may be more extensive than that of nicotinic receptors.

## D. OPIOID PEPTIDES

In 1975, several groups succeeded in isolating a morphinelike substance from the brain which was shown to consist of two pentapeptides, methionine enkephalin and leucine enkephalin. Soon after this, it was discovered that the sequence of five amino acids of met-enkephalin was contained within the 91 amino acids of a peptide called β-lipoprotein. Since then several fragments of the lipoprotein molecule have been found to possess morphinelike activity. The list of these peptides has grown rapidly. The currently known peptides include α-endorphin, β-endorphin, γ-endorphin, enkephalins, dysorphin, and rimorphin.

The distribution of opioid peptides closely parallels that of opiate receptors that are present in several regions of the brain. There is some evidence to suggest that there are separate populations of neurons for each of the opioid peptides. Some peptides coexist with classical neurotransmitters in the same neurons. The opioid peptides are also present in other tissues of the body, such as the gastrointestinal tract, the adrenal gland, the kidney, and the liver. The opioid peptides are considered to be neuromodulators, modifying the activity of neurons within a target region. A typical feature of the peptides indicating their role as neuromodulators rather than neurotransmitters is their relatively long duration of action (over a period of several hours).

The opioid peptides appear to be involved in the analgesia produced by placebo and acupuncture, the euphoric effects of morphine, and the regulation of emotional behavior. The role of the peptides in memory processes appears to be quite complex. They have been found both to facilitate and to inhibit retention and memory. Several laboratories (Belluzzi and Stein, 1977; Stanbli and Huston, 1980) found that high doses of enkephalin or morphine cause memory facilitation, while a number of other studies (Martinez and Rigter, 1980) have demonstrated amnesia following administration of low doses of opiates. These opposite results may be explained on the basis of an inverted-U dose response of peptides as commonly found with other hormones.

Izquierdo *et al.* (1981) found that training resulted in decreased β-endorphin immunoreactivity in the brain following training, suggesting that training causes the release and the metabolism of β-endorphin. Electroconvulsive shock to animals was also shown to cause the release of β-endorphin, suggesting that the amnesic effect of ECS may be related to β-endorphin (Dias *et al.*, 1981; Izquierdo, 1982). This observation was supported by the administration of naloxone after training but prior to ECS, which decreased the amnesic effect of ECS (Carrasco *et al.*, 1982). It has been suggested that endogeneous peptides impair memory retention by inhibiting the adrenergic system, both central and peripheral. Adrenal demedullation blocks the effects of enkephalin on memory retention.

## E. HORMONES

Research on the effects of hormones on memory is currently one of the fastest growing areas in psychopharmacology with the bulk of the literature on this topic appearing in the 1970s and the 1980s. Hormones exert their influences both at cellular and subcellular levels. Most hormones act through more than one of the known mechanisms. In many instances, specificity of hormone action depends upon where rather than how hormones act. Steroid hormones such as corticosteroids, estrogen and androgen enter the target cells from the circulation. Once inside the cell they bind to specific protein molecules called hormone receptors forming an active complex. This complex is translocated to the nucleus where it binds to the genome and thereby regulates the transcription of specific genes.

The catecholamines and peptide hormones bind to receptors located on the surface of the cells in the cell membrane. The binding process initiates a series of events that result in changes of cellular activity. Many of these hormones activate the enzyme adenylate cyclase which stimulates conversion of adenosine triphosphate (ATP) to cAMP. Cyclic AMP in many tissues activates protein kinases which bring about changes in cellular activity.

Training is accompanied by a variety of neurohumoral and hormonal changes that persist for some time and are believed to modulate the early phases of memory consolidation (Izquierdo et al., 1981). Some of these changes have been measured directly, but most have been inferred from pharmacological experiments. Adrenocorticotropic hormone (ACTH), vasopressin, and melanocyte-stimulating hormone (MSH) have been considered as facilitators of memory, while corticosteroids have been shown to have a depressor effect on memory consolidation.

Since peripherally administered hormones generally do not pass the blood–brain barrier, the mechanism of their action is not clear. A variety of mechanisms have been proposed:

1. Passage of minute amounts of hormones through the blood–brain barrier.
2. Passage of metabolic products of hormones through the blood–brain barrier.
3. Influence on the brain region which is poorly protected by the blood–brain barrier such as area póstrema.
4. Alteration in the permeability of the blood–brain barrier.
5. Activation of peripheral receptors influencing the control mechanism.

### Adrenocorticotropic Hormones

There are indications that ACTH aids consolidation of long-term memory by facilitating incorporation of amino acids into brain proteins. Jakoubek *et al.* (1971) showed that high doses of ACTH increased the incorporation of leucine into protein of mouse cerebral hemispheres, but not in the spinal cord. Rudman *et al.* (1974) also showed that ACTH or β-MSH increased the incorporation of lysine, tyrosine, and leucine into the mouse brain. There is widespread support for the possibility that ACTH and similar peptides increase the incorporation of amino acids into proteins without the mediation of adrenocortical hormones.

Several studies have suggested that ACTH enhances the memory retrieval process. $ACTH_{4-10}$ (which has little or no adrenocortical activity) retards the extinction of avoidance learning in normal rats. Adrenocorticotropic hormone also facilitates passive avoidance performance in rats.

The effects of amnesic agents may be blocked by ACTH peptides. Keyes (1974) reported that ACTH administered 4 hr after training reversed ECS–induced amnesia for passive avoidance behavior in rats. Rigter *et al.* (1974) observed a reversal of $CO_2$-induced amnesia in a similar task when ACTH was given to retention testing.

Several studies suggest (Rigter and Riezen, 1975) that ACTH and ACTH-like peptides facilitate attentional processes or reverse specific attentional deficits rather than facilitate retrieval processes. The few studies in which $ACTH_{4-10}$ has been administered to healthy human volunteers are consistent with the above hypothesis. In humans, $ACTH_{4-10}$ retarded the onset of electroencephalographic signs of habituation in a reaction time task, improved performance on a continuous reaction time task, and improved performance on the digit span and visual reproductive portions of the Wechsler Memory Test without, however, improving the immediate or short-term verbal memory portions.

The mechanism of ACTH's action on the brain is not known. There is some evidence that ACTH may act directly on cells in the brain. It has been shown that elevated plasma ACTH stimulates electrical activity in the septum, the sensory–motor cortex, the thalamus, the midbrain reticular formation, and the amygdala and inhibits activity in the median eminence, the lateral hypothalamus, and the hippocampus. These effects appear to be direct, since they occur in adrenalectomized animals.

Dunn and Gispen (1977) proposed that the novelty of the initial training experience acts as a stressor for the animal, thus causing secretion of ACTH and possibly other pituitary hormones. Aside from its action on the adrenal cortex and other peripheral tissues, these hormones directly influence cerebral metabolism, possibly manifested by an increased rate of protein synthesis. These biochemical responses then facilitate the adaptation of the brain to the novel environment.

## Vasopressin

Vasopressin is a nonpeptide synthesized in the anterior hypothalamus, but stored and released by the posterior lobe of the pituitary gland into the circulation and perhaps into the cerebrospinal fluid (where it has been found in humans). There is stronger evidence for ACTH than for vasopressin being a memory consolidation facilitator. The major evidence for vasopressin's memory consolidating effect is as follows:

1. Animals in which the posterior lobe of the pituitary gland has been removed show a premature and excessively rapid extinction of conditioned avoidance behavior which can be corrected by lysine vasopressin [but also by ACTH and L-melanocyte-stimulating hormone (L-MSH)].

2. Animals in which the pituitary gland is removed have difficulty acquiring a conditioned avoidance response. This acquisition difficulty can be remedied by lysine vasopressin (as well as by ACTH and L-MSH).

3. Although both ACTH and lysine vasopressin correct the impaired acquisition of a shuttlebox response in hypophysectomized rats, the response will deteriorate as soon as ACTH treatments stop, but will remain stable when vasopressin treatments are stopped.

4. One injection of desglycinamide lysine vasopressin (DGLVP), which lacks the endocrine and autonomic activities of lysine vasopressin, will preserve a conditioned avoidance response for many days whether administered during acquisition or during extinction, whereas ACTH will preserve the conditioned avoidance response for only a short time.

5. Injection of lysine vasopressin into rats immediately after the acquisition of a one-trial conditioned avoidance response facilitates retention of response, whereas rats into whom antibodies against vasopressin have been placed intracerebroventricularly are almost devoid of conditioned avoidance behavior at the time of the retrieval test.

6. A large subcutaneous injection of DGLVP (100 mg/lb of the animal) will protect animals against the amnesic effect of puromycin when administered from 20 hr prior to training to 12 hr after training.

7. DGLVP diminishes $CO_2$-induced amnesia for a one-trial conditioned avoidance response when subcutaneously injected either 1 hr before acquisition or 1 hr before the retrieval processes.

Despite the foregoing evidence, there is other evidence suggesting that the avoidance response can be acquired even in the absence of vasopressin and that vasopressin does not always facilitate memory consolidation. Carey and Miller (1982) compared active and passive avoidance behavior between rats of the Brattleboro strain and normal rats. The Brattleboro strain in the homozygous state has a specific and completely hereditary inability to synthesize vasopressin with resulting diabetes insipidus. The rats with diabetes insipidus performed as well as or superior to normal rats in three different learning situations. Laczi *et al.* (1982) reported that patients suffering from central diabetes insipidus showed impairment of short-term and long-term memory functions as compared with healthy individuals. There was no impairment in attention span or concentration. A single IM injection or subchronic intranasal administration of either lysine-vasopressin or arginine-vasopressin normalized the disturbed memory functions in diabetes insipidus patients. Vasopressin also improved functions in healthy individuals.

## Melanocyte-Stimulating Hormone

Melanocyte-stimulating hormone is known to cause pigmentary changes in amphibians and other lower vertebrates. Several reviews have concluded that present day effects of MSH in mammals are vestigial rather than adaptive. Adrenocorticotropic hormone shares the first 13 amino acids with α-MSH. Melanocyte-stimulating hormone, like ACTH, seems to improve various types of learning. This improvement has been attributed to its effects on various systems, such as attention and short-term memory. Recent data seem to indicate that the effect of MSH, ACTH, and their analogues is to improve selective attention and stimulus processing.

## Growth Hormone

An examination of the 24-hr secretory pattern of GH in man generally shows that the amount of GH released during slow-wave sleep (SWS) represents a substantial majority of the total amount of GH secreted in a 24-hr period. The biological significance of the association between GH and SWS is unknown. It was reasoned that since SWS always precedes the occurrence of REM sleep episodes, elevated levels of plasma GH may play some role in triggering REM sleep. Since REM sleep has recently been implicated in consolidation of long-term memory, the influence of GH on consolidation of memory would be through promoting REM sleep. The results from cat and rat studies (Drucker-Colin *et al.*, 1975) indicate that injection of GH prior to sleep caused increases in the amount of REM sleep. In addition to these studies, there are parallels between endogenous plasma GH levels and the spontaneous occurrence of REM sleep. During the early postnatal period, basal levels of GH are much higher than in adulthood. Young infants average greater than 50 ng/ml plasma GH during waking and sleep compared with a peak nighttime level of 15–10 ng/ml in adults. The percentage of REM over a 24-hr period in infants is typically four to five times that of normal adults. Conversely, in old age, REM time often diminishes to less than half that of young adults. This diminution has been correlated with a reduction or total absence of the normal SWS release of GH. Subsequent research with hypophysectomized animals indicates that the presence of high levels of plasma GH may be a sufficient, but not a necessary, factor for the occurrence of REM sleep.

Several studies of radioactive GH uptake (Drucker-Colin *et al.*, 1975) indicate that GH enters the brain tissue and influences various metabolic activities, including protein synthesis.

Morgane and Stern (1974) have suggested the following possible mechanism of GH influencing sleep and memory (see Figure 5.1).

## F. SUMMARY

Most of the neuropeptides so far studied appear to influence memory processes in some manner. The findings, however, are not clear-cut and are complicated by the discovery of increasing numbers of neuropeptides. Some of the neuropeptides extensively studied for their influence on memory include catecholamine, serotonin, acetylcholine, opiate peptides, and some of the pituitary hormones.

A variety of evidence suggests that central as well as peripheral adrenergic systems can modulate memory storage. For example, peripheral posttraining injections of adrenaline or noradrenaline can enhance or impair retention in an inverted-U dose-related manner. That is, low doses of adrenaline will enhance while high doses will impair memory retention. Memory retention also appears to be well correlated with the posttraining release of peripheral adrenaline and noradrenaline and central noradrenaline. Drugs such as amphetamine, which increase catecholamine levels, enhance learning and retention whereas reserpine, which decreases catecholamine levels, impairs performance.

The role of serotonin in memory formation appears to be opposite to that of noradrenaline and dopamine. Elevated levels of brain serotonin impair learning and performance whereas low levels enhance memory retention. Patients with carcinoid syndrome and medullary carcinoma of the thyroid have high levels of circulating serotonin and show disturbances of recent memory. A variety of substances such as nicotine and uric acid, which alter serotonin metabolism, influence memory and learning.

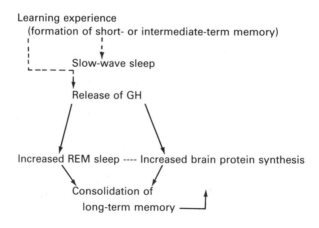

FIGURE 5.1. Influence of growth hormone on sleep and memory.

A great deal of attention has been focused on the cholinergic system because of its presumed involvement in Alzheimer's disease, Huntington's chorea, and tardive dyskinesia. Technical difficulties in measuring acetylcholine turnover in the brain have so far hindered a clear understanding of the relationship between the cholinergic system and these diseases. Anticholinergic drugs such as scopolamine impair performance in animals on various laboratory tasks. Cholinergic agonists (such as arecholine, choline, pilocarpine) and anticholinesterases (physostigmine, DFP, phosdine) enhance performance in animals. However, use of these drugs in normal and demented humans has shown inconsistent results. Extensive trials of acetylcholine precursors, such as lecithin and choline, have produced significant improvement in learning and memory in only a small percentage of cases. Similarly, cholinergic agents (such as physostigmine) have produced only minimal improvement in memory of patients with Alzheimer's disease. Significant improvement in memory usually occurs in patients with early stages of Alzheimer's disease. The lack of improvement in later stages of the disease is explained on the basis of extensive loss of cholinergic neurons from degenerative process.

Opiate peptides appear to be involved in the analgesia produced by placebo and acupuncture, the euphoric effects of morphine, and the regulation of emotional behavior. The peptides appear to influence memory processes in an inverted-U dose-response relationship. Low doses of enkephalin have been shown to impair memory formation whereas high doses cause memory facilitation. Electroconvulsive shock to animals causes release of β-endorphin, which may be responsible for some of the postshock amnesic effect. It has been suggested that the opiate peptides impair memory retention by inhibiting the adrenergic system in the same way that demedullation blocks the effects of enkephalin on memory retention.

Learning is accompanied by a variety of hormonal changes that persist for some time and are believed to modulate the early phases of memory consolidation. Some of these changes have been measured directly but most have been inferred from pharmacological experiments. Adrenocorticotropic hormone, vasopressin, and melanocyte-stimulating hormone have been considered as facilitators of memory, while corticosteroids have been shown to have depressor effects on memory consolidation.

## G.  REFERENCES

Baratti CM, Huygen P, Mino J, et al: Memory facilitation with post trial injections of oxotremerine and physostigmine in mice. *Psychopharmacology* 1979; 64:85–88.

Belluzzi J, Stein L: Enkephalin may mediate euphoria and drive-reduction reward. *Nature* 1977; 266: 556–558.

Boyd WE, Graham-White J, Blackwood G, et al: Clinical effects of choline in Alzheimer senile dementia. *Lancet* 1977; 2:711.

Caltagirone C, Albanese A, Gainotti G: Oral administration of chronic physostigmine does not improve cognitive or amnesic performances in Alzheimer's presenile dementia. *Int J Neurosci* 1982; 16:247–249.

Caltagirone C, Albanese A, Gainotti G: Acute administration of individual optimal dose of physostigmine fails to improve amnesic performancces in Alzheimer presenile dementia. *Int J Neurosci* 1983; 18:143.

Carey, R, Miller M: Absence of learning and memory deficits in the vasopressin-deficit rat. *Behav Brain Res* 1982; 6:1–13.

Carlton P: Some effects of scopolamine, atropine and amphetamine in three behavioral situations. *Pharmacologist* 1961; 3:60.

Carrasco M, Dias R, Izquierdo I: Naloxone reverses retrograde amnesia induced by electroconvulsive shock. *Behav Neural Biol* 1982; 34:352–357.

David D, Yamamura H: Cholinergic under-activity in human memory disorders. *Life Sci* 1978; 23:1729–1734.

Davis K, Mohs R, Tinklenberg J, *et al*: Physostigmine: Improvement of long-term memory processes in normal humans. *Science* 1978; 201:272–74.

Deutsch J: Cholinergic synapse and the site of memory. *Science* 1971; 174:788–794.

Dias R, Perry M, Carrasco M, *et al*: Effect of electroconvulsive shock on beta-endorphin immunoreactivity of rat brain, pituitary gland, and plasma. *Behav Neural Biol* 1981; 32: 265–268.

Drucker-Colin R, Spanis C, Hunyadi J, *et al*: Growth hormone effects on sleep and wakefulness in the rat. *Neuroendocrinology* 1975; 18:1–8.

Dunn A, Gispen W: How ACTH acts on the brain. *Biobehav Rev* 1977; 1:15–23.

Essman WB: Some neurochemical correlates of altered memory consolidation. *Trans NY Acad Sci* 1970; 32:948–973.

Essman WB: Nicotine-related neurochemical changes: Some implications for motivational mechanisms and differences, in Dunn W (ed): *Smoking Behavior*. Washington D.C.; Winston, 1973, pp 51–65.

Flood J, Smith G, Jarvik M: A comparison of effects of localized brain administration of a catecholamine and protein synthesis inhibitors on memory processing. *Brain Res* 1980; 197:153–165.

Glen A, Whalley L: *Alzheimer Disease: Early Recognition of Potentially Reversible Deficits*. Edinburgh; Churchill Livingston, 1979.

Gold P, Van Buskirk R: Effects of α and β-adrenergic receptor antagonists on post-trial epinephrine modulation of memory. *Behav Biol* 1978; 24:168–184.

Gold P, McCarty R, Sternberg D: Peripheral catecholamines and memory modulation, in Marsan CA, and Matthies H (eds): *Neuronal Plasticity and Memory Formation*. New York, Raven, 1982, pp 327–338.

Izquierdo I: Beta-endorphin and forgetting. *Trends Pharmacol Sci* 1982; 3:455–457.

Izquierdo I, Perry M, Dias R, *et al*: Endogenous opioids, memory modulation and state dependency, in Martinez J (ed): *Endogenous Peptides and Learning and Memory Processes*. New York, Academic Press, 1981, pp 269–290.

Jakoubek B, Semiginovsky B, Dedicova A: The effect of ACTH on the synthesis of proteins in spinal motoneurons as studied by autoradiography. *Brain Res* 1971; 25:133–141.

Jensen R, Martinez J, Vasquez B, *et al*: Amnesia produced by intraventricular administration of diethyldithiocarbamate. *Neurosci Abstr* 1977; 3:235.

Keyes JB: Effect of ACTH on ECS-produced amnesia of a passive avoidance task. *Physiol Psychol* 1974; 2:307.

Laczi F, Valkusz Z, Laszlo F, *et al*: Effects of lysine-vasopressin and 1-deamino-8-D-arginine-vasopressin on memory in healthy individuals and diabetes insipidus patients. *Psychoneuroendocrinology* 1982; 7:185–193.

Liljequist R, Mattila M: Effect of physostigmine and scopolamine on the memory functions of chess players. *Med Biol* 1979; 57:402–405.

Martinez J, Rigter H: Endorphins alter acquisition and consolidation of an inhibitory avoidance response in rats. *Neurosci Lett* 1980; 19:197–201.

Martinez J, Jensen R, Messing R, *et al*: Central and peripheral actions of amphetamine on memory storage. *Brain Res* 1980a; 182:157–166.

Martinez J, Vasquez B, Rigter H, *et al*: Attenuation of amphetamine induced enhancement of learning by adrenal demedullation. *Brain Res* 1980b; 195:433–443.

McGaugh JL: Drug facilitation of learning and memory. *Annu Rev Pharmacol* 1973; 13:229–241.

Miczek KA, Grossman S: Punished and unpunished operant behavior after atropine administration to VMH of squirrel monkeys. *J Comp Physiol Psychol* 1972; 81:318–330.

Mollenauer S, Plotnick R, Bean J: Effects of scopolamine on smell discrimination in the rat. *Physiol Psychol* 1976; 4:357–360.

Morgane PG, Stern WC: Rhythms of the biogenic amines in the brain and sleep, in Scheving L, et al (eds): *Chronobiology*. Tokyo, Igaku Shoin, 1974, pp 506–11.

Morley, B, Russin R: The effects of scopolamine on extinction and spontaneous recovery. *Psychopharmacology* 1978; 56:301–304.

Oei TP, King MG: Catecholamine and aversive learning: A review. *Neurosci Biobehav Rev* 1980; 4:161–173.

Overstreet DH: Pharmacological approaches to habituation of the acoustic startle response in rats. *Physiol Psychol* 1975; 5:230–238.

Petersen RC: Scopolamine-induced learning failures in man. *Psychopharmacologia* 1977; 52:283–289.

Remington G, Anisman H: Genetic and autogenic variations in locomotor activity following treatment with scopolamine or d-amphetamine. *Dev Psychobiol* 1976; 9:579–585.

Rigter H, Riezen H: Anti-amnesic effect of $ACTH_{4-10}$: Its independence of the nature of the amnesic agent and the behavioral test. *Physiol Behav* 1975; 14:563–566.

Rigter H, Van Riezen H, DeWied H: The effect of ACTH- and vasopressin analogues in $CO_2$-induced retrograde amnesia in rats. *Physiol Behav* 1974; 13:381–388.

Ross J, McDermott L, Grossman S: Disinhibitory effects of intrahippocampal or intrahypothalamic injections of anticholinergic compounds in the rat. *Pharmacol Biochem Behav* 1975; 3:631–639.

Rudman D, Scott J, DelRio E, *et al*: Melanotropic activity in regions of rodent brain. *Am J Physiol* 1974; 266:682–686.

Singh HK, Ott T, Mathies H: Effects of intrahippocampal injections of atropine on different phases of a learning experiment. *Psychopharmacologia* 1974; 38:247–258.

Sitaram N, Weingartner H, Caine E, *et al*: Choline-selective enhancement of serial learning and encoding of low imagery words in man. *Life Sci* 1978; 22:1555–1560.

Smith C, Swash M: Possible biochemical basis of memory disorder in Alzheimer disease. *Ann Neurol* 1978; 3:471–475.

Stanbli U, Huston J: Avoidance learning enhanced by post trial morphine injection. *Behav Neural Biol* 1980; 28:487–490.

Van der Poel AM: The effects of some cholinolytic drugs on a number of behavior parameters in the T-maze. *Psychologia* 1974; 37:45–58.

Warburton D, Brown K: Faciliation of discrimination performance by physostigmine sulphate. *Psychopharmacologia* 1972; 27:275–284.

Warburton D, Brown K: Effects of scopolamine on a double stimulus discrimination. *Neuropharmacology* 1976; 15:659–663.

Woolley DW: A method for demonstration of the effects of serotonin on learning ability, in Mikhelson M, Longo V (eds): *Pharmacology of Conditioning, Learning and Retention*. Oxford, Pergamon Press, 1965, pp 231–236.

# Memory in Degenerative Diseases of the Nervous System

A large number of degenerative processes affect the brain causing impairment of cognitive and emotional functions. Identifiable patterns of neurological deficits are produced by different degenerative diseases as they affect different parts of the brain. However, deficits in cognition and emotions are much more global and their presence rarely localizes a lesion in specific parts of the brain. Albert and associates (1974) suggested that most of the degenerative diseases of the CNS may be divided functionally into two broad groups depending on whether they predominantly affect the cerebral cortex or the subcortical structures. The terms cortical and subcortical dementia imply patterns of impairment in cognitive and emotional functions.

Dementia is an old term first used by Pinel, a French psychiatrist, in the early 19th century to refer to patients with intellectual deterioration. The term was abandoned for several decades because of its broad implications and was replaced by terms reflecting deficits in specific cognitive functions. The recent use of this term by neurologists to describe overall cognitive deficits in various CNS diseases has popularized this term. More specific meanings have been assigned to this term over the years. Recently, Cummings et al. (1980) defined dementia as an acquired persistent impairment of intellectual functions with compromise in at least three of the following spheres of mental activity: language, memory, visuospatial skills, emotion or personality, and cognition (abstraction, calculation, judgment, etc.). It is apparent that this use of the term is very different from the one used by Pinel. However, it still remains very global and future refinements can be expected.

Degenerative diseases primarily affecting the cerebral cortex (i.e., Alzheimer's and Pick's diseases) give rise to a functional deficit called "cortical dementia." In this group of diseases, there is little or no involvement of the motor system, and posture, gait, speed, muscle tone, and reflexes are generally preserved. Language functions appear to be the most affected and include such symptoms as aphasia and difficulty in naming objects. Memory deficits include impairment of learning and impaired recall of old memory. There is deterioration in visuospatial skills, mathematical calculations, and judgment. Overall IQ declines with the progress of the disease. Personality changes such as lack of interest in the environment and disinhibition are common. Aphasia, amnesia, and agnosia characterize cortical dementia.

Degenerative diseases primarily affecting subcortical structures produce functional deficits called subcortical dementia. The motor system is extensively involved affecting posture, gaits, and muscle tone. Language functions are only mildly affected (Metter *et al.*, 1983). Impairment of other cognitive functions includes general slowness of mental processes and forgetfulness. Overall IQ changes are less than that found in cortical dementia. Personality changes and depression are common.

In addition to the overall clinical picture of cortical and subcortical dementia, there are specific features that are unique to each of the degenerative diseases since they affect the brain differently. It is important to identify the nature and extent of each deficit in order to recommend restrictions on daily activities and plan a comprehensive rehabilitation program. Although the neuropsychological tests are not able to clearly identify degenerative diseases, efforts are being made to determine the specific neuropsychological profiles of each of the diseases. The amount of psychological information varies a great deal for different diseases. Some diseases have been studied extensively with neuropsychological methods while other diseases have little or no specific data with regard to cognitive and emotional functions.

The following pages in this chapter contain descriptions of a selective group of degenerative diseases that have been studied at least minimally with neuropsychological methods. Although specific data are not available for the rest of the diseases, an extrapolation of neuropsychological findings from other diseases that are fairly similar in neuropathology and clinical characteristics may be a temporary solution for our lack of information.

## A. ALZHEIMER'S DISEASE

Alzheimer described the characteristics of this disease in 1907 from his observation of a 51-year-old woman in an insane asylum. This woman was suspicious, had impaired memory, and could not find her way around the hospital. She also had difficulty in recalling names and in comprehending spoken words. She exhibited no deficit in reflexes, motor coordination, or gait. Her condition gradually deteriorated and she died 4½ years after hospitalization. At autopsy, her brain was grossly atrophic. Microscopic studies revealed cell loss, neurofibrillary degenerative changes, and senile plaques throughout the cerebral cortex.

Until recently, the diagnosis of Alzheimer's disease was reserved for dementia beginning before the age of 65, the cases discovered after the age of 65 being labeled as senile dementia. This age restriction, however, is no longer accepted since the neuropathological changes in both conditions are similar. Alzheimer's disease is known to begin in the 4th or 5th decade as well as 6th and 7th decade of life.

## Incidence

Alzheimer's disease is the most common cause of dementia in later life and its incidence increases with age. Several studies (Roth 1978; Gruenberg 1978) found an overall incidence of 1.4%. The prevalence of the diseases is about 2.3% in the age group of 65 to 70 years old, 3.9% in 70 to 80 years old, and 22% beyond age 80.

## Clinical Characteristics

The course of the disease is slowly progressive and death usually occurs within 6 to 12 years after the onset. Remissions do not occur and plateau periods are rare. In an occasional case, death may occur within a year after the onset of the disease. The most characteristic initial change is in the recent memory which becomes progressively worse until no new learning occurs. Gradually, remote memory, language, and all other cognitive functions deteriorate. The patient loses the ability to read, write, and calculate and eventually loses the ability to speak intelligently. Emotional lability, increased irritability, paranoid delusions, and hallucinations appear one to three years after the onset of the disease. Focal neurological signs such as limb rigidity, flexion posture, and loss of sphincter control appear later, 8 to 12 years after the onset.

At present a definitive diagnosis of Alzheimer's disease can be made during life only by cortical biopsy. However, the clinical course of the disease is fairly characteristic and a reliable clinical diagnosis can be made within two to three years after the onset of the disease.

## Etiology

The etiology of Alzheimer's is not known. There are several theories but none of them have yet been proved. Premature aging has been considered as one of the possibilities because of the presence of similar pathological findings in intellectually normal older people. Other theories include aluminum intoxication (Crapper et al., 1976), disordered immune functions (Behan and Feldman, 1970; Nandy, 1978), and deficits in the formation of cellular filaments (Yunis *et al.*, 1981). Genetic predisposition has also been demonstrated in some cases. The most complete genetic study has been Heston's study of 125 autopsy-proven cases of which some 40% were found to be familial (Heston, 1981). The risk in relatives of probands with late onset of Alzheimer's disease and in parents unaffected by the disease was no greater than the risk in the general population. When the proband was less than 70 years old at the onset of the disease and had at least one affected parent, the risk was enormously increased, reaching nearly 50% by the age of 80 years.

## Neuropathology

The brain of patients dying from Alzheimer's disease is quite atrophic, often weighing less than 1000 g (Tomlinson, 1977). The atrophy is most pronounced in the temporoparietal and anteriofrontal regions. The occipital cortex and the primary motor and sensory areas are generally spared.

Histological examination reveals great neuronal loss, neurofibrillary tangles, senile plaques, granulovascular degeneration, and astrocytic gliosis. The disease process is not equally diffuse. The changes are most severe in the temporoparietal–occipital junction area involving the postcingulate gyrus and the temporolimbic region, including the hippocampus, the entorhinal areas, and the amygdala. Neurofibrillary tangles are not unique to Alzheimer's. They are also present in other conditions such as Down's syndrome, postencephalitic Parkinson's disease, and hereditary cerebellar ataxia. Loss of cells and other degenerative changes in the nucleus basalis of Maynert have been found in Alzheimer's. However, degenerative changes in the nucleus basalis also occur in other conditions such as Parkinson's disease.

Identical changes occur in age-matched controls without dementia. However, changes are much less abundant in controls. Terry *et al.* (1981) found that brain weight and cortical thickness were no different in Alzheimer's disease than in controls, indicating that dementia was not due to massive loss of parenchyma. The loss of dendrites and synaptic spines was much more exaggerated in Alzheimer's than in controls, however, indicating perhaps that loss of functional connections among neurons may be one of the underlying pathologies in Alzheimer's dementia. The diagnosis of Alzheimer's thus depends on an identifiable clinical pattern and characteristic neuropathological findings.

Studies of neurotransmitters and the enzymes involved in their metabolism have recently added to our understanding of Alzheimer's disease. Choline acetyltransferase, the enzyme that synthesizes acetylcholine, is decreased in Alzheimer's. The greatest decrease occurs in the cerebral cortex, the hippocampus, and the amygdala. A reduction in the activity of gamma-aminobutyric acid, substance P, and somatostatin have also been reported. A decrease in cortical noradrenergic innervation has been shown in some patients dying of the presenile form of Alzheimer's, but not in the elderly patients dying of Alzheimer's disease.

## Cognitive and Emotional Changes

There is a progressive deterioration of intellectual functions, language, memory, and visuospatial skills. There are marked changes in personality and daily habits. Depression and paranoid ideation are not uncommon. The rate of deterioration varies with the rapidity of the pathological process. In some acute cases severe loss of memory may occur within a year whereas the majority of the cases progress slowly over a period of 6 to 12 years. There are no arrest or plateau periods. Several authors have divided the course of the disease into 3 stages (Lishman, 1978; Berg *et al.*, 1982). Stage I (lasting from 1 to 3 years from the onset of the disease) shows minimal deficits in memory, language, visuospatial skills, intellectual functions, and personality. In stage II, recent and remote memories are more severely impaired. In addition, fluent aphasia, spacial disorientation, acalculia, and ideomotor apraxia become more apparent. This stage may last from 2 to 10 years. Stage III (beginning 8 to 10 years after the onset of the disease) shows severe deterioration of memory functions, intelligence, and complete inability to care for oneself.

### Memory Impairment

Memory impairment is always the initial presenting problem. This deficit is primarily in the short-term memory which impairs the ability to learn new material. The new information is rapidly lost from short-term memory and little or no information is passed to long-term storage and recall. Long-term memory impairment also begins in the first stage of the disease and the person manifests progressive difficulty in recalling remote information.

Several studies have tried to investigate the mechanisms involved in the production of memory deficits. The following multistage model is commonly utilized to investigate the memory impairment:

$$\text{Stimulus} \xrightarrow[\text{Registration}]{\text{Initial}} \text{Encoding} \xrightarrow{\text{Consolidation}} \substack{\text{Maintenance} \\ \text{in storage}} \xrightarrow{\text{Retrieval}} \text{Output}$$

Memory impairment could result from problems at any one stage of this presumed process. For example, short-term memory deficits could occur from impairment in the perception of a stimulus causing faulty initial registration and encoding. Problems in the long-term memory could result from a rapid loss of material from the short-term store. This material would thus not have the opportunity to be transferred to long-term storage. Also, problems in the mechanism of long-term storage and in the retrieval mechanism will result in long-term memory deficit.

Miller (1971) performed several experiments to determine the mechanism of short-term memory problems in Alzheimer's disease. In one experiment, impairment of initial encoding of information was explored. It has been noticed that verbal material is coded predominantly by its acoustic characteristics in short-term memory, but that semantic coding may also play a small part. This means that a group of words that are alike in acoustic characteristics will produce a large amount of mutual interference and confusion resulting in impaired recall. Lists of acoustically similar and semantically similar words were presented to a group of patients and controls. The overall performance of Alzheimer's disease patients was much lower than the controls. The acoustic similarity of the words contributed partly to the lowered performance of the patients. The semantic similarity of the words did not seem to contribute to the lowered short-term memory performance. The overall results indicated that Alzheimer's patients may have some difficulty in the encoding of incoming material, at least in terms of acoustic characteristics.

In the second experiment, the question of retention in short-term memory was explored. Twenty lists of common words, 12 words in each list, were presented verbally to patients and controls. The subjects were asked to recall the words after each list. The normal subjects showed the normal U-shaped curve, recalling more words from the beginning and the end of the list and fewer from the middle of the list.

It is hypothesized that when subjects listen to a list of words, items at the beginning and at the end of the list are most easily recalled giving rise to a U-shaped curve. The items from the beginning of the list are recalled easily because they have been transferred to the long-term store before the short-term store becomes overloaded with incoming material. The items at the end of the list will tend to be lost because they will be squeezed out of short-term store before they can be transferred to long-term storage. The above experiment indicated that there was a rapid loss of material from short-term storage causing problems in the recall of the beginning of the list as well as the end of the list.

A third experiment was designed to determine if the recall problems in the above experiment were related to a difficulty in the transfer of information between the two storage systems. It was further hypothesized that if the rate of presentation of words was slowed down, earlier items would not be crowded out of short-term so quickly by the arrival of later items, and the subjects would have a greater opportunity to renew traces in short-term memory by rehearsal. These two factors would allow traces in the short-term memory to remain active for much longer and have a better opportunity for transfer to long-term storage.

In this experiment, words were presented at a slower rate (3 sec apart in contrast to 1.5 sec apart in the above experiment). Normal subjects showed a better recall of the initial part of the list, but patients showed no difference. The result indicated that the patients, in addition to the lowered capacity in short-term storage, also had an impairment in the transfer of information to long-term storage.

Several other studies have highlighted problems of Alzheimer's patients in encoding and storage processes. Miller (1971) tested a group of patients on a tachistoscope with an array of six letters for a brief exposure followed by a "visual noise" masking the stimulus. The patients were less able to extract information from this brief exposure than the controls. This difficulty may have been the result of impaired attention and/or easy distractibility.

Dichotic listening experiments (Inglis 1957, 1959) also indicate that the short-term memory problems of patients may result from impaired encoding processes. In these experiments, different strings of digits are presented simultaneously to each ear. In immediate recall, subjects typically report information received from one ear before that received by the second ear. It is hypothesized that the information received by the second ear is held in a temporary short-term memory storage. The recall of second-ear information would be impaired if difficulties existed in the mechanisms of short-term storage. Several studies of dichotic listening (Caird and Hannah, 1964) report little difference between control and demented patients in the immediate recall from the first ear, but the demented patients are significantly worse in the second recall, indicating problems in short-term storage.

Miller (1973) noticed that even after repeated presentations, demented patients were less able to reproduce a short list of words.

Long-term memory problems may result from at least two broad deficits: poor encoding in long-term storage and retrieval problems. Miller and Hagen (1975) presented a list of words to subjects three times. After an interval during which an effort was made to distract the subject to avoid rehearsal, retention was tested in three ways: a straightforward test, a recognition test in which subjects had to identify correct words from a list of alternatives, and a partial information condition. In the partial information condition, subjects were given the initial letter of the words as a cue. For control subject, the partial information condition did not improve their recall, but a significant improvement was noted in demented patients. The demented patients did much worse than the control on straightforward recall and on recognition tests.

The improved performance of demented patients with partial information cuing suggests that the problems may be in the retrieval process rather than in the encoding process. Several investigators (Squire et al., 1978) have suggested that in demented patients encoding results in weak traces of memory that are enhanced by partial cuing. Warrington and Weiskrantz (1970) suggested that successful retrieval may depend not only on the ability to recall the correct words, but also on the ability to inhibit the recall of incorrect words. The partial information may enhance recall because it gives a cue for the correct word without providing an alternative which may be incorrectly recognized as is the case with the recognition test. There is, however, no conclusive evidence so far to support this hypothesis.

## IQ Changes

Several studies (Bolton et al., 1966; Cleveland and Dysinger, 1944) indicate that there is an overall decline in intelligence quotient in Alzheimer's disease. Scores on performance tests are decreased to a greater extent than those on the verbal tests. It was argued that the performance subtests on the Wechsler Intelligence Scale are timed and the lower scores on performance items may result from a generalized slowness of response manifested by Alzheimer's disease patients. However, similar results are obtained on tests that are not timed such as the Mill Hill Vocabulary Scale and the Progressive Matrices (Kendrick and Post, 1967; Orme, 1957). The performance tests require manipulation of visuospatial skills. The verbal items of the WAIS require well-rehearsed responses whereas the performance items present unfamiliar situations and require new responses. It may be that performance deficits in Alzheimer's disease patients reflect some inability to adjust to and deal with new and unfamiliar tasks.

Efforts have been made to analyze subscales of IQ tests to determine specific factors that may be contributing to the performance deficits of Alzheimer's disease patients. The results of these studies (Dixon, 1965; Gustafson and Hagberg, 1975) are variable and inconclusive, significant factors ranging from 1 to 14. Similarly, studies comparing the patterns of IQ decline in normal aging and Alzheimer's have not been conclusive. Impairment of visuospatial skills occur early in the course of the disease. The patients are unable to copy simple drawings, especially three-dimensional figures one to two years after the onset of the disease. Problems in mathematical calculations become apparent by midstage of the disease.

### Language Impairment

In a systematic analysis of a group of patients, Ernst *et al.* (1970) found that a poverty of vocabulary in narrative speech was the only common consistent finding in Alzheimer's disease patients. Impairment in naming objects is found in normal aging as well as in dementia. However, the demented group is more disabled than the normal controls. The capacity to name objects improves in demented patients after the use of the objects is demonstrated, but not in normal controls. Miller (1975) compared a group of demented patients with normal controls in a fluency test in which each subject produced as many words as they could beginning with the letter "S" within a period of 5 min. The demented patients produced fewer words than the controls. This tendency is explained on the basis of slow production of words by demented patients. The nature of the difficulties in naming objects in dementia appears to be different from the one found in aphasia resulting from specific local lesions. Misidentification of objects is at least partly responsible for the naming difficulty in demented patients, whereas aphasics are able to correctly identify an object but cannot seem to find a word to name it.

Language impairment begins early in the course of the disease. Initially, there are difficulties in word finding and circumlocution, imparting an empty quality to verbalization. Naming of low-frequency items fails first, followed by difficulty in naming more common objects.

Comprehension of spoken language is also progressively impaired. In the later stages of the disease a variety of speech disturbances may appear such as echolalia (tendency to repeat words and phrases spoken to the patient), palilalia (tendency to repeat words and phrases initiated by the patient), and logoclonia (repetition of the final syllable of a word). In the terminal stage, vocalization is reduced to the production of repetitive sounds unrecognizable as language and mutism may eventually occur.

*Apraxia.* This usually appears in the middle phase of Alzheimer's disease. Two types of apraxia may be recognized: ideational apraxia (failure to correctly pantomime the sequence of events of a complex motor act such as filling and lighting a pipe) and ideomotor apraxia (inability to do on command an act that can be performed spontaneously).

*Agnosia.* One third of the patients studied by Sjogren *et al.* (1952) showed visual agnosia. Rockford (1971) demonstrated that in some demented patients, poor ability to name objects was due to impaired visual recognition and not from aphasic anomia.

### Personality Changes

Personality may be relatively preserved but disinterest and/or disinhibition appears within a few years after the onset of the disease. Changes occur in personal habits, motivation, and in social and interpersonal relationships. Patients become careless in their daily habits and personal hygiene. Poor judgment about small matters becomes evident. The person gets lost in familiar surroundings. Apathy, suspiciousness, paranoia, and depression may become predominant manifestations of the disease.

## B. PICK'S DISEASE

In 1892, Arnold Pick first described the clinical and gross pathological features of this disease in a 71-year-old man with a three-year history of progressive dementia. The usual onset of the disease is between 40 and 60 years of age, but it may begin as early as age 21 and as late as 80 years. It affects women somewhat more than men. Its incidence is very much less than Alzheimer's disease, which is at least 10 to 15 times more frequent than Pick's disease. Most of the cases of Pick's disease are sporadic and only about 20% are recognized as familial. The etiology and pathogenesis of Pick's disease are unknown. Disorders of zinc metabolism and primary axonal disorder have been implicated in some studies.

### Clinical Characteristics

Pick's disease has many of the clinical features of Alzheimer's disease and is difficult to distinguish from it. The course of the disease is generally similar, covering a period of 6 to 12 years and ending in death.

Some of the distinguishing characteristics from Alzheimer's, however, are early development of partial or full Kluver-Bucy syndrome. This syndrome in monkeys can be produced by surgical ablation of both temporal lobes, including the amygdala and the hippocampus. These monkeys developed emotional blunting with loss of fear, altered food preferences (gluttony), mandatory exploration of environmental stimuli as soon as they are noticed, prominent oral exploratory behavior, sensory agnosialike behavior involving vision and hearing, and altered sexual activity (hypersexuality). Aphasia tends to appear early. Memory and visuospatial abilities are preserved until the middle or later stages of the disease.

## Neuropathology

The brain is reduced in size, often weighing less than 1000 g. Atrophy is most common in the temporal and/or frontal lobes whereas in Alzheimer's disease the most prominent changes are in the posterior parts of the cerebral hemispheres. Atrophic changes in Pick's disease show left-sided dominance in 50%, right-sided dominance in 20%, and bilateral in 30%. The anterior and medial temporal area and the orbitofrontal cortex show the most severe atrophy.

Histology reveals two characteristic findings: intracytoplasmic Pick's bodies and inflated neurons. The Pick's bodies are intracellular dense structures, approximately of the same size as the nucleus. In addition, neuronal loss, astrocytic hyperplasia, and microglial cell proliferation are present. Unlike Alzheimer's, no apparent selective involvement of neurotransmitters occurs (White, *et al.*, 1977).

## Cognitive and Emotional Changes

The course of the disease, like Alzheimer's, may be divided into three stages: Stage I (mild), from one to three years; Stage II (moderate) from three to six years; and Stage III (severe) lasting from six to twelve years.

### Stage I

Memory is generally preserved in the initial stage of Pick's disease. Early changes occur in personality and are characterized by lack of tactfulness, concern, and deterioration of social behavior. Judgment is impaired. Language abnormalities are manifested by semantic anomia and circumlocution. Some of the manifestations of Kluver-Bucy syndrome may be apparent. Visuospatial orientation and calculation abilities are relatively intact. The motor system is normal. Thus, the primary changes during the first stage are personality changes.

Early personality changes may lead to a psychiatric diagnosis. Mood disturbances such as depression, euphoria, apathy, irritability, and jocularity may occur. Personality deterioration often includes lack of concern and regard for social norms, sexual indiscretion, and socially inappropriate behavior,

## Stage II

This stage is characterized by further deterioration of personality and language. Visuospatial skills, the motor system, memory, and calculating abilities may remain unimpaired. The impairment of language and speech is fairly marked and is manifested by word-finding difficulties, circumlocution, verbal paraphrasia, and progressive comprehension difficulties. Pure word deafness or auditory agnosia occurs in some cases and worsens comprehension problems. Visuospatial skills remain intact long after the patient is impaired in language and behavior.

## Stage III

There is a progressive involvement of all cognitive functions including memory, visuospatial skills, calculating abilities, and the motor system.

## C. PROGRESSIVE SUPRANUCLEAR PALSY

Steele and associates (1964) first described nine cases that resembled the patients with Parkinson's disease but had more extensive involvement of the brain. The initial symptoms reported by these patients were feelings of unsteadiness, vague visual difficulties, and unclear speech. The disease had its onset in the sixth decade and was rapidly progressive with the development of supranuclear ophthalmoplegia (affecting chiefly vertical gaze), pseudobulbar palsy, dysarthria, rigidity of neck and upper trunk, and other symptoms of cerebellar and pyramidal involvement. Death occurs within five to seven years. These patients resembled the patients with Parkinson's disease with regard to their masked faces, gait difficulties, and postural instability. However, parkinsonism in an elderly patient with retrocollis and paresis of vertical gaze invariably supports the diagnosis of progressive supranuclear palsy.

The pathological examination shows severe degenerative changes of multiple sites. The most involved are the globus pallidus, the subthalamic nucleus, the pretectal region, the superior quadrigeminum, the red nucleus, the tegmentum of the midbrain and the pons, the substantia nigra, the locus coeruleus, the oculomotor, trochlear, and vestibular nerve nuclei, and the dentate nuclei of the cerebellum. The cerebral and cerebellar cortices are remarkably spared. Microscopically, degenerative changes predominate with cell loss and swelling of the nerve cells.

## Cognitive and Emotional Changes

Cognitive and mental changes are characteristic of subcortical dementia. Personality changes such as apathy and mood changes occur early in the course of the disease and cognitive changes are generally mild and become manifest only later in the course of the disease. Slowness of thoughts, forgetfulness, impaired calculation, and abstraction are common. Depression has also been reported in some cases. Albert and associates (1974) noticed the following problems in his group of patients:

1. A general slowness of thinking was very characteristic of all patients. Most of the patients performed poorly on time-limited tests, but the performance improved when more time was given. For example, most patients were able to repeat six to seven digits forward and five digits backward when no time limit was set on recall. This observation indicates that immediate recall and short-term memory were unimpaired.
2. Similarly, memory for remote events was unimpaired. Most patients recalled past events correctly if sufficient time was allotted to respond. The patients usually answered incorrectly if they were pressured to respond quickly.
3. Impaired ability for calculation and concrete level of abstraction was common. Interpretation of proverbial phrases by the patients tended to be simple and concrete.
4. Short attention span was common. Some of the forgetfulness on the part of these patients may be explained on the basis of the attention problems.
5. Verbal and perceptual capacities were strikingly preserved. No aphasia or apraxia was noted.
6. The personality changes included apathy, occasional irritability or euphoria, with inappropriate laughing or crying, or brief outbursts of rage.
7. Depression was also noted in some patients.

Jackson *et al.* (1983) reported 16 cases of progressive nuclear palsy that were previously wrongly diagnosed as Parkinson's disease. Seven of the patients who were tested with neuropsychological tests showed an IQ range from mild mental retardation to above average: full scale IQ from 80 to 111; verbal IQ from 68 to 119; performance IQ from 59 to 115. The Wechsler Memory Scale scores ranged from 83 to 122.

## D. HUNTINGTON'S DISEASE

This is an autosomal dominant condition that usually becomes manifest in adult life. It is characterized by progressive movement disorder, extrapyramidal symptoms, and intellectual deterioration. The most characteristic movement disorder are choreiform movements. These are spontaneous, short, rapid, uncoordinated jerks resulting from the contracting of single isolated muscles. The muscles involved may be in the proximal or distal parts of extremities. Simultaneous contraction of two or more muscles may result in complex movement of upper or lower extremities (dancelike gait).

Extrapyramidal symptoms such as rigidity and akinesia may be an early manifestation in some patients with an earlier onset instead of chorea.

Slight clumsiness or restlessness associated with overt twitching of fingers and grimacing of face are usually the first manifestations in most cases. Chorea becomes more striking as the disease progresses and ultimately involves all the muscles of the body including the lips, tongue, and cheeks. Muscle strength and ability to initiate voluntary movements are unimpaired. However, carrying out continuous movements are frequently impaired by the superimposition of involuntary jerks.

The most significant pathologic feature is a primary loss of neurons in the caudate and the putamen nuclei. These structures are grossly shrunken and atrophic. Small neurons are affected primarily whereas larger neurons degenerate later on. The cerebral cortex shows moderate atrophy of the gyri, most marked in the frontal lobe. Microscopically, there is a definite loss of neurons in all layers of the cortex, more in some layers than others. Degenerative changes also occur in other parts of the brain including the subcortical white matter, the thalamus, and the hypothalamus.

## Cognitive and Emotional Changes

George Huntington (1872) was aware of the early mental changes as he stated, "as the disease progresses the mind becomes more or less impaired, in many amounting to insanity, while in others mind and body gradually fail until death relieves them of their suffering."

Personality changes are the earliest manifestations in the majority of the cases before the chorea begins. The personality changes include general untidiness, loss of interest in work and social activities, increased irritability, and mood changes. Caine et al. (1978) noted that patients themselves were aware of changes in their temperament. They occasionally felt out of control. Increased irritability was the most common complaint. They were often quick to anger and experienced rapid changes in their mood.

Psychiatriac disorders are quite common and some patients are hospitalized in psychiatric hospitals before the manifestation of chorea. In a survey of English psychiatric hospital admissions, Dewhurst et al. (1969) found that 57 of 102 patients with Huntington's disease had onset of the disease predominantly with psychiatric syndromes, 16 with principally neurological symptoms, and 29 had mixed appearance. The psychiatric symptoms included anxiety, irritability, depression, violence, and delusions. Trimble and Cummings (1981) noted that a schizophrenialike syndrome may occur in one third of the patients before the onset of chorea. This syndrome is associated with persecutory delusions and hallucinations (McHugh and Folstein, 1975). Affective disorders resembling unipolar or bipolar illness may also manifest prior to chorea. Suicide rate is high and may account for 7.8% of males and 6.4% of females death in this disease (Reed *et al.*, 1958).

Impairment of cognitive functions is usually apparent after the onset of chorea (McHugh and Folstein, 1975). It includes impairment of intellectual functions, memory disturbances, and slowing of overall cognition. Aphasic and apraxic disturbances, typical of cortical involvement, are usually absent but may appear in the later stages of the disease.

The results of intelligence tests have been variable, resulting primarily from the studies carried out in different stages of the disease. The studies carried out in the early stages of the disease show little or no change in the intellectual potential. For example, Aminoff *et al.* (1975) found that intellectual potentials of Huntington's disease patients were similar to those of normal individuals of advancing age. Josiassen *et al.* (1982) noted deficits in both the verbal and performance subtests of the Wechsler Intelligence Scale especially on digit span, arithmetic, and picture arrangement. Similarly, McHugh and Folstein (1975) reported a 21-point difference between verbal and performance scores. Caine *et al.* (1978) found that there was no significant difference between the means of verbal and performance IQ scores (94 and 91). Eight of his patients had mean verbal IQ scores higher than their mean performance scores, while seven had higher performance scores. The significant impairment found in some patients was on two subtests: paired associate learning sequencing.

Memory disturbances occur early in the course of the disease (Butters *et al.*, 1978). There are difficulties in recalling remote information as well as recently learned material (Albert *et al.*, 1981; Butters *et al.*, 1979; Butters and Cermak, 1980). Initial registration of information is only mildly impaired, but there appears to be a marked deficit in elaborating information for effective encoding and recall (Caine *et al.*, 1977; Weingartner *et al.*, 1979). Caine *et al.* (1978) found that Huntington's disease patients showed a marked lack of self-generated activity such as inability to retrieve stored information spontaneously. Left alone, most patients were content to sit and do nothing. Caine felt that as the disease progressed, it became increasingly more difficult to generate ideas, perform the required planning and organization, and establish the necessary cognitive framework to carry out a task over several days. When presented with planned specified tasks, they participated eagerly and with substained interest.

These patients have difficulty in recalling information on request. However, recognition of information from a multiple choice format is easy for them, indicating that the information is not forgotten but is irretrievable at a desired time.

Caine *et al.* (1977) tested a group of patients on the following tests: (1) verbal presentation of 48 words categorized in 12 categories with 4 words per category; (2) a serial-learning task using 10 random high and low-imagery words; (3) digit repetition task; (4) card sorting; and (5) selective reminding. In the first test, patients were tested on immediate recall of category names, free recall after 10 min, then cued recall using the category name as cues and finally recognition testing of the same list by mixing stimulus words with new distractor words from the same categories. The results indicated that the pattern of memory disorder was similar in the most and the least affected patients. The least affected patients scored within normal limits. Immediate and delayed free recall were slightly impaired but not significantly. Patients could not master the serial-learning task despite repeated trials. The digit span test with forward repetition was minimally reduced but backward repetition was significantly reduced. There was no difference from normal controls on card-sorting tests.

The conclusions of this study are as follows: (1) mild impairment of registration of new material, not related to attention problem; (2) significant difficulty with encoding new information especially in a categorical or serial context; and (3) marked impairment in consistently retrieving stored information. This may be the result of an inability of patients to establish necessary self-generated cues to access stored material. Caine *et al.* (1977) also tested six right-handed Huntington's disease patients, using the parietal lobe battery. They found that the patients had more difficulty in drawing figures when given verbal commands than when they copied from visual presentation. The figures were much more disorganized in severely affected patients than mildly affected ones. Mildly affected patients showed few rotational errors and maintained good configurations of stick figures, while advanced disease patients made more rotational errors and broke the main configurations. Block construction scores were moderately reduced in all patients. Clock-setting ability was intact in some patients, but was affected in most patients.

## E. WILSON'S DISEASE

Wilson's disease is an autosomal recessive condition resulting in an abnormal copper metabolism. Less copper is taken up by the liver and more copper reaches the circulation in loosely bound form. This copper becomes deposited in the various organs of the body, binds to normal tissue proteins, and thus causes destruction of the tissues, especially that of the brain, liver, and kidneys.

In the central nervous system, the most severe involvement is that of the basal ganglia which may shrink and develop cavitation. Microscopically, there is a marked loss of neurons and swelling of astrocytes. In addition, focal areas of degeneration can be seen throughout the brain including the cerebral cortex and the cerebellum. Large amounts of copper are deposited in all areas of the brain.

Clinically, two neurologic pictures are equally characteristic. The acute form, originally described by Wilson, usually begins in late childhood or early adolescence. It is characterized by spasticity, rigidity, dysarthria, slurring of speech, and dysphagia. Early appearance of marked dystonia is one of the important features that differentiates it from the more chronic form.

The chronic form is often referred to as pseudosclerosis. The earliest feature is a tremor which may be a flapping tremor (wrist involvement) or wingbeating (shoulder involvement) in one or both arms. Sleep usually aborts these tremors which are present at rest. The disease is progressive, involving the head and the trunk. Liver and kidney functions are altered.

## Cognitive and Emotional Changes

Wilson (1912) identified slowness of mentation, listlessness, emotionalism, and childishness as the common features of this disease. In children, a failure to make progress in school may often be an early sign of this disease. In adults, paranoid psychosis with hallucinations may develop early in the course of the disease (Beard, 1959). Cognitive changes include slow cognition, forgetfulness, and impaired memory (Knehr and Bearn, 1956).

Goldstein *et al.* (1968) tested 22 Wilson's disease patients with the Wechsler Adult Intelligence Scale (WAIS), the Wechsler Memory Scale (WMS), the Bender Gestalt, and the Minnesota Multiphasic Personality Inventory (MMPI). The disease had existed from a few months to several years. Pretreatment scores of IQ, memory, and Bender Gestalt Tests were essentially within normal limits. These patients were retested 16 to 73 months after treatment with penicillamine. There was improvement in some of the subtests of the WAIS such as information, comprehension, similarities, and block design. Memory subtests of the WMS also showed improvement. In some patients, the change in the test scores was quite dramatic. For example, in one patient the memory quotient increased from 79 in 1960 to 99 in 1966. In spite of these changes, no patterns of scores emerged to suggest any specific or general area of impairment that could be found in common in these patients, indicating a heterogeneity of the sample with regard to cognitive and memory functions.

The pretreatment profile on the MMPI showed mild depression and mild suspiciousness, but no evidence of psychosis or neurosis. With continued treatment, the MMPI profile showed improvement in most cases.

Psychiatric symptoms may precede the diagnosis of Wilson's disease. In the above sample, two of the patients had been hospitalized for psychiatric treatment, one of them receiving electroshock treatment before the diagnosis of Wilson's disease. In a third patient, a hypomanic-paranoid reaction developed at a time when the neurological symptoms were improving.

Knehr and Bearn (1956) studied seven patients, (ages 17 to 54, and duration of illness from 3½ to 23 years) using a battery of tests designed to study disorganization of thinking and impairment of cerebral functions. The results showed some loss in the capacity for conceptual thinking in all cases. Involvement of the cerebral cortex in the disease process was also suggested by a lowered flicker frequency threshold and a prolonged afterimage time.

There was no deficit in the accuracy of simple visual patterns perception and the duration of visual span attention.

## F. HALLERVORDEN–SPATZ SYNDROME

In 1922 Hallervorden and Spatz reported an unusual extrapyramidal syndrome in 5 of the 12 siblings in one family. The syndrome began between the ages of 7 and 9 producing dystonia and athetosis leading to death between 16 and 17 years of age. It is probably an autosomal recessive genetic disease. Three clinical variants of this disorder have been described: a late-infantile type with onset in the second year of life; the classic juvenile type usually beginning in the first decade of life; and a rare adult type that becomes manifest in middle age or later.

Pathological studies indicate cortical involvement with widened sulci and narrowed gyri especially in the frontal and temporal regions. Basal ganglia, which are pigmented by a brownish pigment especially in the globus pallidus, contain iron. Microscopic examination shows severe changes in the pigmented areas with loss of neurons, moderate fibrillary gliosis, and demyelination. Neuronal loss and gliosis are minimal in the cerebral cortex.

### Cognitive and Emotional Changes

Mental changes typically follow the appearance of motor symptoms, but occasionally may be the initial presenting symptoms. Personality changes, depression, moodiness, and episodes of rage occur early in the course of the disease (Rezdilsky et al., 1968). Progressive failure of cognitive and memory functions is a prominent feature of the illness in the majority of the cases. Psychomotor retardation and progressive deterioration of functions gradually develop in memory, attention, concentration, abstraction, visual–spatial skills, and mathematical calculations (Dooling, et al 1974).

Mental confusion and paranoid schizophrenia has been reported in a few cases. Sacks et al. (1966) described a patient longitudinally who manifested fits of rage and depression, progressive deterioration of intelligence, and impairment of memory and judgment.

## G. PARKINSON'S DISEASE

Parkinson's disease is a degenerative disease affecting primarily the pigmented nuclei of the brain stem. Although most cases are idiopathic, some cases result from encephalitis and arteriosclerosis. It is a sporadic disease usually occurring between the ages of 50 and 65 years. Its prevalence in the general population is approximately 1 per 1000. The disease is slowly progressive from 1 to 30 years (average 8 years) resulting in death from respiratory and urinary complications.

## Clinical Characteristics

It is characterized by four groups of signs: tremors, akinesia, rigidity, and loss of normal postural reflexes. Tremors consist of rhythmically alternating contractions of a given muscle group and its antagonists. Distal parts of an extremity are most commonly involved such as in pillrolling tremors of hands. Tremors may begin in one arm or leg and may remain unilateral for several years. These tremors are present during rest and disappear on purposeful movements.

Akinesia and bradykinesia include slowness in initiation and execution of all voluntary movements, marked poverty of spontaneous movements, a loss of normal associated movements resulting in masklike facies, and diminished swinging of arms in walking and running.

There is an increased muscle tone and rigidity. The rigidity to passive movements is widespread and is often more prominent at larger joints such as the elbows.

The disease often begins insidiously with mild stiffness of the arms. The tremors usually appear later. The stiffness spreads to other muscle groups causing adductions of arms, flexion of elbow, dorsal kyphosis, flexion of knees, and slow gait with small shuffling steps.

The disease is progressive in virtually all patients. Degree and rate of progression vary from individual to individual and within a single individual at different times.

## Pathology

The most severe lesion is found in the zona compacta of the substantia nigra which shows nerve cell loss and degenerative changes with inclusion bodies (Lewy bodies) and glial scarring. Nerve cell loss is also seen in the globus pallidus. Atrophic changes occur throughout the cerebral cortex but are especially apparent in the frontal lobe. Histologically, these atrophic changes in the cerebral cortex are similar to the ones seen in Alzheimer's disease.

## Cognitive and Emotional Changes

Earlier studies of Parkinson's disease were focused on the disorders of the motor system and cognitive changes were not recognized. Slowness in mentation and performance was attributed to generalized slowness of movements. Estimates of cognitive impairment were also biased by the types of tests utilized and the stage of the disease at which these patients were studied.

Consequently, estimates of dementia as low as 3% and as high as 93% were reported in different studies (Boller *et al.*, 1980).

When do the cognitive deficits begin during the course of the disease? There are no longitudinal studies to answer this question specifically. However, cross sectional studies indicate that dementia is more prevalent and becomes more severe as the disease advances. Cognitive changes are typical of subcortical dementia and include slowness of abstraction and mathematical abilities. However, in some cases, deficits characteristic of cortical degeneration are present including aphasia, agnosia, and apraxia.

Do cognitive impairments in Parkinson's disease result from subcortical degeneration or are they the result of a combined degenerative process in both cortical and subcortical areas? Alvord (1971) first suggested that dementia in Parkinson's disease may be the result of the simultaneous occurrence of Alzheimer's disease. Boller *et al.* (1980) found that the prevalence of Alzheimer's was much higher in Parkinson's disease patients. In this study, 33% of the Parkinson's disease patients were found to suffer from Alzheimer's type of dementia. This is six times greater than that found in an age-matched population (5.1%).

Several studies indicate that Parkinson's disease patients matched with normal controls show greater deficits in memory, perception, and psychomotor speed (Reitan and Boll, 1971). Mortimer *et al.* (1982) argued that if cognitive impairment results from the same subcortical lesion that causes motor symptoms, there should be a correlation between the severity of the motor symptoms and the degree of neuropsychological deficits. On the other hand, if cognitive deficits are due to cortical lesions, the relationship between the motor and cognitive disorders might be weak or absent. In this study, 60 Parkinson's disease patients were tested for motor disorder—rigidity, tremor, and bradykinesia. Neuropsychological tests included the WAIS, the WMS, the Bender Gestalt, finger-tapping test, and the Zung self-rating scale. The results supported an association between the severity of motor symptoms and the degree of the neuropsychological impairment, suggesting that some of the cognitive deficits may result from the same subcortical lesions that cause the motor symptoms. Bradykinesia and tremors were related significantly with selected cognitive functions such as visuospatial perceptions and memory. There was a decline in intellectual functions with increased bradykinesia. Muscle rigidity was not related to cognitive decline. Despite marked impairment of verbal memory, the degree of memory loss was not significantly correlated with the severity of the motor symptoms. The authors concluded that both subcortical and cortical lesions may be involved in overall dementia of Parkinson's disease patients.

Various other cognitive deficits have been reported in Parkinson's disease such as impairment of abstract reasoning (Reitan and Boll, 1971), concept formation and shifting mental set (Albert, 1978), and high-speed memory scanning (Wilson, *et al.*, 1980).

Studies suggest a progressive downward course with regard to cognitive, motor, and social abilities (Diller and Riklan, 1956). However, many patients do not suffer such a course. In a study of 42 Parkinson's disease patients, Mathews and Haaland (1979) concluded that mild decrements in cognitive, motor, and memory functions can be demonstrated after three to five years of the disease. Intelligence tests frequently report a decrease in overall IQ. Even when the IQ scores are within normal limits, a comparison with past performance indicates some decline (Diller and Riklan, 1956). Loranger and Goodell (1972) tested the IQ of 41 men and 22 women who had moderate to severe Parkinson's disease before a treatment trial of L-dopa. There are extreme variations among the scores of the various subtests. A difference of 20 points was found between the verbal and performance IQ (performance being lower). In another study, Mathews and Haaland (1979) found a similar pattern of IQ scores, but explained that the lower performance scores were the result of a general slowing of motor functions rather than real cognitive deficits. However, memory tests and tests of intellectual functions which are independent of motor functions also show impairment of cognitive functions in Parkinson's disease patients.

Depressed mood is more common in patients with Parkinson's disease than in patients with other chronic illnesses (Celesia and Wanamaker, 1972). Clinical depression is apparent in at least 40% to 60% of patients with Parkinson's disease sometime during the course of the illness (Brown and Wilson, 1972). Mayeux *et al.* (1981) noticed that depression in Parkinson's disease patients was often accompanied by intellectual impairment. In a group of 55 patients, 47% were found to be depressed on Beck's self-inventory. The severity of depression was not significantly related to sex, degree of disability, or levodopa therapy. There was a significant correlation between the depression and intellectual impairment. A reduction in brain monoamine has been implicated in some studies as a cause of the depression (Brown and Wilson, 1972). Dopaminergic neurons from the tegmental area project to the cingulate, the entorhinal, and the frontal cortex. Nigral dopaminergic fibers project to the globus pallidus, the midbrain tegmentum, and the thalamus. The substantia nigra receives input from the neurostriatum and the frontal cortex. There is a widespread dopaminergic deficiency that could result in depression.

There is a significant improvement in cognitive functions following the introduction of levodopa therapy. However, even at the optimal level of levodopa therapy, Parkinson's disease patients do not achieve the level of cognitive performance shown by nonparkinsonian individuals. Loranger *et al.* (1972) showed that with levodopa therapy initial improvement in memory functions was not permanent. Parkinson's disease patients who received levodopa therapy for less than two years performed significantly better on six of nine measures of a memory test than those patients who were treated for four years. Patients with serious motor disability did more poorly on memory tests than less disabled patients. Levodopa dosage levels did not correlate significantly with changes in any of the memory measures. Improvement in cognitive functions following levodopa therapy appears to be limited in time. A gradual decline in cognitive functions occurs as the disease progresses.

## H. AMYOTROPHIC LATERAL SCLEROSIS AND PARKINSONIAN DEMENTIA COMPLEX OF GUAM

Parkinsonian dementia complex is a degenerative disease of the central nervous system which is endemic in Guam and the Mariana Islands. The incidence of this disease is much higher in the native population indicating genetic and some environmental factors specific to the islands. The disease affects more males and has its onset usually in the fifth and sixth decades of life. It is progressive and death occurs within ten years from the date of onset.

Pathologically, depigmentation of the substantia nigra and the locus coeruleus is often found. The presence of severe cortical atrophy, especially in the frontal and temporal lobes, is quite striking. Microscopically, there is severe neuronal destruction, neurofibrillary tangles, and gliosis in the cerebral cortex of patients dying from the disease.

Elizan and associates (1966) analyzed neurological features of 104 cases in Guam and compared them with those of classical amyotrophic lateral sclerosis (ALS) in the literature. Guam ALS is indistinguishable from classical ALS. However, Guam ALS has a younger age of onset, especially in the females, and a more protracted course. Five of the original ALS cases developed parkinsonism and 27 of the original 72 Parkinson's disease patients developed ALS. Thus a total of 32 cases had clinical features of both ALS and Parkinson's disease during the seven-year follow-up period.

### Cognitive and Emotional Changes

In original Parkinson's disease patients, functional deficits of subcortical dementia were the most common initial symptoms. Memory deficits and disorientation for time, place, and person were the presenting signs of dementia in almost all cases. There was a progressive deterioration of intellectual functions: slow comprehension, poor calculations, and concrete abstraction. Personality changes were present in about a third of the cases and included apathy, irritability, agitation, childishness, and violent behavior. Some of the patients became very depressed whereas others remained indifferent to their illness. Hallucinations were reported in three cases during the last phases of the illness.

## I. IDIOPATHIC CALCIFICATION OF BASAL GANGLIA

Idiopathic calcification of basal ganglia (ICBG) is considered a familial disorder with autosomal dominant or autosomal recessive modes of inheritance. Several clinical forms of the disease have been recognized: a childhood form with onset in infancy resulting in death in the first few years of life; a young adult form with onset between 20 and 40 years of age, usually manifesting as schizophrenialike syndrome; and a later onset form, between 40 and 60 years of age, usually presenting as a movement disorder such as choreatic movements or parkinsonism.

The calcification of the basal ganglia in 70% to 80% of the cases can be related to pseudohypoparathyroidism, idiopathic to hyperparathyroidism, postoperative hypoparathyroidism, or rarely to hyperparathyroidism. In the remainder of the cases no abnormality of calcium metabolism has yet been defined.

### Cognitive and Emotional Changes

Cognitive and emotional changes are characteristic of subcortical dementia. Memory for recent events is impaired. Poor attention, short concentration, impaired calculation, and concrete abstraction become evident as the disease progresses (Boller *et al.*, 1980).

A variety of psychiatric symptoms including schizophrenialike disorder have been noted. The familial cases appear to suffer from a progressive organic syndrome with mental symptoms. Schizophreniform disorder with delusions and hallucinations and depression have also been reported in some cases.

## J. SPINOCEREBELLAR DEGENERATIONS

Spinocerebellar degenerations are a heterogeneous group of degenerative diseases involving the cerebellum and its afferent and efferent fibers. These are various specific clinical entities that are inherited in an autosomal dominant or autosomal recessive manner. Each of the clinical entities involves varying degrees of the cerebellum, brain stem, basal ganglia, and spinal structures. The clinical picture is usually consistent in one family, but one or more members of the same family may have an entirely different presentation of the disease.

The classifications of this group of diseases are usually based on typical clinical manifestations and the age of onset of symptoms. However, categorization of these diseases is arbitrary and nonspecific since many gradations of symptoms between various entities exist. A commonly used classification is as follows (Greenfield, 1954):

1. Diseases that predominantly affect the cerebellum, i.e., cerebellar cortical degeneration and cerebellar degeneration.
2. Diseases predominantly affecting the spinal cord, i.e., Friedreich's disease and hereditary spastic ataxia.

3. Diseases predominantly affecting the brain stem and the cerebellum, i.e., olivopontocerebellar degeneration.

In Friedreich's ataxia, the primary area of pathology is in the spinal cord and the peripheral nerves. The spinocerebellar, lateral corticospinal tracts, and posterior columns are selectively involved. The primary sensory neurons undergo neuronal loss with secondary demyelination occurring in the posterior columns of the spinal cord. Neuronal loss also occurs in Clarke's column, which is the cell nucleus of origin for the spinocerebellar tracts. The anterior horn neurons of the spinal cord may also be lost. Neuronal loss may occur in the cerebellar cortex and the deep cerebellar nuclei. The cerebral cortex is histologically normal. Demyelination and gliosis do not extend above the level of the medulla.

Cerebellar involvement includes loss of Purkinje's cells, granular cells, and cells in the dentate and other deeper nuclei.

Involvement of the cerebrum may be an early or a terminal phenomenon, causing cognitive and memory deficits.

### Cognitive and Emotional Changes

In Friedreich's disease, dementia is not a prominent feature. Minor intellectual difficulties, mood irritability, paranoid ideation, and even frank hallucinations may occur.

In type I olivopontocerebellar atrophy, dementia with early loss of recent memory is common.

Impairment of intellectual functions is observed at times in spinocerebellar degeneration. Greenfield (1954) quoted Bell and Carmichael as having found mental deficiency in 23% of 242 families with Friedreich's ataxia and in 27.5% of 76 families with spastic paraplegia. Sjogren (Davies, 1949) noted progressive dementia in 58% of cases of Friedreich's ataxia. Gilman and Sorenstein (1964) reported several cases of familial amyotrophic dystonic paraplegia. Two of the cases that had been tested with IQ tests showed moderate mental retardation.

### K. SUMMARY

Various degenerative diseases produce identifiable patterns of neurological deficits since they affect different areas of the brain. The deficits in cognitive and emotional functions, however, are much more global and their presence rarely localizes a lesion in specific parts of the brain. Several broad classifications have been suggested for localization of lesion. For example, left-hemispheric lesions are likely to influence predominantly language functions whereas lesions in the right hemisphere would impair visuospatial skills. Albert *et al.* (1974) suggested a distinction between cortical and subcortical lesions: degenerative diseases primarily affecting the cortex (i.e., Alzheimer's and Pick's diseases) give rise to a functional deficit called "cortical dementia," whereas brain stem lesions produce subcortical dementia. In cortical dementia, there is little or no deficit of the motor system, posture, gait, speed, muscle tone, and reflexes. Language functions are most affected and are manifested by aphasia and difficulties in naming objects. Memory deficits include impairment of new learning and impaired recall of old memories. There is a deterioration in visuospatial skills, mathematical calculations, and judgment. Overall, IQ declines with the progress of the disease. Aphasia, amnesia, and agnosia characterize cortical dementia.

Degenerative diseases predominantly affecting subcortical structures (i.e., progressive supranuclear palsy, Huntington's disease) produce functional deficits called subcortical dementia. The motor system is extensively involved affecting posture, gait, and muscle tone. Language functions are only mildly affected. Impairment of cognitive functions includes general slowness of mental processes and forgetfulness. Overall IQ changes are lesser than found in cortical dementia.

In addition to the overall clinical picture of cortical and subcortical dementia, there are specific features that are unique to each of the degenerative diseases since they affect the brain differently. It is important to recognize the specific deficits associated with each disease since the degree of disability and prognosis vary in each disease. Undue restrictions on patients' activities and vocation may be avoided if specific deficits in cognitive functions can be identified and working conditions adjusted to them.

Neuropsychological data have been available only for a selected group of diseases. There are many rare diseases that have not been studied with modern methods and provide only clinical impressions of cognitive deficits. Similarities between the diseases with regard to sites of lesions may help clinicians to extrapolate some of the neuropsychological findings from well-studied diseases to rarer ones.

## L. REFERENCES

Albert ML: Subcortical dementia, in Katzman R, Terry R, Bick K (eds): *Alzheimer's Disease: Senile Dementia and Related Disorders*. New York; Raven Press, 1978, pp 173–180.

Albert ML, Feldman RG, Willis AL: The "subcortical dementia" of progressive supranuclear palsy. *J Neurol Neurosurg Psychiatry* 1974; 37:121–130.

Albert ML, Butters N, Brandt J: Patterns of remote memory in amnesic and demented patients. *Arch Neurol* 1981; 38:495–500.

Alvord EC Jr: The pathology of Parkinsonism. Part II. An interpretation with special references to other changes in the aging brain, in McDowell FH, Markham CH (eds): *Recent Advances in Parkinson's Disease*. Philadelphia; FA Davis, 1971, pp 131–161.

Aminoff M, Marshall J, Smith E, *et al*: Pattern of intellectual impairment in Huntington's chorea. *Psychol Med* 1975; 5:169–172.

Beard AW: The association of hepatolenticular degeneration with schizophrenia. *ACTA Psychiatr Neurol* 1959; 34:411–428.

Behan PO, Feldman RG: Serum proteins, amyloid and Alzheimer's disease. *J Am Geriatr Soc* 1970; 18:792–797.

Berg L, Hughes C, Cuben L, et al: Mild senile dementia of Alzheimer type: Research diagnostic criteria, recruitment, and description of a study population. J Neurol Neurosurg Psychiatry 1982; 45:926–968.

Boller F, Mizutani T, Roessmann V, et al: Parkinson disease, dementia and Alzheimer disease: Clinicopathological correlations. Ann Neurol 1980; 7:329–335.

Bolton N, Brutton PG, Savage R: Some normative data on the WAIS and its indices in an aged population. J Clin Psychol 1966; 22:184–188.

Brown G, Wilson W: Parkinsonism and depression. South Med J 1972; 65:540–545.

Butters N, Cermak L: Alcoholic Korsakoff's Syndrome. New York, Academic Press, 1980.

Butters N, Sax D, Montgomery K, et al: Comparison of the neuropsychological deficits associated with early and advanced Huntington's disease. Arch Neurol 1978; 35:585–589.

Butters N, Albert M, Sax D: Investigations of the memory disorders of patients with Huntington's disease. Adv Neurol 1979; 23:203–212.

Caine E, Ebert M, Weingartner H: An outline for the analysis of dementia. The memory disorder of Huntington's disease. Neurology 1977; 27:1087–1092.

Caine E, Hunt R, Weingartner H, et al: Huntington's dementia, clinical and neuropsychological features. Arch Neurol 1978; 35:377–384.

Caird WK, Hannah F: Short-term memory disorders in elderly psychiatric patients. Dis Nerv Syst 1964; 25:564–568.

Celesia G, Wanamaker W: Psychiatric disturbances in Parkinson's disease. Dis Nerv Syst 1972; 33:577–583.

Cleveland S, Dysinger D: Mental deterioration in senile psychosis. J Abnorm Soc Psychol 1944; 39:368–372.

Crapper, DR, Krishnan SS, Quittkat S: Aluminum, neurofibrillary degeneration and Alzheimer's disease. Brain 1976; 99:67–80.

Cummings JL, Benson DF, LoVerme S Jr: Reversible dementia. JAMA 1980; 243:2434–2439.

Davies DL: The intelligence of patients with Friedreich's ataxia. J Neurol Neurosurg Psychiatry 1949; 12:34–38.

Dewhurst K, Oliver J, Trick K, et al: Neuropsychiatric aspects of Huntington's disease. Confin Neurol 1969; 31:258–268.

Diller L, Riklan M: Psychosocial factors in Parkinson's disease. J Am Geriatr Soc 1956; 4:1291–1300.

Dixon JC: Cognitive structure in senile conditions with some suggestions for developing a brief screening test of mental status. J Gerontal 1965; 20:41–49.

Dooling EC, Schoene W, Richardson E Jr: Hallervorden-Spatz syndrome. Arch Neurol 1974; 30:70–83.

Elizan TS: Amyotrophic lateral sclerosis and parkinsonism–dementia complex of guam. Arch Neurol 1966; 14:356.

Ernst B, Dalby MA, Dalby A: Gnostic-praxic disturbances in presenile dementia. ACTA Neurol Scand 1970; 46(suppl 43):99–100.

Gilman S, Sorenstein S: Familial amyotrophic dystonic paraplegia. Brain 1964; 87:51.

Goldstein NP, Ewert J, Randall R, et al: Psychiatric aspects of Wilson's disease (hepatolenticular degeneration): Results of psychometric tests during long-term therapy Am J Psychiatry 1968; 124:1555–1561.

Greenfield JG: Spinocerebellar Degenerations. Oxford, England, Blackwell Scientific Publications, 1954.

Gruenberg E: Epidemiological studies, in Katzman R, Terry RD, Bick KL (eds): Alzheimer Disease, Senile Dementia and Related Disorders. New York, Raven Press, 1978, pp 323–326.

Gustafson L, Hagberg B: Dementia with onset in the presenile period: A cross-sectional study. ACTA Psychiatry Scand (suppl) 1975; 257:1–36.

Hallervorden H, Spatz M: Eigenartige erkrankung im extrapyramidalen system mit besonderer beteiligung des globus pallidus und der substantia nigra. Zentralbl Gesamte Neurol Psychiatr 1922; 79:254.

Heston LL: Genetic studies of dementia: With emphasis on Parkinson's disease and Alzheimer's neuropathology, in Mortimer JA, Schulman LM (eds): The Epidemiology of Dementia. New York, Oxford University Press, 1981, pp 101–114.

Huntington G: On Chorea. *Med Surg Reporter* 1872; 26:317–321.

Inglis J: An experimental study learning and memory function in elderly psychiatric patients. *J Ment Sci* 1957; 103:796–803.

Inglis J: Learning, retention and conceptual usuage in elderly patients with memory disorder. *J Abnor Soc Psychol* 1959; 59:210–215.

Jackson J, Jankovic J, Ford J: Progressive supranuclear palsy: Clinical features and response to treatment in 16 patients. *Ann Neurol* 1983; 13:273–278.

Josiassen R, Cury L, Roemer R, *et al*: Patterns of intellectual deficit in Huntington's disease. *J Clin Neuropsychol* 1982; 4:173–183.

Kendrick D, Post F: Differences in cognitive status between healthy, psychiatrically ill and diffusely brain-damaged elderly subjects. *Br J Psychiatry* 1967; 113:75–81.

Knehr CA, Bearn AG: Psychological impairment in Wilson's disease. *J Nerv Ment Dis* 1956; 124:251–255.

Lishman WA: *Organic Psychiatry*. London, Blackwell Scientific Publications, 1978.

Loranger AW, Goodell H: Intellectual impairment in Parkinson syndrome. *Brain* 1972; 95:405–412.

Mathews CG, Haaland K: The effect of symptom duration on cognitive and motor performance in Parkinsonism. *Neurology* 1979; 29:951–956.

Mayeux R, Stern Y, Rosen J, *et al*: Depression, intellectual impairment and Parkinson disease. *Neurology* 1981; 31:645–650.

McHugh P, Folstein M: Psychiatric syndromes of Huntington's chorea: A clinical and phenomenologic study, in Benson D, Blumer D, (eds): *Psychiatric Aspects of Neurologic Disease*. New York, Grune and Stratton, 1975, pp 267–285.

Metter EJ, Reige W, Hanson W, *et al*: Comparison of metabolic rates, language and memory in subcortical aphasias. *Brain Lang* 1983; 19:33–47.

Miller E: On the nature of memory disorder in presenile dementia. *Neuropsychology* 1971; 9:75–81.

Miller E: Short- and long-term memory in patients with presenile dementia (Alzheimer's disease). *Psychol Med* 1973; 3:221–224.

Miller E, Hagen D: Some characteristics of verbal behavior in presenile dementia. *Psychol Med* 1975; 5:255–259.

Mortimer JA, Pirozzolo FJ, Hansch EC, *et al*: Relationship of motor symptoms to intellectual deficits in Parkinson disease. *Neurology* 1982; 32:133–137.

Nandy K: Brain-reactive antibodies in aging and senile dementia; in Katzman R, Terry RD, Bick KL (eds): *Alzheimer Disease, Senile Dementia and Related Disorders*. New York, Raven Press, 1978, pp 503–507.

Orme JE: Non-verbal and verbal in normal old age, senile dementia and elderly depression. *J Gerontol* 1957; 12:408–413.

Reed H, Lindsay A, Silversides JL, *et al*: The uveoencephalitic syndrome or Vogt-Koyanagi-Harada disease. *Can Med Assoc J* 1958; 79:451–459.

Reitan RM, Boll TJ: Intellectual and cognitive functions in Parkinson's disease. *J Consult Clin Psychol* 1971; 37:364–369.

Rezdilsky B, Cummings J, Huston A: Hallervorden-Spatz disease—Late infantile and adult types, report of two cases. *ACTA Neuropathol* 1968; 10:1–16.

Rockford G: A study of naming errors in dysphasic and demented patients. *Neuropsychology* 1971; 9:437–443.

Roth M: Epidemiological studies, in Katzman R, Terry RD, Bick KL (eds): *Alzheimer's Disease, Senile Dementia and Related Disorders*. New York, Raven Press, 1978, pp 337–339.

Sacks OW, Aguilar MJ, Brown WJ: Hallervorden-Spatz disease. Its pathogenesis and place among the axonal dystrophies. *ACTA Neuropathol* 1966; 6:164–174.

Sjogren R, Sjogren H, Lindgren A: Morbus Alzheimer and morbus Pick. *ACTA Psychiatr Neurol Scand* 1952; (supple 82):1–152.

Squire L, Wetzel C, Slater P: Anterograde amnesia following ECT: An analysis of the beneficial effects of partial information. *Neuropsychologia* 1978; 16:339–348.

Steele JC, Richardson JC, Olszewski J: Progressive supranuclear palsy. *Arch Neurol* 1964; 10:333–359.

Terry RD, Peck A, De Teresa R, *et al*: Some morphometric aspects of the brain is senile dementia of the Alzheimer type. *Ann Neurol* 1981; 10:184–192.

Tomlinson BE: The pathology of dementia; in Wells CE (ed): *Dementia* ed 2. Philadelphia, FA Davis, 1977, pp 113–153.

Trimble MR, Cummings J: Neuropsychiatric disturbances following brainstem lesions. *Br J Psychiatry* 1981; 138:56–59.

Warrington E, Weiskrantz L: Amnesic syndrome: Consolidation or retrieval? *Nature* 1970; 228:628–630.

Weingartner H, Caine E, Ebert M: Encoding processes, learning and recall in Huntington's disease. *Adv Neurol* 1979; 23:215–216.

White P, Goodhardt M, Keet J, *et al*: Neocortical cholinergic neurons in elderly people. *Lancet* 1977; 1:668–670.

Wilson RS, Kasniak A, Klawans H, *et al*: High speed memory scanning in Parkinsonism. *Cortex* 1980; 16:67–72.

Wilson SA: Progressive lenticular degeneration: A familial nervous disease associated with cirrhosis of the liver. *Brain* 1912; 34:295–509.

Yunis JY, Bloomfield CD, Ensrud K: All patients with acute nonlymphocytic leukemia may have a chromosonal defect. *N Engl J Med* 1981; 305:135–139.

CHAPTER 7

# Memory in Cerebrovascular Disorders

---

The brain is about 1/50 of the total body weight in an adult, but it uses 1/5 of the resting cardiac output amounting to 1000 ml of blood per minute, extracting from it 500 to 600 ml of oxygen and 75 to 100 mg of glucose each minute. This basal need of the brain remains the same whether the person is asleep, awake, excited, or happy. During exercise, cardiac output increases to increase the blood flow to the muscles, but the brain blood flow remains the same since the brain adjusts its own blood supply under varying conditions of cardiac output. Thus physical exercise, standing on the head, or ingesting a heavy meal have no effect on the overall flow of blood to the brain.

The brain requires a continuous supply of oxygen and glucose for its proper functioning. Neuronal metabolism suffers within 6 sec after the blood supply to the brain is interrupted. Brain activity ceases within 2 min and brain damage begins 5 min after circulation stops.

There are regional variations in the blood flow through the brain. At rest, the flow is higher in the frontal areas than the parietal and the temporal areas. This pattern of flow changes in response to changes in mental activities. During excitement and anxiety, the baseline flow becomes exaggerated. Motor activities increase the blood flow in the corresponding primary cortical regions.

Some increase of blood flow also occurs in the opposite cortex. Listening to a speech increases the blood flow in the left (and to a lesser extent in the right) temporal auditory cortices and Wernicke's area on the left. The regional blood flow differences caused by physical and mental activity have no effect on overall brain blood flow. There is a close relationship between the blood flow and the metabolism. The increase in the flow is activated by the increased metabolic requirement of the region.

There are very modest changes in the blood flow and the metabolism of the brain with age. There is a progressive but slight decrease in the blood flow and in the consumption of oxygen and glucose with increasing age. This change is noticeable mainly in the frontal lobes. There is little or no overall or local decrease in other areas of the brain.

## A. CHRONIC ISCHEMIA OF THE BRAIN

The typical, insidious, slowly progressive changes in cognitive and memory functions of old age are not due to atherosclerosis. Use of the term "cerebral atherosclerosis" to describe cognitive deterioration in the elderly is probably the most common medical misdiagnosis. It was hypothesized that the atherosclerotic changes in old age probably caused a progressive ischemia that gave rise to cognitive deficits. It is now well recognized that atherosclerosis of the brain vessels does not cause dementia directly, but it is related to old-age dementia in a complex manner.

Atherosclerosis is the usual cause for the occlusion of the carotid arteries. Common carotid artery occlusion occurs in less than 1% of the cases of carotid artery syndrome. It is more common on the left side. Because of the rich collateral circulation, unilateral occlusion of the common carotid artery produces few symptoms. Some patients may develop bilateral carotid artery stenosis or occlusion. The effects will depend on the efficiency of the collateral flow from the basilar artery system. It may cause quadriplegia or be asymptomatic. However, even in asymptomatic cases, ophthalmic pressures are equally reduced in both eyes.

### Cognitive and Emotional Changes

Neuropsychological studies of patients before and after carotid surgery have not shown any conclusive results. Kelley *et al.* (1980) compared 35 patients with carotid artery stenosis with 17 controls who were selected from the group that underwent peripheral vascular surgery and had no impairment of carotid circulation. These subjects were tested preoperatively and postoperatively with neuropsychological tests including the Stanford Binet Intelligence Test, the Wechsler Memory Scale, and several other tests for receptive and expressive language functions, left–right discrimination, and perceptual analysis. Personality changes were tested with the State-Trait Anxiety Inventory and Minnesota Multiphasic Personality Inventory (MMPI). The experimental subjects underwent endarterectomy. The preoperative mean scores of both groups were similar on the various neuropsychological tests. Postoperatively, only endarterectomy patients showed mean improvement on several of the measures such as the Wechsler Memory Scale and on the Word Association tests.

On tests of personality, the two groups did not differ preoperatively. However, postoperatively, both groups showed a significant reduction in State-Trait Anxiety Inventory and the MMPI Schizophrenia Scale. Further analysis of the sample indicated that the endarterectomy patients who showed cognitive improvement postoperatively were younger, better educated, and had lower admitting systolic blood pressure.

In another study (Haynes *et al.*, 1976), 17 patients who had at least 50% carotid artery stenosis were compared with 9 control patients on neuropsychological tests. The tests included subtests of the Wechsler Adult Intelligence Scale to test verbal comprehension and perceptual organization. Personality changes were assessed with the Minnesota Multiphasic Personality Inventory and the State-Trait Anxiety Inventory. After endarterectomy, patients improved in verbal comprehension and perceptual organization tasks. They also showed a decrease in time taken to complete perceptual motor tasks, a decrease in aphasic signs, and a significant reduction in anxiety, suspicion, confusion, and disorientation.

## B. TRANSIENT ISCHEMIC DISORDER

The term transient ischemic attack (TIA) is used to describe sudden episodes of focal neurological deficits that result from an inadequate supply of blood to specific brain areas. The episodes usually resolve within 24 hr without leaving any residuum.

The episodes lasting longer than 24 hr, up to a week or two but with complete recovery, are called "reversible ischemic attacks." These conditions seem to represent a continuum from a mild cerebrovascular insufficiency to a complete loss of blood supply to the damaged area.

The clinical picture is characterized by numbness of fingers, vision impairment, speech disturbances, vertigo, tinnitus, and facial parathesias. It has been suggested that very brief TIAs may occur in some patients during sleep without any awareness.

Neurological examination performed between the attacks is normal. However, during the attack, the examination indicates an evolving cerebral infarction. Various estimates indicate that about 36% have infarction within the month and 50% within 12 months of onset of TIA. Another third continue to suffer from recurrent TIAs, while the rest cease to have TIAs spontaneously. There is as yet no way of telling which patient belongs to which group.

### Cognitive and Emotional Changes

There is a paucity of information regarding the effect of a focal or general reduction of cerebral blood flow on learning and memory. The studies of individuals after varying periods of cardiac arrest and resuscitation indicate that a few minutes of complete ischemia produces no apparent change in learning capacity or in retention of information. After 8 min, there is a severe impairment of new learning, but the retention of previous knowledge remains intact. It is possible that transient ischemia may cause one or more strategically located lesions such as in the hippocampal formation system resulting in a loss of the ability to form new memories.

By definition TIA leaves no residuum. However, many patients may present with symptoms of failing memory, personality changes, inability to think quickly, and difficulty in recalling remote information. In the studies at Bayler-Methodist Center for Cerebrovascular Research, where predominantly vascular cases are referred, measurable impairment of intellectual functions occurred in about 50% of the patients with vertebrobasilar insufficiency (Fields *et al.*, 1970).

## C. LARGE CEREBRAL INFARCTIONS

Large cerebral infarctions are caused by occlusion of major cerebral arteries. Single unilateral infarction usually produces a well-defined focal syndrome. Occlusion of the middle cerebral artery or its branches are among the most commonly involved. Left-hemispheric infarction typically causes aphasia and apraxia. Right middle cerebral artery infarction produces less well-defined cognitive deficits such as problems in visuospatial orientation, visuomotor performance, abnormalities in language melody, and dressing disturbances.

### Angular Gyrus Syndrome

This deserves special emphasis since it is usually difficult to distinguish from Alzheimer's disease. It results from occlusion of the posterior portion of the middle cerebral artery (Benson *et al.*, 1982). It is characterized by aphasia, agraphia, and Gerstmann's syndrome. It shares many clinical features with Alzheimer's disease and is easily confused with it. Gerstmann's syndrome includes acalculia, agraphia, difficulty in distinguishing right from left, and finger agnosia. Constructional disturbances are common. Although any individual component of Gerstmann's syndrome may occur in lesions of other locations, when four of the above components occur together, they reliably indicate dominant angular gyrus dysfunction. Focal damage to the posterior dominant hemisphere causes fluent aphasia, including Wernicke's aphasia, transcortical sensory aphasia, and anomic aphasia, depending upon the location and the extent of the lesion. If the angular gyrus is involved, the patient may show alexia with agraphia and/or Gerstmann's syndrome. The fluent aphasia is characterized by spontaneous fluent verbal output which is paraphasic and empty and the patient has impaired comprehension of language. Focal neurological signs are not usually prominent and standard CT scans do not disclose focal abnormalities.

Several clinical features may differentiate it from Alzheimer's disease. Amnesia is nearly always an initial symptom in Alzheimer's disease and memory disturbances remain prominent throughout the course of the disease. Angular gyrus syndrome patients, although always complaining about their memory problems, are usually referring to word-finding difficulties. They preserve memory in daily behavior, including the ability to carry out complex tasks such as learning new routines, shopping, and cooking. They show little tendency to become lost or spatially disoriented. An abrupt onset or stepwise progression is suggestive of vascular process whereas Alzheimer's is an insidious onset and progresses slowly. Table I shows some of the distinguishing features of the two diseases.

The anterior cerebral arteries supply a major portion of the frontal lobes and anterior four fifths of the corpus callosum. Occlusion of this artery causes an interhemispheric disconnection syndrome as a result of destruction of the callosal fibers (Geschwind and Kaplan, 1962). Writing with the right hand is usually normal, but left-hand writing is incorrect, both to dictation and spontaneously. Objects placed in the left hand (concealed from vision) are named incorrectly, but the patient could select the object afterward with the left hand by touch or point to it. He could also draw the object with the left hand. Even while giving an incorrect verbal description, he could demonstrate correctly the use of the object being held in the left hand. If the object was placed in one hand (concealed from vision) the patient cannot select it from a group of items or draw it with the other hand. The patient's performance of verbal commands with the left hand is frequently incorrect.

Occlusion of the left anterior cerebral artery causes transient mutism followed by transcortical aphasia. Alexander and Schmitt (1980) described two cases of left anterior cerebral artery occlusion. The clinical features varied in the two cases. In one case, there was a marked inability to generate word lists, moderate impairment of reading comprehension, and unintelligible writing with the nondominant left hand. Reading aloud was minimally impaired.

**TABLE I.** Distinguishing Features between Alzheimer's Disease and the Angular Gyrus Syndrome

|  | Alzheimer's disease | Angular gyrus syndrome |
|---|---|---|
| History | Insidious onset<br>Progressive course | Abrupt onset |
| Orientation for place | Impaired | Intact |
| New learning | Impaired | Intact except for verbal tests |
| Awareness of deficit | Absent | Present |
| Paraphasias | Little relation to target word | Within category |
| Reading | Reading aloud often spared until late | Impaired |

In the second case, there was marked inability to generate word lists. Auditory comprehension was intact, but responses occurred with increased latencies. Automatic speech was normal, although an initiating cue was required. Writing with the dominant right hand was limited to production of name and address.

Posterior cerebral artery occlusion produces contralateral hemianopia. In addition, right-sided lesion may be associated with visual hallucinations, environmental disorientation, and difficulties in facial recognition (DeRenzi *et al.*, 1969). Left posterior artery occlusion produces contralateral hemiparesis, hemisensory loss, mild anomia, and alexia without agraphia. Bilateral occlusion produces severe amnesia and cortical blindness. There appears to be a differential specialization between the two hemispheres in the process of visual recognition. The right side is more involved in discriminating and comparing sensory data and the left side is more involved in mediating the higher cognitive function of identification of the meaning of visual sensations.

## D. MULTI-INFARCT DEMENTIA

Multi-infarct dementia results from the occlusion of large, medium size and small arteries. However, the clinical features of infarcts produced by the occlusion of large and medium size arteries are fairly characteristic and easy to recognize. Occlusion of small arteries also produces small infarcts both in the cortex and the subcortical regions, but these infarcts, depending on their number and location, may or may not give rise to any apparent deficits in the sensory and motor areas. Changes may become evident in cognitive functions, memory, and personality. These changes may be confused with pure psychiatric disorders. Cognitive and memory impairments occur in a stepwise fashion. Clinical manifestations of cortical, subcortical, or a mixed type of dementia are usually apparent.

Lacunar state and Binswanger's disease are two pathological subentities causing vascular dementia.

### Lacunar State

In severely hypertensive patients, multiple "little strokes" may occur in all parts of the brain. Small multiple lacunar infarctions develop in the basal ganglia and pons from thrombotic-hemorrhagic lesions. As these infarcts heal, cavities with a lacunar appearance result ranging between 2 to 15 mm in size (hence, the name). As the number of lacunae increases, the lacunar state develops with progressive dementia. Neurological signs result predominantly from the damage of the basal ganglia and the brain stem and include bradykinesis, rigidity, dysarthria, dysphagia, and small-stepped gait (frequently resembling Parkinson's disease).

Dementia is a prominent feature in 70% to 80% of the cases with lacunar state (Brown and Wilson, 1972). The characteristics of dementia are variable depending upon the location of most lacunae. It is usually characterized by impaired mentation, marked slowness of psychomotor performance, recent memory disturbances, confusion, and perseveration. Personality changes include apathy and loss of tactfulness.

### Binswanger's Disease

Otto Binswanger described eight patients who were demented and were found to have pronounced atrophy of the white matter at autopsy. Pathologically, brains of these patients show multiple infarctions in the white matter of the cerebral hemisphere and are probably of vascular origin. Lacunar infarcts may also be present in the basal ganglia and the thalamus, but the cortex and subcortical arcuate fibers are largely spared.

Clinically, this disease runs a long progressive course. Cognitive and memory impairments resemble those found in lacunar state.

## E. SUMMARY

The brain is about 1/50 of the total body weight in an adult but it uses 1/5 of the resting cardiac output, amounting to 1000 ml of blood per minute, extracting from it 500 to 600 ml of oxygen and 75 to 100 mg of glucose each minute. This basal need of the brain remains the same whether the person is asleep, awake, excited, or happy. The brain adjusts its own blood supply under varying conditions of cardiac output. There are regional variations in the blood flow through the brain. For example, the flow is higher in the frontal areas than in the parietal and the temporal areas. Motor activities increase the blood flow in the corresponding primary cortical regions.

The brain requires a continuous supply of oxygen and glucose for its proper functioning. Neuronal metabolism suffers within 6 sec after the blood supply to the brain is interrupted. Brain activity ceases within 2 min and brain damage begins in 5 min after the circulation stops. Vascular diseases such as atherosclerosis, spasm, occlusion, or hemorrhage interrupt normal blood flow and cause varying degrees of deficits in cognitive and memory functions.

There are very modest changes in the blood flow and the metabolism of the brain with age. There is a progressive but slight decrease in the blood flow and the consumption of oxygen and glucose with increasing age. This change is noticeable mainly in the frontal lobes. There is little or no overall or local decrease in other areas of the brain. The use of the term "cerebral atherosclerosis" to describe the cognitive deterioration in the elderly is probably the most common medical misdiagnosis.

Atherosclerosis is the usual cause for occlusion of the carotid arteries. Because of the rich collateral circulation, unilateral and sometimes even bilateral occlusions may cause little or no symptoms. Neuropsychological studies of patients before and after carotid surgery to improve brain blood flow have not shown any conclusive results. Several studies indicate some improvement in cognitive functions after endarterectomy especially in patients who are younger, better educated, and have lower admitting systolic blood pressure.

By definition, transient ischemic attacks leave no residuum. However, many patients may present with symptoms of failing memory, personality changes, inability to think quickly, and difficulty in recalling remote information.

Occlusion of large cerebral arteries results in large infarction with fairly well-defined focal syndromes. Left-hemispheric infarction typically causes aphasia and apraxia. Right middle cerebral artery infarction produces less well-defined cognitive deficits such as problems in visuospatial orientation, visuomotor performance, and abnormalities in language melody. Angular gyrus syndrome resulting from occlusion of the posterior portion of the middle cerebral artery should be differentiated from early Alzheimer's disease. Patients suffering from this syndrome have word-finding difficulty and frequently complain about their memory. These patients manifest no problem in daily behavior, including the ability to carry out complex tasks such as learning new routines, shopping, and cooking. An abrupt onset or a stepwise progression is suggestive of vascular process whereas Alzheimer's disease has an insidious onset and progresses slowly.

Occlusion of small arteries may produce small multiple infarcts both in cortical and subcortical regions. In the absence of physical symptoms, cognitive and personality changes resulting from multiple infarcts may be confused with pure psychiatric disorders.

## F. REFERENCES

Alexander MP, Schmitt MA: The aphasia syndrome of stroke in the left anterior cerebral artery territory. *Arch Neurol* 1980; 37:97–100.

Benson DF, Cummings JL, Saisy T: Angular gyrus syndrome simulating Alzheimer disease. *Arch Neurol* 1982; 39:616–620.

Brown G, Wilson WP: Parkinsonism and depression. *South Med J* 1972; 65:540–545.

DeRenzi E, Scotti G, Spinnler H: Perceptual and associative disorders of visual recognition. *Neurology* 1969; 19:634–642.

Fields WS, Maslenikov V, Meyer J: Joint study of extracranial arterial occlusion. V. Progress report of prognosis in operated and nonoperated patients with transient cerebral ischemia attacks and cervical carotid artery lesion. *JAMA* 1970; 211:1993–2003.

Geschwind N, Kaplan E: A human cerebral disconnection syndrome. *Neurology* 1962; 12:675–685.

Haynes CD, Gideon DA, King GD, *et al*: The improvement of cognition and personality after carotid enartrectomy. *Surgery* 1976; 80:699.

Kelley MP, Garron DC, Javid H: Carotid artery disease, carotid enartrectomy and behavior. *Arch Neurol* 1980; 37:743.

CHAPTER 8

# Memory in Chronic CNS Infections

General paresis of the insane was the first mental illness that was clearly attributed to the chronic infection of the brain. Availability of treatment with penicillin halted the progress of dementia in most of the cases and confirmed the infectious nature of the disease and is mostly of historical interest. However, many other bacteria and viruses have been shown to be related to degenerative changes in the brain, causing progressive dementia.

## A. CNS SYPHILIS

*Treponema pallidum*, a spirochete, is transmitted almost exclusively through direct contact with the infectious lesion. Chancre, a primary lesion, occurs at the site of the contact six to eight weeks later. A systemic secondary reaction develops in the form of a skin rash and generalized lymphadenitis. Occasionally, syphilitic meningitis may occur in the early stages of the disease. Late CNS manifestations of syphilis include general paresis, meningovascular syphilis, symptomatic syphilitic meningitis, and multiple gummas. These late manifestations may become evident from a few to 20 to 30 years after the initial infection. During the latent period, there is usually a subclinical inflammation of the meninges.

The clinical presentation of general paresis tends to be atypical and can manifest in an array of neurological signs and symptoms: tremor of the tongue and hands, quivering of facial muscles, dysarthria, ataxia, apraxia, and convulsive seizures. If untreated, general paresis progresses to cause aphasia, hemiparesis, cranial nerve palsy, and death within three to four years.

## Pathology

There is achronic spirochetal meningoencephalitis which destroys neurons in the cerebral cortex. At autopsy the brain is atrophic, particularly in the anterior portion of the frontal and temporal lobes. Over the atrophic area, the meninges are opaque, thickened, and adherent to the underlying cortex. Cerebral sulci are widened. Microscopically there are widespread degenerative changes of the parenchyma.

## Cognitive and Emotional Changes

Dementia is an early manifestation of CNS syphilis. Forty to sixty percent of the patients suffer from "simple progressive dementia"; 20% to 40% suffer from dementia with manic features; 6% show major depression; and 3% to 6% manifest paranoia or paranoid psychosis (Bruetsch, 1959).

During the early stages of the disease, the primary changes are in the personality, mood, and memory impairment. Early personality changes and poor judgment appear to be related to the damage of the frontal lobes. The person becomes irritable, inattentive, absent-minded, and does not grasp events transpiring around him. Early memory changes are manifested in the impairment of recent memory.

In the later stages of the disease, the person tends to confabulate, loses insight into his condition, and judgment becomes poor. Recent, as well as remote, memory becomes impaired.

Psychiatric features are multiform and general paresis can mimic all forms of psychosis. The most common type of psychotic picture is that of simple deterioration of cognitive and mental functions. Paranoia and paranoid psychosis with unsystematized delusions are also common. In the later stages, confusion, disorientation, aphasia, and other neurological complications lead to death.

## B. CHRONIC VIRAL INFECTIONS

In some viral infections illness may not manifest until many years after exposure to the responsible virus. Kuru was the first chronic degenerative disease of man known to be caused by a slow virus infection, with incubation period measured in years and with a progressive accumulative pathology always leading to death. These observations established the fact that slow virus infection could produce chronic degenerative diseases in man after a long delay of months and years, with apparent inflammatory responses regularly associated with acute viral infections. Thereafter, several other degenerative diseases of man were linked with slow virus etiology, such as subacute sclerosing panencephalitis, progressive multifocal leukoencephalopathy, and transmissible spongioform encephalopathies.

## C. SUBACUTE SCLEROSING PANENCEPHALITIS

The disease is associated with infection by measles virus (or measleslike virus). It was first described by Dawson in 1934. Pathological studies in long-standing severe cases shows unduly hard brains. There is a perivascular infiltration in the cortex and white matter with plasma and other mononuclear cells. There are patchy areas of demyelination and gliosis in the white matter and deeper layers of the cortex. The neurons of the cortex, basal ganglia, pons, and inferior olives show degenerative changes. The electron micro-scopic picture shows inclusion bodies that show a positive staining section by the fluorescence antibody method for measles virus.

Children under twelve are predominantly affected. The disease has a gradual onset without fever. Forgetfulness, inability to keep up with school work, and restlessness are early symptoms. Temper outbursts, distractibility, sleeplessness, and occasional hallucinations are frequent. In a course of weeks or months, incoordination, ataxia, and myclonic jerks of muscles of trunks and extremities become manifest. There is an associated impairment of read-ing, writing, and visuomotor performance. In the terminal stage, a rigid quad-riplegia simulating complete decortication appears.

## D. PROGRESSIVE MULTIFOCAL LEUKOENCEPHALOPATHY

This is a progressive degenerative disorder caused by papova viruses and occurs primarily in patients suffering from malignant neoplasms such as cancer of the lungs and breasts, chronic lymphocytic and myelogenous leu-kemias, Hodgkin's disease, and lymphosarcoma. A few cases occur in the absence of malignant disease.

The pathological examination shows multiple areas of demyelination in various parts of the CNS, a mild to moderate degree of perivascular infiltra-tion, and hyperplasia of astrocytes into bizarre giant forms that resemble neoplastic cells. Eosinophilic intranuclear inclusions are seen in the oligo-dendroglial cells. These inclusions are composed of viruslike particles. It is postulated that the demyelination is due to destruction of the oligodendroglia by a virus.

The clinical features are quite diverse and are related to the location and the number of the lesions. Hemiplegia, other focal signs, and mental symp-toms are common. A progressive decline in cognitive functions is associated with impaired memory, poor concentration, and language disturbances. The disease usually progresses to death within two to four months, but cases lasting up to a year or longer have been observed.

## E. TRANSMISSIBLE SPONGIOFORM ENCEPHALOPATHIES

A transmissible infectious agent appears to cause, in animals and man, a group of diseases that show common neuropathological findings. Although the agent has been labeled a virus, it is unlike the known viruses. It has been difficult to purify this agent since it is resistant to X irradiation, ultraviolet exposure, and chemical treatment. It does not induce inflammation and does not evoke antibody response. Transmission of the spongioform encephalopathy from human to several species of primate such as pigs, cats, and mice has been achieved. Two of the neurological diseases recognized in man are kuru and Creutzfeldt-Jacob disease.

### Kuru

This disease has been found exclusively among the Fore tribe in the New Guinea Highlands. When the incidence of kuru was highest, it affected 1% of the tribal people and was a leading cause of death. Eighty percent of the adults affected are women. It usually manifests with cerebellar dysfunction, incoordination, chorea, myoclonus, strabismus, and dementia. The disease is progressive and is fatal within 12–24 months. The pathological examination reveals widespread neuronal loss and intense astrocytic and microglial proliferation.

Dementia occurs late in the course of the disease and is rarely severe. Behavioral changes and psychomotor retardation are common (Gajdusek, 1977).

### Creutzfeldt–Jakob Disease

This is a rare disease, approximately one case per million world-wide population. Onset is frequently in the sixth and seventh decade of life. This late occurrence in life causes some difficulty in the differential diagnosis from Alzheimer's and Pick's diseases. An occasional case as young as 20 years old has been reported. The pathological examination reveals loss of nerve cells in the cortex, the basal ganglia, and the spinal cord.

There is a gradual development of pyramidal signs such as muscle stiffness and weakness with reflex changes and superimposition of extrapyramidal signs (tremors, dysarthria, slowness of movements) and characteristic changes in the EEG. The disease is rapidly progressive resulting in death within a few months to a year.

During the initial stage, there is a feeling of mild fatigue, poor concentration, forgetfulness, and occasional depression (McAllister and Price, 1982).

After several weeks and months, signs of cortical dementia become increasingly evident with progressive intellectual deterioration, aphasia, apraxia, agnosia, and amnesia. Hallucinations and delusions also occur in the later stages of the disease.

## F. LONG-TERM SEQUELAE OF BACTERIAL MENINGITIS IN CHILDREN

With rapid and intensive treatment of meningitis, 95% to 98% of the children are able to survive. This decrease in mortality has been accompanied by a significant increase in permanent and serious neurological and mental sequelae. A considerable number of children are left with evidence of brain damage, emotional instability, impaired memory, restlessness, and poor concentration.

The follow-up studies of surviving children have shown somewhat contradictory results. This is primarily due to the variability of the samples, types of control, and above all the varying sensitivity of the methodology used for the assessment. Sell *et al.* (1972) reported psychological sequelae in two groups of children. In one group, 21 postmeningitic children who were between 2 months and 3 years of age at the onset of the disease were paired with near-age sibling controls. The mean IQ on the Wechsler Intelligence Scale for Children was 86 and that of the controls was 97. Six of the patients had 1 SD (= 15 points) below their controls. In two patients the difference in IQ exceeded 2 SD. Six patients had IQ scores higher than their controls, but none by 15 points. In the second group, normal survivors of meningitis were compared with the peers in their classrooms. The tests included the Illinois Test of Psycholinguistic Abilities, the Frostig Developmental Test of Visual Perception, and the Peabody Picture Vocabulary Test. The result indicated that the normal survivors functioned at a significantly lower level in perceptual discrimination and vocabulary.

Tejani *et al.* (1982) followed 22 children who had recovered from *Haemophilus influenzae* type B meningitis. These children were divided into two groups depending upon the age of the children at the time of the illness. Group A included 13 children who developed meningitis between the ages of 2 months and 2 years. Group B included nine children who developed meningitis after 4 years of age. Only two children, one in each group, had neurological or auditory sequelae. Fifteen of the children were tested psychometrically, using siblings as controls. The tests used for the preschool children were the Weschler Preschool, the Primary Scale of Intelligence Test, and the Frostig Developmental Test of Visual Perception. The children over 6 years of age were tested with the Wechsler Intelligence Scale for Children, the Bender Gestalt, and the Wide Range Achievement Tests. The results are outlined in Table I.

TABLE I. Results of Psychometric Testing of Children Following Recovery of
*Haemophilus Influenza* Type B Meningitis[a,b]

|  | Group A | | | Group B | | |
| --- | --- | --- | --- | --- | --- | --- |
|  | VIQ | PIQ | FSIQ | VIQ | PIQ | FSIQ |
| Patients | 95.5 | 103.37 | 97.0 | 93.7 | 100.8 | 97.0 |
| Controls | 98.2 | 100.3 | 101.6 | 90.1 | 95.1 | 91.5 |

[a]From Tejani *et al.* (1982).
[b]See text for explanation of groups A and B and specific tests given.

Analysis of the data indicated no significant difference between the patients and their controls. Only one patient in group A had an IQ 2 SD below his control. On the Frostig Test, seven patients in group A scored over 100 and eight patients had a score of 95 (normal mean = 100). On the Wide Range Achievement Test, seven older children were reading below their age-appropriate level, but so also were their controls. On the Bender Gestalt, four of the seven older patients, as well as their controls, showed a lag in perceptual age. The authors concluded that there was no significant difference between the patients and the controls, thus contradicting the findings of earlier studies (Sell *et al.*, 1972).

Sell (1983) reported preliminary results of a follow-up study of 50 children that began in 1975–1976. These children had recovered from *H. influenzae* meningitis. In 1981, results were as follows: normal in all respects, 50%; normal except behavior problems, 9%; overall significant handicaps, 28%. The major significant handicaps included hearing loss, language disorder, vision impairment, mental retardation, motor abnormalities, and seizures.

## G. SUMMARY

General paresis of the insane was the first mental illness that was clearly attributed to the chronic infection of the brain. Since then many other bacteria and viruses have been shown to be related to degenerative changes in the brain, causing progressive dementia. Some of the slow viral infections that cause chronic CNS infections are of particular importance since they produce chronic degenerative changes after a long delay of months and years. Slow viruses have been linked to several degenerative diseases such as subacute sclerosing panencephalitis, progressive multifocal leukoencephalopathy, and transmissible spongiform encephalopathies. Although the clinical features and causes of these diseases are quite diverse, they are characterized by progressive decline in cognitive functions and memory impairment.

Meningeal infection in childhood may have long-lasting effects. Although the majority of the children suffering from bacterial meningitis in infancy are able to survive with rapid and intensive treatment, they frequently suffer from varying degrees of cognitive and memory impairments. The long-term follow-up studies indicate that at least one fourth of these children may suffer from significant handicaps including hearing loss, language disorders, vision impairment, mental retardation, motor dysfunctions, and seizures.

## H.  REFERENCES

Bruetsch WL: The schizophrenic patients with increase of the protein content of the cerebrospinal fluid. *Am J Psychiatry* 1959; 115:545.

Dawson JR: Cellular inclusion in cerebral lesions of epidemic encephalitis. *Arch Neurol Psychiatr* 1934; 31:685.

Gajdusek DC: Unconventional viruses and the origin and disappearance of kuru. *Science* 1977; 197:943–960.

McAllister T, Price TR: Severe depressive pseudodementia with and without dementia. *Am J Psychiatry* 1982; 139:626–629.

Sell SH: Long-term sequelae of bacterial meningitis in children. *Pediatr Infect Dis* 1983; 2:90–93.

Sell SH, Webb W, Pate J, *et al*: Psychological sequelae to bacterial meningitis: Two controlled studies. *Pediatrics* 1972; 49:212–217.

Tejani A, Dobias B, Sambursky J: Long-term prognosis after *H. influenza* meningitis: Prospective evaluation. *Dev Med Child Neurol* 1982; 24:338–343.

CHAPTER 9

# Memory in Chronic Diseases

---

## A. CHRONIC ANOXIA OF THE BRAIN

Chronic anoxia of the brain may result from inadequate cerebral perfusion and from poor oxygen-carrying capacity of the blood. A large number of chronic diseases of the lungs, the cardiovascular system, and the blood can produce chronic anoxia and impairment of cerebral metabolism leading to disturbances of cognitive and memory functions. The clinical manifestations of anoxia vary with the duration and the rate at which anoxia develops. Acute sudden anoxia causes confusion, disorientation, and delirium. Amnesia for the duration of the acute condition, such as cardiac arrest, may persist after the recovery. In some cases, acute anoxia of sufficient duration will result in extensive brain damage and dementia. Chronic anoxia produces slow changes in cognitive functions and personality. Impairment of recent memory functions are frequently more apparent than impairment of cognitive abilities. Changes in personality usually begin with increased irritability and decreased interest in social activities and career achievements.

## B. CARDIAC DISEASES

Cerebral perfusion appears to be directly related to cardiac output. Regardless of the status of the cerebral blood vessels, cerebral symptoms will occur if the cardiac output falls below a critical level. Cardiac symptoms are common when cardiac arrhythmias, especially ventricular arrhythmias, are present.

These patients show progressive encephalopathy as a consequence of their diminished cardiac outputs. The symptoms frequently include inattention, irritability, confusion, somnolence, and loss of recent memory. Improvement in mental functions is frequently obtained with treatment that restores the cardiac output.

## C. LUNG DISEASES

Chronic obstructive lung disease causes disability in millions of people. There are slowly progressive changes in cognitive functions and personality. The changes include inattentiveness, slowness of mental functions, drowziness, lethargy, and forgetfulness. Austen *et al.* (1957) described several cases with chronic obstructive lung disease who fell asleep while at work, eating, or in conversation with family and friends. They were also forgetful, irritable, and easily confused. Their disorientation in time and place, their diminished capacity to recall events, and their failure to think quickly and coherently appeared to be the result of inattention and reduced awareness.

Several studies have shown that an improvement in pulmonary functions will reverse the impairment in cognitive functions. Krop *et al.* (1973) tested 22 patients having chronic obstructive pulmonary disease with a neuropsychological test before and after four weeks of continuous oxygen therapy. These patients were compared with a group of patients with similar severity of airway obstruction but who demonstrated a partial pressure of arterial oxygen greater than 55 mm Hg. The neuropsychological tests included the Wechsler Adult Intelligence Scale, the Wechsler Memory Scale, the Bender Gestalt, and the MMPI. The results indicated that the performance of the experimental group improved significantly in several areas such as full-scale IQ, performance IQ, memory quotient, and Bender Gestalt drawings. The experimental group also showed significant improvement in mean scores for hypochondriasis, depression, hysteria, and the social introversion categories of the MMPI after treatment.

## D. ANEMIAS

Chronic slow blood loss, hemoglobinopathies, failure of abnormal erythropoiesis, or excessive red cell destruction all produce a decrease in the oxygen-carrying capacity of the blood and consequently an impairment of the cognitive and emotional functions. Mental status changes include short attention span, poor recent memory, emotional lability, and restlessness.

Haruda *et al.* (1981) described a case of a 10-year-old boy with sickle cell anemia who had a recurrent organic mental syndrome with lethargy, drooling, and slurred speech. On two occasions symptoms and signs cleared up promptly with exchange transfusion and his neurological condition remained stable when his hemoglobin S was 19.4%.

## E. CHRONIC RENAL FAILURE

Patients with chronic renal failure have symptoms attributable to anemia, bone disease, hypertension, and changes in mental functions. As the severity of the renal failure increases, symptoms of cerebral dysfunction become more apparent. The patients feel sluggish and drowsy during the daytime. They exhibit impaired ability to focus attention, erratic short-term and long-term memory, difficulty in performing mental arithmetic, or expressing ideas in more than simple language. They manifest emotional irritability, social withdrawal, bizarre behavior, compulsions, paranoias, delusions, and occasionally hallucinations.

Ginn (1975) tested a group of patients who were on maintenance dialysis. The tests were selected to evaluate the following functions: (1) sustained attention and alertness; (2) speed of decision making and response selection; (3) short-term recognition memory; and (4) mental manipulation of symbols. Most of the patients performed below average on these tests. Auditory short-term recognition memory seemed to be the area that was most impaired and was especially sensitive to treatment by dialysis. Regardless of the absolute value of the original level of performance immediately before dialysis, subjects showed a temporary improvement in the level of performance on the morning following the dialysis and a regression to a lower level immediately prior to the next dialysis.

Lederman and Henry (1978) reviewed 42 cases including nine from their own service for clinical and pathological characteristics. Nineteen of the patients showed psychiatric symptoms and 98% exhibited symptoms of progressive dementia including difficulty in concentration, reduction in attention span, and poor memory. Mental symptoms were early manifestations in 20 of the 42 patients. One young woman developed severe agitation, confusion, outbursts of profanity, hostility, violent behavior, religious delusions, and vivid visual hallucinations.

The elderly with renal impairment are more prone to suffer from cognitive and emotional symptoms. This may be due to the additional physiological changes that occur with age in renal functions. There are decreases in cardiac output, changes in renal vasculature, and a decrease in glomerular filtration. Although this decrease is not sufficient to cause azotemia, it results in a blunted response of the kidney to stress. Minor alterations in the fluid and electrolyte balance may cause some cognitive and emotional impairment.

## Pathophysiology

Olsen (1961) investigated the histologic changes in the brain of patients who died from uremia. Of the 104 autopsies, 33 had suffered from a chronic kidney disease and 71 had developed acute renal failure. In 68 cases, uremia had lasted 21 days or less. Only 14 patients had had serum urea under 200 mg/100 ml. Neuronal degeneration was discovered in almost all autopsies. The localization of the pathological changes, however, was not constant. Various structures such as the sensory nuclei of the brain stem, the reticular formation and the cerebral cortex were most frequently affected. The cases with chronic uremia showed the most pathological changes. There were no inflammatory changes in any part of the brain. Besides uremia, other factors such as cerebral ischemia and thrombotic vascular disease contributed to the extreme variability of the clinical and pathological pictures.

Impairment of renal functions results in a variety of metabolic abnormalities, including rise in blood urea nitrogen and serum creatinine, hyponatremia, hyperkalemia, hypocalcemia, metabolic acidosis, and hypermagnesemia. The pathological findings in the brain have been attributed to uremia, brain edema, depressed oxygen consumption of the brain, cerebral acidosis, and electrolyte imbalance. However, none of the factors alone has been shown to be pathognomonic of brain pathology in chronic renal failure.

### Dialysis Dementia

This syndrome was first described by Alfrey *et al.* (1972) and has since been reported by hemodialysis centers around the world. The syndrome is slowly progressive with deterioration of cognitive functions, speech disturbances, involuntary movements, myoclonic jerks, and multifocal seizures with characteristic EEG changes. The condition may occur irrespective of the etiology of renal failure, the type of hemodialysis used, or the age of the patient. The duration of dialysis has been reported as short as nine months and as long as six years before the occurrence of this syndrome. Burks *et al.* (1976) reported 12 cases of a similar syndrome. All patients showed progressive dementia. The psychological symptoms that were present in eight of the cases included paranoia, paranoid delusions, and hallucinations.

No distinct pathological changes are found in the brains of patients dying of dialysis dementia. The etiology of this syndrome remains unknown. Numerous factors have been suggested, including aluminum intoxication (Alfrey *et al.*, 1972), plasticizers, viral infection, and depletion of trace metals.

### F. CHRONIC LIVER DISEASES

Chronic liver disease such as cirrhosis can give rise to hepatic encephalopathy. This condition is characterized by changes in mental status and occurrence of neurological abnormalities such as increased muscle tone, hyperreflexia, ataxia, and flapping tremor. The mental status changes include poor attention, impaired recent memory, mood changes, and psychiatric disorders. In some patients neuropsychiatric symptoms may be the initial presenting symptoms and the diagnosis of liver disease may be delayed. Summerskill *et al.* (1956) noted that 8 of their 17 patients with chronic liver cirrhosis had presented initially with neuropsychiatric symptoms. Four had been admitted to mental hospitals and three others had sought psychiatric opinions.

The overall clinical picture is variable and fluctuates with the disease condition and is sometimes characterized by complete remission. Hypersomnia is common, associated with overpowering attacks of sleep during the day. Personality changes include intensification of previous personality trends, inhibition of behavior, irritability, violent outbursts, lack of concern for family members, and loss of achievement motivation. Affect may fluctuate between depression and euphoria. Hypomania and paranoia may occur in some patients.

Amnesia is usually present for the duration of stupor and coma. In cases of prolonged coma, amnesia may include anterograde and retrograde extensions. Summerskill *et al.* (1956) reported a patient who, after emerging from three weeks of coma, had no recollection either of the preceding surgical operations or of her life for several years previously. Most patients show a progressive impairment of recent and remote memory.

Reed *et al.* (1967) indicated that widespread cerebral damage can be associated with portal systemic shunting in patients with chronic liver disease. They emphasized that any neuropsychiatric syndrome developing in such patients should be considered to be related to the liver disease and to the portal systemic collateral circulation. In 21 patients who received portacaval anastomosis, six developed acute psychosis that was related to postoperative depression of hepatic functions.

The major neuropathological changes include a diffuse but patchy cortical laminar or pseudolaminar necrosis and polymicrocavitation at the corticomedullary junction and in the striatum (Adams and Cole, 1965). There is a diffuse increase in the size and the number of protoplasmic astrocytes, many of which contain intranuclear inclusions of glycogen, an uneven degeneration of nerve cell and medullated fibers in the cerebral cortex (especially in the deeper layers), the cerebellum, and the lenticular nuclei.

Neuropsychiatric disturbances are almost the same whatever the underlying pathology of the chronic liver disease may be. It appears that mental symptoms are due to cerebral intoxications by intestinal contents which have failed to be metabolized by the liver. Several compounds such as ammonia, short-chain fatty acids, mercaptans, and false neurotransmitter amines have been proposed as solely or partially responsible for the symptoms (Soeters and Fischer, 1976). These patients are sensitive to the intake of proteins. Large ingestion of proteins worsens the mental condition. Other associated metabolic disturbances and fluid and electrolyte imbalance worsen the mental balance.

## G. FLUID AND ELECTROLYTE DISTURBANCES

Disturbances of fluid and electrolytes are common in the elderly. Chronic diseases of the kidney, liver, adrenal, and heart, to which elderly are more predisposed, frequently give rise to fluid and electrolyte disturbances. The functions of the brain are quite sensitive to the water and electrolyte contents of its environment. Cognitive and emotional functions are commonly impaired with the disturbances of fluid and electrolytes. Mental status changes include poor concentration, recent memory impairment, progressive weakness, lethargy, disorientation, and an occasional psychosis.

Hypernatremia is often seen in association with extracellular volume depletion resulting from dehydration. The mechanism of thirst defending against dehydration may be normally impaired in the elderly. The hyperosmolarity of the serum associated with hypernatremia may cause shrinkage of the brain and mental symptoms. At a serum sodium level greater than 154 mEq/liter central nervous system depression is frequently present. Serum sodium levels higher than 166 mEq/liter may give rise to acute confusional state and coma.

Water intoxication in the elderly or in psychiatric patients from excessive drinking or from nonjudicious use of intravenous fluids, may cause acute hyponatremia. Mental symptoms correlate well with the rapidity of the development of hyponatremia. In acute situations brain edema may result. A slow fall in serum sodium level is less consequential since the central nervous system undergoes internal adaptation that involves loss of intracellular potassium and/or sodium. Chronic hyponatremia (serum sodium level <115 mEq/liter) gives rise to lethargy, impairment of memory, and other cognitive functions.

Potassium depletion may occur from chronic starvation, gastrointestinal diseases, excessive use of diuretics, adrenocorticotropic hormone (ACTH) and adrenal steroids, and diseases of the kidney and the endocrine glands. Judge (1971) noticed that a frequent cause of hypokalemia in the elderly is an inadequate intake of potassium in the diet. Mental symptoms frequently include weakness, lethargy, apathy, drowsiness, confusion, irritability, and impaired cognitive functions.

## H. ENDOCRINE DISORDERS

The brain itself can be considered as a target organ for the endocrine hormones. The hormones exert positive and negative feedback effects on hypothalamic and pituitary secretions. Thyroid hormone is essential for normal development of the brain. The gonadotropin-releasing hormone facilitates sexual behavior in the ovariectomized or the hypophysectomized female. Adrenocorticotropic hormone has been shown to have a number of effects on behavior such as influencing motivation, learning, and memory.

Since a wide variety of chemical substances are recognized as hormones, including amino acid derivatives, polypeptides, proteins, and steroids, no single mechanism of action would seem adequate to explain all of the effects of hormones on target cells. Currently, two mechanisms of action have been clearly recognized:

1.  One mechanism involves an interaction between a hormone and its receptor on the surface of the target cell. This mechanism of action

does not require the entry of the hormone inside the cell to exert its effect on the cell. The interaction on the surface of the cell sets in motion chemical changes inside the cell. Amino acid derivatives (e.g., norepinephrine) and polypeptides (glucagon, ACTH) appear to utilize this mechanism to influence target organs.

2. The second mechanism involves the entry of the hormones (e.g., steroid hormones) into the target cell where they combine with receptor protein in the cytoplasm.

Receptor sites in the brain have been demonstrated in animal studies for various types of steroid hormones. Nonsteroid hormones, such as protein and polypeptide hormones, may be blocked by the blood–brain barrier. Nevertheless, these hormones have some known effects on the brain. It is suggested that the peptide hormones reach the brain via excretion in the CSF or via the perivascular organs.

## Hyperthyroidism

Occurrence of mental and cognitive disturbances in thyrotoxicosis has long been known (Graves, 1835). Although fatigue, anxiety, and irritability are frequent accompaniments of hyperthyroidism, the incidence of psychosis varies with the types of patients studied. For example, Johnson (1928) found 24 patients with psychosis among 2000 patients who were referred for thyroidectomy. Liz and Whitehorn (1949) estimated that at least 20% of their hyperthyroid patients seen in the outpatient clinic manifested psychotic symptoms. Bluestone (1957) searched a large mental hospital population and found only one psychotic patient per 1000 patients, whose psychotic symptoms could be attributed to thyrotoxicosis. Bursten (1961) found ten patients with psychotic symptoms among 54 patients with hyperthyroidism who were hospitalized for treatment in a general hospital. Types of psychosis include schizophrenia, bipolar affective disorder, and brain syndromes. All varieties of schizophrenia have been reported, paranoid type being the most common. Manic episodes are described to be the most common type of affective disorder. Some investigators have observed that manic components such as boisterousness, pressure of speech, and hyperactivity are also associated with schizophrenia. With the treatment of hyperthyroidism, manic components clear up and schizophrenic features become more apparent.

Artunkal and Togrol (1964) studied 20 women with thyrotoxicosis on the Minnesota Multiphasic Personality Inventory. The paranoid and schizophrenic scales of the MMPI were above normal but returned to normal after treatment of the thyrotoxicosis, suggesting that the psychological symptoms may be directly linked to the toxic state.

Robbins and Vinson (1960) found a group of ten patients with thyrotoxicosis who manifested impairment of intellectual functions. The intellectual functions, however, improved with treatment of the thyrotoxicosis. Whybrow *et al.* (1969) found a mild impairment of cognitive functions (as tested by the Trailmaking and the Proteus Maze tests) in 17 hyperthyroid patients. They felt that deficits in cognitive functions resulted from overarousal which led to distractibility and poor concentration. However, a careful examination may reveal cognitive impairments of which the patients are unaware in the form of difficulty with simple arithmetic and difficulty with recent memory (Whybrow *et al.*, 1969).

## Hypothyroidism

Diminished activity of the thyroid gland has a profound effect on the functions of the central nervous system. In most cases hypothyroidism develops slowly and the diagnosis may be missed until major physical, neurological, and psychological symptoms become apparent. The physical symptoms of myxedema are characteristic with pale, puffy complexion, baggy eyelids, dry skin, and nonpitting edema of face and limbs. Neurological signs include peripheral neuropathy, myopathy, cranial nerve abnormalities, ataxia, and seizure disorder.

Psychiatric problems are common among hypothyroid patients. Psychosis occurs in 5 to 15% of the patients. Asher (1949) reported 14 cases of myxedema with psychosis. Although these cases were not clearly classified into the specific types, most of the patients had paranoid ideas. Treatment with thyroid produced complete recovery in nine patients, two were partially recovered, one showed no change, and two died.

Memory and other cognitive functions are affected in all cases. In the early stages, most patients are aware of the slowing of their mental functions. Subjective feelings of "thick in the head" and "feeling in a fog" are common. Further diminution of thyroid function leads to psychomotor retardation, poor concentration, and memory and intellectual impairments.

Reitan (1953) indicated that the intellectual performance of myxedema patients fell between that of the neurotic and organic brain damage patients. Olivarous and Roder (1970) emphasized that the symptoms of myxedema are easily confused with presenile dementia and organic psychosis in older patients. A long-standing hypothyroidism may lead to dementia and psychosis with nonspecific neurological symptoms. In a study of several hypothyroid patients, Whybrow *et al.* (1969) reported that all the patients complained of poor recent memory and difficulty in concentration and difficulty in simple arithmetic. Several of the women complained that they could no longer remember recipes for cooking without constant reference to a book. Others had come to rely on their children to remember where they had placed things in the house. Five persons were markedly depressed and one was frankly psychotic with depression and paranoid features. Performance on some of the intellectual functions (the Proteus Maze and the Trailmaking tests) was lowered. The patients showed a profound difficulty with the psychological tests that required constant attention, abstraction, and memory. Most of these difficulties in cognitive functions improve with treatment (Schon *et al.*, 1961).

The MMPI profile of many myxedema patients shows marked elevation of the depression scale and a subpeaking of the scales collectively called "psychotic triad"—schizophrenia, psychasthenia, and paranoia.

## Cushing's Syndrome

This syndrome covers a group of disorders which have in common a sustained, excessive profusion of cortisol and, to a variable extent, of adrenal androgens. These patients are obese, plethoric, and have purple striae on the abdomen and thighs, mild diabetes, virilism, and moderate hypertension.

Psychiatric disturbances are very frequent. Michael and Gibbons (1963) reported that up to half of the patients with Cushing's syndrome suffer from severe psychiatric symptoms. Fifteen to twenty percent of these manifest psychosis. Depression is most frequently encountered and is usually associated with psychomotor retardation. Classical schizophrenic disorder is rare. Similarly, acute organic brain syndrome is uncommon. A wide range of other psychiatric disorders are present, such as acute anxiety, agitation, irritability, and hypersensitivity. Fatigue often becomes prominent in the later stages of the disease and colors the symptomatology of the other psychiatric disorders.

Poor concentration, memory impairments, and disturbances of intellectual functions are associated with organic brain syndrome. The mental symptoms improve and frequently disappear completely with the successful treatment of Cushing's syndrome.

## Addison's Disease

Addison's disease was first described by Addison in 1855. Until recently, the commonest cause of the disease was bilateral destruction of the adrenal gland by tuberculosis. The remaining cases were caused either by primary atrophy or by rare diseases such as secondary neoplasm. It is a disease of the middle life and affects men two and three times more often than women. The main clinical characteristics include asthenia, weight loss, hypotension, hypoglycemia, and diminished resistance to stress. The most striking biochemical changes include loss of sodium, retention of potassium, and extracellular dehydration. The electrolyte changes are associated with increased excitability of the central nervous system. The electroconvulsive seizure threshold is decreased by 15% in both adrenalectomized rats and mice.

In an extensive monograph on Addison's disease and a review of 108 cases, Rowntree and Snell (1931) noted that mental symptoms were "about what would be expected in complete exhaustion." They pointed out that the striking asthenia involved the psychic and mental attitude as well as musculature. The patient exhibited inability to concentrate or exert mental effort.

Other characteristics of the disease included restlessness, irritability, insomnia, constant drowsiness in some patients and apprehension. Progression of the disease was associated with disorientation, confusion, hallucinations, and delusions.

Hartman *et al.* (1933) emphasized the presence of irritability, depression, and marked changes in personality from a cheerful, friendly person to a withdrawn, seclusive person. Engel and Margolin (1941) found a high incidence of neuropsychiatric disorder in 16% of 25 patients with Addison's disease admitted during a ten-year period to a general hospital. Three of the patients developed psychosis. In other cases personality changes were apparent. Cleghorn (1951) reported the following symptoms in 25 cases:

| Symptoms | Number of Patients |
| --- | --- |
| Apathy | 21 |
| Negativism | 20 |
| Seclusiveness | 12 |
| Depression | 12 |
| Irritability | 12 |
| Suspiciousness | 4 |
| Agitation | 2 |
| Paranoia with delusions | 1 |

Stoll (1953) noticed frank abnormalities in 27 of 29 patients. Mood changes and memory defects were common. The predominant mood was euphoria in 50%, apathy in 25%, and depression in 25%. Most patients showed a mild to moderate chronic organic brain syndrome with memory defects as the main symptom. Mild transitory periods of confusion, failing recent and remote memory, and loss of mental alertness are quite common.

### Hyperparathyroidism

Hyperparathyroidism may produce physical and mental changes that may go on unrecognized for years. The characteristic clinical picture includes fatigue, weakness, weight loss, renal colic, abdominal pain, bone pain, and mental changes. In a review of 33 cases of histologically proven primary hyperthyroidism, Karpati and Frame (1964) found 14 cases with neuropsychiatric manifestations including headache, apathy, lethargy, depression, confusion, amnesic states, and dementia. Petersen (1968) reported neuropsychiatric symptoms in 36% of his cases.

Functional psychosis is rare. Fitz and Hallman (1952) reported two cases with striking symptoms. The first case manifested paranoia with hallucinations in addition to headache and recurrent episodes of unconsciousness. The second case developed personality changes, confusion, and aggression, and died in delirium and coma.

Organic mental symptoms are fairly common. Petersen (1968) found that 12% of the cases showing symptoms of memory impairment can give rise to a mistaken diagnosis of Alzheimer's disease.

Characteristic mental changes usually begin with fatigue and depression. Increasing tiredness, listlessness, and mental dullness lead to loss of initiative and spontaneity. The patients become home-bound and are unable to carry on their work. Irritability and outbursts of temper are occasionally associated with the depression.

In general, neuropsychiatric symptoms are directly related to the level of serum calcium. Serum calcium levels above 17 mg/dl are always associated with neuropsychiatric symptoms such as poor attention, disorientation, impairment of memory, hallucinations, and delusions. Serum calcium levels lower than 16 mg/dl frequently give rise to fatigue, loss of appetite, depression, and mild memory impairment. Successful treatment of hyperparathyroidism or hypercalcemia, due to other causes, generally ameliorates most of the symptoms.

## Hydrocephalus

Hydrocephalus in infancy is frequently recognized early and is treated with shunts. Improved techniques of operation and better care of shunts have brightened the prognosis of early hydrocephalus. With treatment, the majority of the hydrocephalic children are able to achieve near-normal intellectual potential. Delay in the detection and treatment of early hydrocephalus results in mild to moderate mental retardation.

Adult-onset hydrocephalus, although rare, is a definite entity. Normal-pressure hydrocephalus was first recognized and described by Hakim (1964). Obstruction of the subarachnoid space or an impedance to the drainage of the cerebrospinal fluid into the cortical subarachnoid channels may result in hydrocephalus. Normal-pressure hydrocephalus in adults may be caused by multiple etiology, such as subarachnoid hemorrhage, hypertensive cerebrovascular disease, chronic meningoencephalitis, residual changes following bacterial meningitis, carcinomatosis of the meninges, cerebellar hemangioblastoma, and no apparent causes.

In the early stages of the disease there may be little or no symptoms. The progression of hydrocephalus is associated with the disturbances of various areas of the brain that are damaged by the expanding ventricular system. The clinical symptoms frequently include a triad characterized by gait disturbances (unsteadiness of gait, falling without loss of consciousness), urinary and fecal incontinence, and dementia. Most patients become quiet, withdrawn, and lethargic. The psychomotor retardation in these patients is easily confused with depression and Alzheimer's disease in the elderly. Occasionally, some patients become anxious and agitated. Crowell *et al.* (1973) described two patients in whom normal-pressure hydrocephalus was associated with aggression and hostile behavior. One of the patients shouted obscenities at the ward personnel and tackled, indiscriminately, any woman who came within his reach. He would attempt to wrestle them to the ground and scratch or bite them. The attacks were sudden and explosive in character and were generally suppressed by phenothiazine treatment.

Rice and Gendelman (1973) reported the presence of a variety of psychiatric symptoms such as agitated depression, anxiety, paranoid delusions, ideas of reference, visual hallucinations, and sudden violent and self-destructive behavior.

Cognitive and memory changes include reduced spontaneity, slow mental processes, impaired abstraction, poor performance on tasks requiring sequential analysis, difficulty in complex computation, and disturbances of writing and drawing. Forgetfulness and impairment of recent and remote memory are characteristic.

Advanced cases may exhibit long periods of mutism, episodes of severe hypokinesia, and sometimes catatoniclike immobility.

## I. SUMMARY

Chronic diseases of the lungs, cardiovascular system, and blood can produce chronic anoxia of the brain from inadequate cerebral perfusion and from poor oxygen-carrying capacity of the blood. Electrolyte imbalance, chronic renal failure, and endocrine disorders also cause impairment of cerebral metabolism leading to disturbances of cognitive and memory functions. The clinical manifestations vary with the duration and the rate at which anorexia and metabolic disturbances develop. Acute and sudden changes cause confusion, disorientation, and delirium whereas chronic changes produce slowly progressive impairment of cognitive functions and personality. Early symptoms frequently include inattention, irritability, somnolence, and memory disturbances. Impairment of recent memory functions are frequently more apparent than impairment of other cognitive abilities.

Chronic diseases of the kidneys, liver, adrenal, and heart, to which elderly are more predisposed, frequently give rise to fluid and electrolyte disturbances. Brain functions are quite sensitive to the water and electrolyte contents of its environment. Mental status changes include poor concentration, recent memory impairment, progressive weakness, lethargy, disorientation, and occasional psychosis. Hypernatremia may cause shrinkage of the brain and CNS depression. Chronic hyponatremia usually gives rise to lethargy, impairment of memory, and cognitive dysfunctions. Mental symptoms from hypokalemia frequently include lethargy, apathy, drowsiness, confusion, irritability, and impaired cognitive functions.

Cognitive impairment are also common in endocrine disturbances. In hyperthyroidism, deficits in cognitive functions may result from overarousal, distractibility, and poor concentration. In hypothyroidism, memory and other cognitive functions are impaired in almost all cases. Subjective feelings of "thick in the head," and "in a fog" are common. Cushing's syndrome is frequently associated with poor concentration, memory impairment, and disturbances of intellectual functions. Addison's disease is also associated with lethargy and depression of mental functions.

## J. REFERENCES

Adams R, Cole M: The acquired (non-Wilsonian) chronic hepatocerebral degeneration. *Medicine* 1965; 44:345–396.

Alfrey AC, Mishell JM, Burks J, et al: Syndrome of dyspraxia and multifocal seizures associated with chronic hemodialysis. *Trans Am Soc Artif Intern Organs* 1972; 18:257–261.

Artunkal S, Togrol B: *Psychological Studies in Hyperthyroidism in Brain Thyroid Relationship.* Boston, Little Brown, 1964.

Asher R: Myxedematous madness. *Br Med J* 1949; 2:555–562.

Austen FK, Carmichael MW, Adams RD: Neurologic manifestations of chronic pulmonary insufficiency. *N Engl J Med* 1957; 257:579–590.

Bluestone H: Hyperthyroidism masqueraded as functional psychosis. *Am Pract Digest Treat* 1957; 8:557–558.

Burks JS, Huddlestone J, Alfrey AC, et al: A fatal encephalopathy in chronic hemodialysis patients. *Lancet* 1976; 1:764–768.

Bursten B: Psychosis associated with thyrotoxicosis. *Arch Gen Psychiatry* 1961; 4:267–273.

Cleghorn RA: Adrenal cortical insufficiency: Psychological and neurological observations. *Can Med Assoc J* 1951; 65:449–454.

Crowell RM, Tew JM, Mark VH: Aggressive dementia associated with normal pressure hydrocephalus. *Neurology* 1973; 23:461–464.

Engel G, Margolin S: Clinical correlation of electroencephalogram with carbohydrate metabolism. *Arch Neurol Psychiatry* 1941; 45:890.

Fitz TE, Hallman BL: Mental changes associated with hyperparathyroidism. *Arch Intern Med* 1952; 89:547–551.

Ginn HE: Neurobehavioral dysfunction in uremia. *Kidney Int* 1975; 217(suppl 2):S217–221.

Graves RJ: Newly observed affection of the thyroid gland in females. *Med Surg* 1835; 7:516–517.

Hakim S: *Some Observations on CSF Pressure: Hydrocephalic Syndrome in Adults with "Normal" CSF Pressure*, thesis. Javeriana University School of Medicine, Bogota, Columbia, 1964.

Hartman FA, Beck G, Thorn S: Improvement in nervous and mental states under cortin therapy. *J Nerv Ment Dis* 1933; 77:1.

Haruda F, Friedman JH, Ganti SR, et al: Rapid resolution of organic mental syndrome in sickle cell anemia in response to exchange transfusion. *Neurology* 1981; 31:1015–1016.

Johnson W: Psychosis and hyperthyroidism, *J Nerv Ment Dis* 1928; 67:558–566.

Judge TG: The interrelationship between physical and mental disease in the elderly, in Kay D, Walk A (eds): *Recent Developments in Psychogeriatrics.* London, British Journal of Psychiatry Special Publication #6, 1971, chap 11.

Karpati G, Frame B: Neuropsychiatric disorders in primary hyperparathyroidism. *Arch Neurol* 1964; 10:387–440.

Krop HD, Block AJ, Cohen E: Neuropsychologic effects of continuous oxygen therapy in chronic obstructive pulmonary disease. *Chest* 1973; 64:317–322.

Lederman RJ, Henry CE: Progressive dialysis encephalopathy. *Ann Neurol* 1978; 4:199–204.

Liz T, Whitehorn J: Psychiatric problems in thyroid clinic. *JAMA* 1949; 139:698–701.

Michael RP, Gibbons JL: Interrelationships between the endocrine system and neuropsychiatry. *Int Rev Neurobiol* 1963; 3:243–302.

Olivarus Bde F, Roder E: Reversible psychosis and dementia in myxedema. *Acta Psychiatr Scand* 1970; 46:1–13.

Olsen S: The brain in uremia. *Acta Psychiatr Neurol Scand* 1961; vol 36. (Suppl 156)

Petersen P: Psychiatric disorders in primary hyperparathyroidism. *J Clin Endocrinol Metabol* 1968; 28:1491–1495.

Reed E, Sherlock S, Laidlow J, *et al*: Neuropsychiatric syndrome associated with chronic liver disease and an extensive portal-systemic collateral circulation. *Q J Med* 1967; 36:135–150.

Reitan RM: Intellectual functions in myxedema. *Arch Neurol Psychiatry* 1953; 69:436–449.

Rice E, Gendelman S: Psychiatric aspects of normal pressure hydrocephalus. *JAMA* 1973; 233:409–412.

Robbins L, Vinson D: Objective psychological assessment of the thyrotoxic patient and response to treatment: Preliminary report. *J Clin Endocrinol* 1960; 20:120–129.

Rowntree L, Snell A: *Mayo Clinic Monograph*. Philadelphia, WB Saunders, 1931.

Schon M, Sutherland A, Rawson R: Hormones and neurosis: The psychological effects of thyroid deficiency, in *Proceedings of 3rd World Congress in Psychiatry*. Montreal, McGill University Press, 1961.

Sell SH, Warren W, Pate J, *et al*.: Psychological sequelae to bacterial meningitis: Two controlled studies. *Pediatrics* 1972; 49:212–217.

Soeters PB, Fischer JE: Insulin, glucagon, amino acid imbalance, and hepatic encephalopathy. *Lancet* 1976; 2:880–882.

Stoll WA: *Die Psychiatric des Morbus*. Stuttgart, Addison, Thieme, 1953.

Summerskill WH, Davidson E, Sherlock S, *et al*: Neuropsychiatric syndrome associated with hepatic cirrhosis and extensive portal collateral circulation. *Q J Med* 1956; 25:245–266.

Whybrow PC, Prange AJ Jr, Treadway CR: Mental changes accompanying thyroid gland dysfunction. *Arch Gen Psychiatry* 1969; 20:48–63.

CHAPTER 10

# Memory in Head Trauma

The head is injured in more than two thirds of all automobile accidents and head injury is the cause of death in about 70% of fatal accidents (Partington, 1960). The National Center for Health Statistics estimated 8 to 9 million new cases of head injuries per year (Karlsberk, 1980). Several small studies that have collected data from well-defined geographic localities provide better and more reliable information on the characteristics of these injuries. One such study, carried out by the University of Virginia, collected prospective data on 1248 head injury patients from a well-defined geographic area. There was an overall incidence of 24 head injuries per 10,000 population. Males comprised twice as many cases as females. The incidence was highest in the age group 15 through 19 with 42 head injuries per 10,000 population. The second highest-risk age group was 75 and over with an incidence of 30 per 10,000. The lowest incidence occurred in children 5 through 9 years of age. The majority of the injuries from automobile accidents occurred on small two-lane roads and secondary highways. Of all the patients studied, 93% suffered from some period of unconsciousness following head injury. The majority of the patients (54%) were unconscious for a period of 30 min or less. Twenty-five percent of the patients were still comatose at the time of admission to the emergency department, with a score of 8 or less on the Glasgo Coma Scale (GCS). The remaining patients had altered levels of consciousness, with 49% sustaining only minor injuries with scores of 12 or more on the GCS. Twenty-four percent of all head injuries were associated with skull fracture. Overall mortality in patients with GCS of 8 or less was 70%. However, when gunshot wounds were excluded, mortality was reduced to 48%. Mortality was only 1% in patients with scores of 12 and 13 on the GCS and none in patients with scores of 14 and 15.

Morbidity in survivors of head injury is high. In the University of Virginia study, 14% of all cases were not considered self-sufficient in activities of daily living. In the remaining patients who were able to take care of themselves, recovery of cognitive functions was slow, extending over periods of years. Memory problems were common and caused a major handicap in productive work.

## A. SEVERITY OF INJURY

Damage to the brain may result not only from the direct impact of trauma on the head, but also from secondary complications occurring after the injury. The secondary complications include both intracranial and systemic changes such as brain swelling, intracranial hypertension, delayed intracranial hemorrhage, infection, systemic hypotension, and shock. Although skull fractures are frequently associated with intracranial hemorrhage, a patient with a linear skull fracture may escape all intracranial pathology.

Trauma to the head is capable of producing focal, multifocal, and diffuse damage in any part of the brain. The best guide to the severity of brain damage after head injury appears to be the degree and duration of the altered state of consciousness. The degree and duration of coma in an unconscious patient reflects the severity of diffuse brain damage. The GCS (Teasdale and Jannett, 1974) assesses level of consciousness to motor responses, verbal response, and eye opening. The patients scoring 8 or less on the GCS are regarded as suffering from severe head injury.

After recovery from coma, the best guide to the severity of diffuse brain damage is the duration of posttraumatic amnesia (PTA). Russel and Mathan (1946) correlated the duration of PTA to the severity of the injury in the following way:

PTA $<$ 1 hr = mild injury
PTA 1–24 hr = mild injury
PTA 1–7 days = severe injury
PTA $>$ 7 days = very severe injury

Fortuny (1980) extended the above list to include minor cases of head injury:

PTA $|$10 min = very mild injury
PTA $<$ 10–60 min = mild injury

## B.  FOCAL VERSUS DIFFUSE BRAIN DAMAGE

Since head trauma can produce a lesion at the trauma site, opposite to it, and anywhere in between, it is difficult to classify, at least initially, the focal or diffuse nature of the brain damage. In fact, it is likely that in the

Pathological evaluation of patients who die of diffuse head injuries show very little macroscopic changes. Careful examination of the brain, however, does disclose two lesions regularly associated with diffuse shearing injuries: hemorrhagic lesions in the superior cerebellar peduncle and in the corpus callosum. Disruption of the fornix or hemorrhages in the periventricular regions may also be seen. Microscopic examination will show axons that have been torn throughout the white matter of both cerebral hemispheres.

Groat *et al.* (1945) reported histological alterations in the brains of monkeys six to eight days after they had been struck concussive blows six or eight times. These consisted of differential chromatolytic changes in certain interneuron systems of the brain stem and of other cytolytic changes in the pyramidal cells of the motor cortex.

Severe closed head injuries include a great heterogeneity of intracranial pathology. In a study of 124 cases of head injury with GCS scores of 8 or less, Clifton *et al.* (1980) found that 68% suffered from diffuse brain injury not associated with extracerebral or intracerebral hematoma and without midline shift or ventricular compression. The remaining 32% of the cases had intracranial hematoma including epidural, subdural, and intracerebral. Twenty-four of the patients deteriorated after initial recovery. They developed brain edema, intracranial hypertension, and hemorrhages.

## C. NATURE OF DISABILITY

Residual effects of head injury are often pervasive. Brain damage usually causes an impairment of both physical and mental functions. Physical deficits occur in motor and sensory functions, and include tremors, dyskinesia, ataxia, hemiparesis, and visual and hearing defects. The physical disabilities generally have much less severe impact on the overall disability of the person than the mental deficits (Bond, 1976). The major physical disabilities are often accompanied by mental disabilities, but mental disabilities can occur without physical disabilities.

Diffuse brain injury can affect almost all mental processes including perceptual, cognitive, and emotional. Most persistent of these disabilities are memory deficits, decreased abstraction, poor judgment, short attention span, distractibility, poor eye–hand coordination, poor depth perception, impulsivity, and irritability. Social and vocational disability are frequently the result of a complex interaction between premorbid personality and physical and mental disabilities. These disabilities may have a profound effect upon self-image and self-worth, leading to social withdrawal, apathy, depression, unemployment, and financial problems. Eson and Bourke (1980) indicated that social disability is usually secondary resulting from deficient coping capacities of head injury patients. Premorbid personality disorders have been implicated in the cause of posttraumatic mental disorders. Aita and Reitan (1948), after reviewing 500 cases of head injury suffered in World War II, concluded that posttraumatic psychosis was strongly related to premorbid personality. Tennent (1937) also believed that a constitutional predisposition was a major factor in producing posttraumatic psychosis. Davidson and Bagley (1969), from a review of the literature, concluded that trauma itself may be a direct etiological factor and not simply a precipitant.

## D. RECOVERY OF PHYSICAL AND MENTAL FUNCTIONS

Once the acute phase of head injury is over and the patient is out of coma, recovery of physical and mental functions becomes an important consideration. The Glasgo Outcome Scale (Teasdale and Jannett, 1974) classified recovery into five categories according to overall social outcome:

1. Good recovery—patient resumes a normal life despite minor neurological and psychological deficits.
2. Moderate disability—patient is independent in the chores of daily life. There may be residual neurological and speech deficits such as aphasia, hemiparesis, and ataxia.
3. Severe disability—patient is totally dependent because of cognitive or physical handicaps.
4. Persistent vegetative state—patient is without awareness and speech, and does not respond to external stimuli, but has cycles of wakefulness and sleep.
5. Death—directly related to head injury or consequence of it.

Jannett *et al.* (1979) studied the recovery of 1000 patients according to the above scale. These patients were in coma for at least 6 hr. Six months later, outcome was as follows: good recovery, 23%; moderate disability, 17%; severe disability, 10%; vegetative state, 2%; and death, 48%.

The Glasgo Coma Scale is, however, a very general and broad scale. It reveals little about the subtle changes in cognitive and emotional functions during recovery. More comprehensive neurological examination may be necessary to define the extent of CNS damage and to identify prognostic indicators that predict eventual outcome. Similarly, deficits in perceptual, cognitive, and memory functions require a comprehensive evaluation to detect. The Katz Adjustment Scale—Relative Form (KAS-R) has been used extensively in assessing the social adjustment of patients. The scale has 205 items, with each item rated on a 4-point scale. There are five sections that cover (1) performance at socially expected tasks, (2) relatives' expectations for performance of the tasks, (3) free activities, (4) relatives' rating of performance, and (5) rating of symptoms and social behavior.

Impairment of cognitive functions is often a major cause of impaired functioning at the level of moderate and severe disability (Jannett and Bond, 1975). Tests of memory and learning are more sensitive measures of cognitive changes in head injury patients than tests of intelligence. Mental slowness is one of the most common and persistent intellectual deficits and it lowers the scores on those intelligence tests that are time limited.

Communication disorders are frequent after head injury. Speech and language deficits are closely linked with other cognitive and perceptual functions, such as memory, orientation, and attention, all of which are frequently impaired. Traumatic aphasia (Lauria, 1970) may include:

1. Total aphasia—a severe loss in the capacity of expression and reception of language.
2. Aphasic symptomatology—such as disorders of auditory comprehension, naming, word finding, reading and writing disturbances.
3. Slight loss of language—expressive output is less smooth, articulation impairment, poor comprehension of more difficult grammatical constructs especially when the person is fatigued.

## E. MEMORY DISORDERS FROM HEAD TRAUMA

Memory disorders in the survivors of head injury are only one aspect of the enormous disability that many of these patients suffer. Posttraumatic changes in personality, social relations, and in emotional adjustment influence the patient's motivation and performance on memory tests.

Memory disorders in head injury are discussed under the following main headings: (1) posttraumatic amnesia; (2) retrograde amnesia; and (3) residual memory impairment (recovery of memory).

### Posttraumatic Amnesia

A slight blow on the head may cause a momentary loss of consciousness. A severe head injury may render a person unconscious for hours, days, or weeks before recovery occurs. Emergence from the state of unconsciousness or coma is generally taken to be marked by obeying spoken commands and the return of speech or an equivalent signal from the patient. A period of disorientation and confusion follows. During this period, the patient may be docile, aggressive, talkative, shouting, or delusional. The patient is usually able to retain memories of certain small events occurring during this period, such as a visit from a friend or relative. These are only islands of memory without the context of time or sequence of events. The period of confusion may last three to four times longer than the duration of unconsciousness or coma. The end of the disorientation period generally occurs gradually, but sometimes suddenly, and is marked by the recovery of continuous memory for day-to-day events. The time interval between the injury and recovery of continuous memory is called the period of posttraumatic amnesia (PTA). Thus PTA includes the period of coma and period of disorientation. These two associated with a facile euphoria. Russel (1935) reported a patient who was involved in a motorcycle accident caused by a dog. He subsequently described his injuries resulting from an attack by the dog and further elaborated by suggesting that the dog's owner had also attacked him. These delusions are generally short-lived, but they may persist in some cases leading to false accusations and legal difficulties.

*Traumatic Automatism.*   A blow on the head normally causes concussion. The person falls on the ground, becomes unconscious and motionless. If the blow is minor, recovery is quick. In some cases, a blow on the head may interrupt the memory of the event partially or completely, but does not cause the loss of consciousness or motor activity. The person may continue the routine or repetitive activity. It is determined only sometimes afterward that the person has no memory of the events occurring for some period of time after the blow. This phenomenon is not uncommonly reported by the boxer and football players who may get hit on the head enough to cause a temporary impairment of memory, but they may continue to box or play football.

*Changes in Duration of PTA.*   The period of PTA may vary from a few minutes to weeks or months. It correlates well with the severity of head injury. Minor head injury causes a brief period of PTA, while severe injury results in a prolonged PTA.

In uncomplicated cases of closed head injury, the duration of PTA is related to the degree of diffuse brain damage. However, secondary complicating factors such as intracranial hemorrhage, brain edema, and intracranial hypertension frequently prolong the duration of PTA.

Although the duration of PTA is more or less permanent after recovery, occasionally it is reduced by the appearance of continuous memories extending backward into the period of PTA. Posttraumatic amnesia may also be lengthened in the early days after recovery. Even after the acquisition of continuous memories, lapses of memory may occur.

### Cognitive Deficits during PTA

While the duration of PTA correlates well with a variety of parameters relating to sensory, motor, memory, and psychiatric disturbances, its correlation with deficits on tests of intelligence is somewhat ambiguous. Mandleberg and Brooks (1975) administered the Weschler Adult Intelligence Scale to two groups of head-injured patients, one in PTA and the second out of PTA. Patients tested during the early portion of PTA were able to make appropriate responses to verbal tasks, but they performed poorly on performance tasks, indicating that verbal abilities are fairly intact during PTA while nonverbal skills are disrupted. These performance tasks are to be differentiated from simple repetitive motor skills that are generally intact. The performance tasks recall of certain important links "brings them all together." This phenomenon may seem like a "spontaneous shrinkage of RA."

Retrograde amnesia usually clears up after recovery from head injury except in cases of long PTA. There appears to be some relationship between the severity of head injury and the duration of RA, severe injury causing long RA. Retrograde amnesia, however, could result from minor head injury with concussion. Crovitz *et al.* (1983), in a retrospective study of 1000 college students, found that 24% of the males and 16% of the females had suffered head injury with loss of consciousness sometime in their life, usually in childhood. Thirteen males and 14 females in this group claimed still to have RA of brief durations. There were indications that RA had shrunk with time.

### Mechanism of RA

One widely accepted explanation of RA is that a short time is required for the physiological process of memory consolidation to occur, and head injury interferes with the process. This theory is supported by the occurrence of a very short duration of RA in the majority of cases. Other mechanisms such as damage to the storage site may be the basis of a longer duration of RA. The shrinkage of permanent RA with time has not been documented precisely. It is usually explained on the basis of accelerated forgetting (Williams, 1966) and by displacement of past memories to fill the amnesic period of RA.

### F.  RECOVERY OF MEMORY

The recovery of memory is related to overall recovery of cognitive and neurological functions. Most memory processes seem to improve with time. The recovery is usually rapid initially during the first few months, then the progress slows down. Different memory processes recover at different rates. There are great individual variations with regard to the rate and extent of recovery. Eson *et al.* (1978) examined head injury patients serially, using a scale modeled on a developmental scale. The results indicated that, in general, the course of recovery of adaptive functions is relatively rapid at its onset during PTA, and then appears to slow down to reach asymptote. There are individual differences as to both rate and final outcome. The study of the individual course of recovery suggests that in some cases maximum recovery occurs before the end of six months after injury whereas in others recovery continues beyond that point.

Levine *et al.* (1979) studied 27 patients with severe closed head injury. The goal was to determine the best neuropsychological recovery possible in patients who had sustained the most severe injury, but who had recovered to a testable state. Only 22% of the patients returned to full employment by approximately one year after the injury. Two thirds of the patients became chronically disabled. The overall level of outcome was significantly related to cognitive deficits. The full-recovery patients functioned within normal range of intelligence. The severely disabled exhibited marked impairment of intelligence.

Parker and Serrats (1976) serially examined 118 patients during a period of 1 to 24 months after injury on a test of free recall. They found that the recovery varied with the duration of posttraumatic disorientation (PTD). The patients with a shorter duration of PTD recovered earlier than the patients with a longer PTD. Only 50% of the patients with the longest PTD (>1 month) recovered to normal level by two years after the injury.

Groher (1977) found much early recovery of memory functions on the Wechsler Memory Scale. He noted that if the memory skills were going to recover, they would do so by the end of two months after injury.

Denker (1960) reported the results of a follow-up study of 128 cases of closed head injury in persons of twin births. The injured twins were examined 3 to 25 years after the accident (10 years on the average) on various tests of cognitive and memory functions. Their co-twins of the same sex were used as controls. The group included 36 monozygotic and 81 dizygotic twins. The psychometric study of monozygotic twins indicated that the head-injured twins were significantly inferior to their controls. The inferior results were not associated with any of the pretraumatic factors or mental traits studied, indicating that they were not caused by differences existing before the injuries. In another follow-up study, Smith (1974) found deficits in memory and cognitive functions 10 to 20 years after the head injury.

McKinlay et al. (1981) interviewed close relatives of 55 patients at intervals of 3, 6, and 12 months after severe head injury. The problems in the patients frequently observed by the relatives were poor memory and emotional disturbances. Memory difficulties were reported in 73% of cases at 3 months, 59% at 6 months, and 69% at 12 months. The subjective reports of the patients also focused on difficulties in memory, shortened attention span, and increased fatigability.

## Factors Complicating Recovery

Brain damage resulting from a head injury is not a unitary phenomenon. The resulting dysfunction of mental capacities is widely variable. Multiple factors such as duration of coma, duration of PTA and PTD, presence of skull fracture and intracranial hematoma, focal brain damage, and residual neurological signs correlate with the severity of head injury and with the recovery of mental functions.

### Focal versus Diffuse Brain Damage

Smith (1974) examined 77 patients who had sustained severe closed head injury 10 to 20 years previously. This group comprised patients whose injuries had not been complicated by surface compression, intracranial infection, or brain penetration, either traumatic or surgical. In addition, they had a PTA of at least 7 days. The main object of the study was to determine the influence of the site of impact on the cognitive functions, with the expectation that left-hemisphere damage was likely to cause problems in visual-spatial functions. It was further hypothesized that the primary damage to the brain was the result of contrecoup lesions: right-sided impact on the head causing damage to the left hemisphere and vice versa. The results indicated that cognitive abilities of right-handed men who sustained right-sided impact showed deficits in both verbal and nonverbal skills, indicating that the brain damage was not limited to one hemisphere. These deficits were demonstrable 10 to 20 years after the injury and were not related to the duration of PTA, initial neurological state, or age at which the impact was sustained.

Brooks (1976) compared 55 patients with head injury showing minimal or no neurological signs with 27 patients with moderate to severe neurological signs (such as paralysis, paresis, coordination, and sensory deficits). The difference between the two groups on the Wechsler Memory Scale was minimal. The group with neurological signs performed slightly more poorly than the group with no neurological signs only on a few of the subtests such as information, orientation, and visual reproduction.

Lezak (1979) examined 24 head-injured patients of whom 8 had sustained predominately right-sided, 8 left-sided, and 8 bilateral or diffuse brain injuries. A battery of neuropsychological tests was administered serially on four occasions—within the first six months, within the second year, and the third year post injury. Performances on the tests were classified as within or below normal range. By and large, the site of the injury made little difference in the proportion of within normal performances. On Rey's Auditory-Verbal Learning Test, the right-side (of the brain)-injured patients performed better than the left-side-injured patients at each time interval, but the difference reached statistical significance only in the fourth examination (in the third year). On every measure of the test, the left-side-injured patients performed least well immediately posttrauma, and while their course of recovery varied from measure to measure, they tended to show the least improvement. On the Digit Span Test (reverse) both left-side-injured and bilaterally injured patients tended to perform less well on the verbal tasks than those with right-side or bilateral injuries. However, most performance differences associated with site of injury amounted mostly to trends. The lack of a clear significant difference was explained by Lezak on the basis that brain injuries are rarely ever confined neatly to one area.

Levine et al. (1979) compared head injury patients with and without residual neurological signs (i.e., hemiparesis) on tests of intelligence and memory. The group with neurological signs performed worse than the group without neurological signs. Acute hemiparesis showed a greater trend toward impairment of storage and retrieval of memory processes. An acute aphasia was predictive of residual deficit in verbal IQ but not on performance IQ. The hypothesis of more complete recovery of memory in patients who were spared acute aphasia was not substantiated by statistical comparisons. Oculovestibular deficit was strongly related to intellectual and memory deficits. The median intellectual level in patients with acute oculovestibular deficit was within the borderline range, and all patients with oculovestibular deficit suffered marked impairment of memory.

## Skull Fracture and Intracranial Hematoma

Although a considerable amount of force is necessary to cause a skull fracture, a patient with skull fracture may have no signs or symptoms of central nervous system injury. Conversely, a serious brain injury may occur without skull fracture. A careful search for skull fracture is essential in all cases of head injuries because of its association with occult intracranial hematoma, causing delayed symptoms. Henry and Taylor (1978) found an identical proportion of patients with and without skull fracture who had epidural hematoma. In this study, twice the percentage of patients without skull fracture had subdural hematoma than the patients with skull fractures. Incidence of brain damage, however, was four times greater in those with skull fracture than those without skull fracture. Gallbraith and Smith (1976) found that 81% of the cases with posttraumatic intracranial hematoma were associated with skull fracture. Depressed skull fracture usually results from injury with small objects such as a baseball, edge of a brick, or a pool cue stick. These fractures cause local injuries to the brain. Five to 7% of these have a coexisting intracranial hematoma (Harris, 1979).

Tooth (1947) compared head injury patients with and without skull fracture on the Digit Span Test. On this simple test of memory patients with fractures were slightly (but not significantly) worse than the nonfracture patients. Klove and Cleeland (1972) found no significant difference on tests of memory between the fracture and nonfracture patients.

Brooks (1980) compared 65 patients with skull fracture with 24 nonfracture patients. There was no significant difference between the two groups on the tests of memory given within two years after the injury. The site of the fracture (left versus right) or the type of fracture (linear versus compressed) did not make much difference. The patients who were operated on for hematoma performed better than the nonoperated cases.

## Posttraumatic Amnesia

A fairly large number of studies are in agreement with the notion that the duration of PTA is an important indicator for the outcome of head injury. Tooth (1947) found a significant correlation between performance on the Digit Span Test and length of PTA. Patients with PTA longer than 24 hr were particularly worse than the patients with shorter duration of PTA. Brooks (1976) found that the duration of PTA had a significant influence on simpler tasks of memory such as the Associate Learning and the Logical Memory subtests of the Wechsler Memory Scale. There was some evidence that the maximum effect of PTA was reached within four weeks of PTA, after which the duration of PTA was less influential on cognitive and memory functions.

In a later replication of the study, Brooks (1980) found that in a group of patients with severe head injury, the duration of PTA was an important predictive factor for the outcome of memory impairment on verbal and non-verbal memory tested within two years of injury. Parker and Serrats (1976) argued that the duration of PTD rather than PTA was more important in predicting the rate and the extent of memory recovery.

## G.  NATURE OF IMPAIRED MEMORY IN HEAD TRAUMA

Which of the processes of memory are disrupted by head trauma? What are the underlying mechanisms of such disruptions? These are the ultimate questions requiring answers from future studies. At present, however, our tools to assess all the possible processes involved in memory are too primitive to arrive at a definite answer. The major aspects of memory such as storage of new information, immediate and delayed recall of perceived or stored information, and factors interferring with the storage of memory have been evaluated by the available tests. Studies indicate that during the period of PTD, most patients perform well on tests of immediate recall, but the delayed recall is invariably impaired, indicating problems with retention or storage of information. It has been argued that the impairment in delayed recall during PTA may be the result of poor organization ability of patients rather than a basic problem with memory storage. They found that if they organized the test material in a coherent and logical sequence, retrieval capacity of the patients was improved.

Brooks (1975) tested 30 patients with severe head injury for immediate and delayed recall. These patients were alert, well oriented, and out of PTA at the time of testing which ranged from less than a month to over 12 months after the injury. These patients were compared with a control group of patients with limb injuries. There was no significant difference for immediate recall. In a subsequent study, Brooks (1976) compared 82 patients with 35 controls. The groups did not differ on simple tests of immediate recall, such as ability to repeat sequences and forward repetition of digits. However, on slightly more complex tasks of immediate recall such as Associate Learning (patient is given three trials to learn ten pairs of words, six are related, such as "up and down," and four are unrelated, such as "cabbage and pen"), head injury patients performed significantly worse than the controls. These patients also performed poorly on tests of delayed recall. Brooks (1980) further differen-tiated head injury patients with regard to the duration of PTA and the nature of the memory difficulties. Eighty nine patients were tested on two verbal and one nonverbal tests of immediate and delayed recall. The verbal tests were the Logical Memory and the Associate Learning (subtests of the Weschler Memory Scale) and the nonverbal memory was assessed by Rey's drawings. The patients were divided into three groups on the basis of the duration of PTA: short (PTA <7 days), medium (8 to 27 days), and long (28 or more days). The patients performed progressively worse with increasing duration of PTA on immediate as well as delayed recall of verbal and nonverbal material.

Eson *et al.* (1978) noticed a characteristic pattern of memory recovery on sequential testing of head injury patients. The patients seemed to recover context-free memory responses before they could apply them in context-dependent situations. Thus the patients could recite the days of the week in sequence and tell what day came before or after a specific day before they became well oriented to the current time. Similarly, the patients could identify right and left before they could consistently put their shoes on the right foot.

Levine *et al.* (1979) examined 27 severely head-injured patients who had recovered to varying degrees: 12 good recovery, 10 moderately disabled, and 5 severely disabled. They found an improvement in memory of storage of words on successive trials. The retention curve (memory storage) showed a progressive gain with training for both the good recovery and the moderately disabled groups. The retention curve for the severely disabled group was significantly lower than the other two groups and reached asymptote much before those of the other two groups. Analysis of the total long-term memory retention disclosed that the patients in the good recovery group were significantly better than the patients in the severely disabled group. The good recovery and moderately disabled groups, but not the severely disabled group, showed a significant increment in retrieval from long-term memory storage.

Intrusion errors (incorrect recall of items from previous word list on the current word list) were also analyzed as a possible cause of poor performance on tests of delayed recall. The moderately and severely disabled groups exhibited more intrusion errors than the good recovery group. The results, however, were not statistically significant mainly because of the marked variability within each group.

The authors concluded that about one third of their severe head injury patients showed a deficit in memory storage and/or retrieval. Disruption of long-term memory processes and inefficient screening of intrusion errors was common in patients with moderate and severe disability.

Visual memory loss was documented by Levine and Peters (1976). They found that head injury patients were significantly poor on the task of facial recognition. Their performance on such tasks was less than the second percentile of normative distribution.

The increased cautiousness of head injury patients in making decisions has been investigated by Brooks (1974). He attributed the poor performance of head injury patients on delayed recall partly to their increased caution and stricter criteria for making a decision. This phenomenon may be understood in terms of adaptation of head injury patients to their deficits. They realize that their memory is not as good as it was before the injury and that they are making more mistakes in the recall of past events and making decisions. They cope with this realization by going overboard and becoming overly cautious in making new decisions.

In conclusion, head injury patients show less impairment in recall of already learned material from their past. New learning, however, is slow and is hampered by many problems. Immediate recall for simple tasks is usually unimpaired, but it becomes progressively worse with increasing complexity of the task. Delayed recall is invariably poor for most head injury patients, indicating memory storage problems. The memory storage difficulties are influenced by several factors, which are also the consequences of head injury, such as short attention span, poor organizational ability, and increased cautiousness. Different types of memories such as verbal, visual, and motor appear to be affected to different degrees by head injury.

## H. SUMMARY

Trauma to the head is capable of producing focal, multifocal, and diffuse damage in any part of the brain. The best guide to the severity of brain damage after head injury appears to be the degree and duration of the altered state of consciousness. The degree and duration of coma in an unconscious patient reflects the severity of diffuse brain damage. After recovery from coma, the best guide to the severity of diffuse brain damage is the duration of PTA. Posttraumatic amnesia as brief as ten minutes duration may indicate mild brain injury, whereas PTA of greater than 24 hr usually indicates severe injury.

Diffuse brain injury can affect almost all mental processes including perceptual, cognitive, and emotional. Most persistent of these are memory deficits, decreased abstraction, poor judgment, short attention span, distractibility, poor eye–hand coordination, poor depth perception, impulsivity, and irritability. Social and vocational disability is frequently the result of a complex interaction between premorbid personality and physical and mental disabilities. These disabilities may have a profound effect upon self-image and self-worth, leading to social withdrawal, apathy, depression, unemployment, and financial problems.

Memory disorders in the survivors of head injury may be classified under the following headings: (1) posttraumatic amnesia (PTA); (2) retrograde amnesia (RA); and (3) residual memory impairment (recovery of memory).

A severe head injury may render a person unconscious for hours, days, or weeks before recovery occurs. Emergence from the state of unconsciousness or coma is generally taken to be marked by obeying spoken commands and the return of speech or an equivalent signal from the patient. A period of disorientation and confusion follows. During this period, the patient may be docile, aggressive, talkative, shouting, or delusional. The patient is usually able to retain memories of some small events occurring during this period such as a visit from a friend or a relative. These are only islands of memory without context of time or sequence of events. The period of confusion may last three to four times longer than the duration of unconsciousness or coma. The end of the disorientation period generally occurs gradually, but sometimes suddenly, and is marked by the recovery of continuous memory for day to day events. The time interval between the injury and recovery of continuous memory is called the period of PTA. This PTA includes the period of coma and period of PTD. These two periods are not clearly distinct and gradually merge into one another. The PTD may be characterized by various memory disturbances such as islands of memory, paramnesia, confabulation, and traumatic automatism. Although the duration of PTA is more or less permanent after recovery, occasionally it is reduced by the appearance of continuous memories extending backward into the period of PTA.

The duration of RA is taken as the time between the injury and the last clear memory that the patient recalls before the injury. Retrograde amnesia is usually of very brief duration; RA of long duration is extremely rare and usually requires exploration of psychological causes. Retrograde amnesia may be selective for certain types of memory. Some individuals may fill up the period of RA with islands of memories displaced from the past. Retrograde amnesia may extend to a long period that gradually shrinks during the recovery. Permanent RA is usually of short duration and persists after recovery.

Most memory processes seem to improve with time. The recovery is usually rapid initially during the first few months then the progress slows down. Different memory functions recover at different rates. There are great individual variations with regard to rate and extent of recovery. Maximum recovery usually occurs before the end of six months after injury. Multiple factors such as duration of coma, duration of PTA and PTD, and presence of skull fracture and intracranial hematoma complicate the course of recovery of mental functions.

New learning is impaired by head injury, but the recall of already-learned material is less affected. Immediate recall of simple tasks is usually unimpaired, but it becomes progressively worse with increasing complexity of the task. Delayed recall is invariably poor for most head injury patients.

# I. REFERENCES

Aita JA, Reitan RM: Psychotic reactions in the late recovery period following brain injury. *Am J Psychiatry* 1948; 105:161–169.

Bond MR: Assessment of the psychosocial outcome of severel head injury. *Acta Neurochir* 1976; 34:57–70.

Brooks DN: Recognition memory after head injury: A signal detection analysis. *Cortex* 1974; 10:224.

Brooks DN: Long- and short-term memory in head injury patients. *Cortex* 1975; 11:329.

Brooks DN: Wechsler Memory Scale performance and its relationship to brain damage after severe closed head injury. *J Neurol Neurosurg Psychiatry* 1976; 39:593.

Brooks DN: Cognitive sequelae in relationship to early indices of severity of brain damage after severe blunt head injury. *J Neurol Neurosurg Psychiatry* 1980; 43:529.

Clifton G, Grossman R, Makela M, *et al*: Neurologic course and correlated computerized tomography findings after severe closed head injury. *J Neurosurg* 1980; 52:611–624.

Crovitz H, Horn R, Walter D: Interrelationships among retrograde amnesia, PTA and time since head injury: A retrospective study. *Cortex* 1983; 19:407–412.

Davidson K, Bagley CR: Schizophrenia-like psychoses associated with organic disorders of the central nervous system: A review of the literature, in Herrington RN (ed): *Current Problems in Neuropsychiatry*. London, British Journal of Psychiatry Special Publication No. 4, 1969, pp 113–184.

Denker SJ: Closed head injury in twins. *Arch Gen Psychiatry* 1960; 2:569.

Denny-Brown D, Russell W: Experimental cerebral concussion. *Brain* 1941; 64:93–164.

Eson ME, Bourke R: Assessment of information processing deficits after serious head injury. Presented at the 8th Annual Meeting of the International Neuropsychological Society, New York, 1980.

Eson M, Yen J, Bourke R: Assessment of recovery from serious head injury. *J Neurol Neurosurg Psychiatry* 1978; 41:1036.

Fortuny LA: Measuring the duration of post-traumatic amnesia. *J Neurol Neurosurg Psychiatry* 1980; 35:377–379.

Gallbraith S, Smith J: Acute traumatic intracranial hematoma without skull fracture. *Lancet* 1976; 1:501–503.

Gennavelli TA, Thibault L, Ommaya A: Pathophysiologic response to rotational and translational acceleration of the head, in *16th Stapp Car Crash Conference*. New York, Society of Automotive Engineers, 1972, pp 296–308.

Groat RA, Windle W, Magoun H: Functional and structural changes in the monkey's brain during and after concussion. *J Neurosurg* 1945; 2:26–35.

Groher M: Language and memory disorder following closed head trauma. *J Speech Hear Res* 1977; 20:212.

Harris J Jr: High yield criteria and skull radiography. *J Am Coll Emerg Physicians* 1979; 8:438–440.

Henry R, Taylor P: Cerebrospinal fluid otorrhea and otorhinorrhea following closed head injury. *J Laryngol Otol* 1978; 92:743–756.

Jannett B, Bond M: Assessment of outcome after severe brain damage. A practical scale. *Lancet* 1975; 1:480–487.

Jannett B, Teasdale G, Braakman R: Progress in a series of patients with severe head injury. *Neurosurgery* 1979; 4:283.

Karlsberk WD: The National Head and Spinal Cord Injury Survey: Major findings. *J Neurol* 1980; 53:519.

Klove H, Cleeland CS: The relationship of neuropsychological impairment to other indices of severity of head injury. *Scand J Rehabil Med* 1972; 4:55.

Lauria AR: *Traumatic Aphasia: Its Syndromes, Psychology and Treatment*. The Hague, Mouton, 1970.

Levine HS: Short-term recognition memory in relation to severity of head injury. *Cortex* 1976; 12:175–182.

Levine HS, Peters BH: Neuropsychological testing following head injuries: Prosopagnosia without visual field defect. *Dis Nerv Syst* 1976; 68:21–22.

Levine HS, Grossman RG, Rose JE *et al*: Long-term neuropsychological outcome of closed head injury. *J Neurosurg* 1979; 50:412–422.

Lezak MD: Recovery of memory and learning functions following traumatic brain change. *Cortex* 1979; 15:63.

Mandleberg IA, Brooks DN: Cognitive recovery after severe head injury. I. Serial testing on the WAIS. *J Neurol Neurosurg Psychiatry* 1975; 38:1121–1126.

McKinlay WW, Brooks DN, Bond M, *et al*: Short-term outcome of severe blunt head injury as reported by relatives of the injured persons. *J Neurol Neurosurg Psychiatry* 1981; 44:527.

Parker SA, Serrats AF: Memory recovery after traumatic coma. *Acta Neurochir* 1976; 34:71–77.

Partington MW: The importance of accident proneness in the etiology of head injuries in children. *Arch Dis Child* 1960; 35:215.

Russel WR: Amnesia following head injury. *Lancet* 1935; 2:762.

Russel WR: *Traumatic Amnesia*. London, Oxford University Press, 1971.

Russel WR, Mathan P: Traumatic amnesia. *Brain* 1946; 69:280–300.

Smith E: Influence of site of impact. *J Neurol Neurosurg Psychiatry* 1974; 37:719–726.

Symonds CP: Concussion and its sequelae. *Lancet* 1962; 1:1–5.

Teasdale G, Jannett B: Assessment of coma and impaired consciousness: A practical scale. *Lancet* 1974; 2:81.

Tennent T: Mental disorder following head injury. *Proc R Soc Med* 1937; 30:1092–1093.

Tooth G: On the use of mental tests for the measurement of disability after head injury. *J Neurol Neurosurg Psychiatry* 1947; 10:1.

Williams M: Memory disorders associated with electroconvulsive therapy, in Whitty C, Zangwill O (eds): *Amnesia*. London, Butterworths, 1966, pp 134–149.

Windle WF, Groat R, Fox C: Experimental structural alterations in the brain during and after concussion. *Surg Gynecol Obstet* 1944; 79:561.

CHAPTER 11

# Functional Disorders of Memory

## A.  MEMORY FUNCTIONS IN DEPRESSION

Depression is often associated with two types of memory disturbances: short-term memory impairment and increased recall of unpleasant memories. The short-term memory impairment is frequently present in severe depression. Walton (1958) reported that the depressed patients achieved lower scores on the Wechsler Memory Test. Friedman (1964) found that psychotically depressed patients showed a deficit of short-term memory and the capacity for sustained concentration. Sternberg and Jarvik (1976) compared a group of 26 depressed patients with 26 controls (matched for age, sex, and level of education) on a battery of memory tests before and after 26 days of treatment with antidepressant drugs. The patients were hospitalized for the first time and the diagnosis of depression was made in each case on the basis of a personal interview, the case record, and the Zung Self-Rating Depression Scale. The controls were evaluated by a psychiatric interview and were found to be free of current mental illness. The memory tests included parts of the Cronholm and Molander Test Battery: the 15 Word-Pair Test, the 15 Figure Test, and the 9 Personal Data Test. The results indicated that immediate recall (short-term memory) in all memory tests was significantly lower in depressed patients than the control group. There was, however, no significant difference in long-term memory. The short-term memory deficit was due to impaired registration, not impaired retention. Twenty of the improved patients after treatment showed a significant recovery of short-term memory. The authors suggested that deficits in attention and the alerting mechanism in depression may be responsible for impaired registration and learning.

Most patients with mild and moderate depression do not show short-term memory deficits on objective tests. They do, however, complain of experiencing more memory impairments. Kahn *et al.* (1975) tested 113 psychiatric outpatients and 40 normal controls (all over the age of 50 years). Depressed patients reported more problems with their memory than did normals. Objective assessment revealed no significant difference between the two groups. Popkin *et al.* (1982) compared a group of 18 depressed elderly (mean age 67.72 years) with a group of normal elderly, matched for age and level of education, on a battery of memory tests. The normals and the depressed elderly were evaluated with the Research Diagnostic Criteria for the presence or absence of depression. Memory complaints were assessed with a questionnaire and memory performance was tested with several memory tests: immediate recall of a 20-word list after three minutes of study; delayed recall of the same 20 words; and their delayed recall and recognition 20 minutes later. The results indicated that the two groups did not differ significantly in any of the performance measures. However, the depressed patients reported significantly more complaints about their memory impairment. In addition, the depressed patients who responded favorably to the psychotherapy showed a significant reduction in memory complaints.

Increased recall of unpleasant memories is frequently present in depressed patients. Beck (1976) suggested that the individuals vulnerable to depression are characterized by having a permanent "negative-self schema" which may remain latent until subsequently primed by events. The depression is maintained by distorted negative views of one's self and one's capabilities and preoccupation with unpleasant memories. Fogarty and Hemsley (1983) compared a group of depressed patients (age range 20 to 65 years) with a group of normal subjects on two successive occasions for the accessibility of memories. Each subject was presented with a series of words and was asked to recall a past real life experience associated with each word and briefly to describe their experience. At the end of each experience the subject was asked to give details of each recalled experience and to rate each one for pleasantness and happiness. The depressed patients showed an increased probability of recalled sad memories. Improvement in depression was associated with greater recall of happy memories.

Several studies negate the premorbid vulnerability of depressed patients hypothesis and propose that depressed mood pre se has the temporary effect of rendering positive material less accessible to memory. This hypothesis is usually tested by temporary induction of sad or pleasant affects. Teasdale and Russell (1983) made a group of subjects feel temporarily despondent using the Velten Mood-Induction Task (Velten, 1968). They recalled fewer happy memories or positive adjectives and more unhappy memories or negative adjectives when despondent. Some subjects recalled more happy memories when elated. Unfortunately, these studies are flawed by the fact that the experimental procedure demands that the subject feel sad. This would require suppression (conscious) of all happy memories in order to meet the demands of the experiment.

## Pseudodementia

Elderly patients with severe affective disorders are frequently misdiagnosed as demented. Several studies (Ron *et al.*, 1979; Nott and Fleminger, 1975) have indicated that as many as 20% to 50% of elderly patients discharged from hospitals with a diagnosis of dementia may actually be suffering from primary psychiatric disorders, with pseudodementia. The differential diagnosis of depression from other causes of dementia may at times be quite difficult especially when combined with a marked physical and intellectual decline in the elderly. The presence of Parkinson's disease and the early stages of Alzheimer's disease may also simulate pseudodementia. Evidence of precipitating events, rapid progress, family history of affective disorders, and response to antidepressant treatment may help clarify the diagnosis in difficult cases.

## B. MEMORY FUNCTIONS IN SCHIZOPHRENIA

Chronic schizophrenics have been shown to be slow in perceptual functions (Korboot and Yates, 1973), have deficits in verbal recall and visual recognition (Johnson *et al.*, 1977), and an impaired recall from long-term memory (Calev, 1981).

Earlier studies (Yates, 1966) had advanced the notion that the basic deficit in schizophrenia existed in the early stages of information processing and that the other characteristics of schizophrenics such as thinking and language disorders were secondary outcomes of the basic deficit. This notion was supported by some studies (McGhie, 1970) that demonstrated that schizophrenics were unable to exclude irrelevant information, suggesting the presence of an impairment in the filtering process and an inability to attend selectively to relevant information. This inability is manifested as poor short-term as well as impaired long-term memory.

A second hypothesis of memory impairment focuses on the inability of schizophrenics to organize the information available in the short-term memory, leading to poor consolidation in long-term memory and poor recall. A great deal of research has been focused on the validation of this hypothesis.

Koh *et al.* (1973) compared three groups of subjects: 12 schizophrenics, 12 nonschizophrenic psychiatric patients, and 12 nonhospitalized normals. The schizophrenic patients were young (in their early 20s) with good premorbid adjustment and a brief history of hospitalization (median length of hospitalization, 2.9 months, including previous hospitalization). The memory tasks included free recall of 20 unrelated and 20 categorized words. The schizophrenics were inferior to the other two groups in the recall of both categories of words. The authors attributed the poor recall performance of schizophrenics to their inability to organize information and their inability to build higher-order mnemonic units.

In the second part of the study, 20 young schizophrenics and 20 normals were compared on tests for recognition memory. The schizophrenics were found to perform as well as the normals.

Recent studies make a clear distinction between the memory impairments of young (with a brief history of hospitalization) and older chronic schizophrenics. The young schizophrenics with a recent history of breakdown and a fair premorbid adjustment show little or no deficits in recognition memory and in long-term memory when they are induced to organize the presented material effectively before the recall tests. However, chronic schizophrenics tend to show deficits in all areas such as verbal recall, recognition memory, and long-term memory due to poor organization and encoding of material.

Young as well as older chronic schizophrenics have been shown to have a poor memory on various types of recall tests such as words, sentences, nonsense syllables, paired associates, and free- and cued-recall paradigms (Russell and Beekhuis, 1976). Calev et al. (1983) have shown in a series of experiments that chronic severely disturbed schizophrenics, unlike mild young schizophrenics, suffer from deficits in recognition memory as well as in recall even after they are induced to organize and encode information the same way as normals.

The etiology of the poor postencoding deficit of chronic schizophrenics is not clear. It has been suggested (Calev et al., 1983) that multiple factors may play a role in causing this deficit. For example, the presence of hallucinations and delusions would cause greater output interference during recall; narrow attention and less motivation may contribute to poor recall; and dysfunction in certain brain structures and the chronic use of drugs may induce some deficits in recall.

Rado (1956) advanced the notion of anhedonia in schizophrenics, a basic biologically based pleasure deficit that results in pronounced, pervasive, and refractory dysfunction in activity and in integrity of emotions such as joy, love, and pride. Koh et al. (1981) tested young schizophrenics for recall of affect-laden memories. The subjects were required to sort a list of words repeatedly, each in terms of pleasantness, until a consistent sorting was achieved. Then they were unexpectedly asked to recall the list. Schizophrenics' total recall was comparable to that of normals, but while the normals recalled significantly more pleasant than unpleasant words, such differential recall was absent in schizophrenics.

## C. MEMORY DYSFUNCTION IN AUTISTIC CHILDREN

Boucher (1961) compared memory functions of autistic, normal, and retarded children (ten subjects in each group) matched for age, sex, and nonverbal mental age. The memory tests included four lists of verbally presented paired associates to be learned by the study-test method, a maximum of four trials being given on any list.

The results showed that autistic children of relatively high ability are significantly less able than the controls to recall recent activities in which they had participated. Autistic children's recall was significantly inferior to that of both the control group and the retarded children's group. The recent event in memory correlated with a language measure in the autistic group and with a nonverbal measure in the retarded control group.

Kanner (1944) suggested that all autistic children were average to above average in intelligence, at least in some areas of their intellectual functioning. This criterion of diagnosis has been modified by subsequent studies. It is now known that infantile autism may also be present in moderate to severely retarded children.

The unusual memory abilities of some autistic children is quite striking. These abilities are usually quite specific such as musical talent, reading early, and memorizing large numbers of facts without much effort. For example, a 7-year-old boy was able to recite all the fifty states and their respective capitals in the right order of location and contiguity.

## D. MEMORY IMPAIRMENT IN DISSOCIATIVE DISORDERS

According to the diagnostic criteria of DSM-III, dissociative disorders are characterized by a sudden, temporary alteration in the normally integrated functions of consciousness, identity, or motor behavior so that some part of one or more of these functions is lost.

The most important characteristic of dissociative disorders is a partial or complete loss of memory for a specified period of time. The memory, however, is restored with the resolution of the anxiety and conflict. This distinguishes these disorders from organic causes such as postconcussion amnesia, epilepsy, and intoxication with permanent loss of memory.

DSM-III recognizes four primary and several less common types of dissociative disorders: (1) psychogenic amnesia; (2) psychogenic fugue; (3) depersonalization; and (4) multiple personality.

### Psychogenic Amnesia

This disorder is characterized by sudden inability to recall important personal information. This inability is too extensive to be explained by ordinary forgetfulness.

The amnesia may take several forms such as localized, generalized, systematized, or continuous. Localized amnesia is referred to as a loss of memory for a short period of time (a few hours or less), whereas generalized amnesia covers a much larger segment of time or the whole of the past life.

In systematized amnesia, the patient loses memory for a specific event such as the birth of a baby or the death of a friend. Memories for other events occurring during the same period of time are retained. In continuous amnesia (anterograde), memory is lost for all events as soon as they occur for a specific period of time. The patient at all times is aware of his inability to recall the amnesic event or the period.

## Psychogenic Fugue

This disorder is characterized by a sudden, unexpected trip away from home or one's customary place of work with an inability to recall one's past and an assumption of a new identity (partial or complete).

During the state of fugue, the person is amnesic about his past. After assuming a new identity, the individual may work on a job and carry on his daily life quietly without experiencing the conflicts that precipitated the fugue. The person does not seem to be experiencing any psychiatric problem. At the termination of the fugue, the memory for the past life before the onset of fugue is restored, but the memory for the events occurring during the state of the fugue is temporarily lost.

## Depersonalization Disorder

Depersonalization refers to the feeling that one's own self is unreal or temporarily lost. (This is frequently distinguished from "derealization" in which only the environment appears to be unreal.) There is no loss of memory but a dissociation of feelings about one's self or the environment. The person is fully aware of himself and his environment. However, there is a dreamlike sense of one's self and a feeling of unreality. The person may feel detached from his own body and other mental operations. This disorder occurs in different degrees of intensity and for variable durations. The frequency of recurrence may be quite frequent or only occasional. The periods of depersonalization may last from a few minutes to hours, occurring several times a day. Occasionally, the disorder may continue uninterruptedly for days.

The feelings of depersonalization and derealization are common in young adults under conditions of stress, anxiety, and bereavement. However, the disorder is more commonly associated with severe psychiatric conditions such as depression and schizophrenia.

## Multiple Personality

This disorder is characterized by the existence of two or more personalities within an individual. At any given time, the person is dominated by one of the personalities that determines his behavior. Each individual personality is complex and integrated with its own unique behavior patterns and social relationships. Transition from one personality to another is sudden.

There is generally an amnesic barrier between the personalities. The initial psychiatric examination rarely reveals any abnormal findings with the exception of possible amnesia for varying periods of time. Without the history and the collateral information, it may be very difficult to assess if the patient leads other lives at other times.

## E. OTHER DISSOCIATIVE DISORDERS

### Dissociative Trance States

These are characterized by alteration in the level of consciousness, produced spontaneously by psychological stress, or induced with suggestion by spiritual healers, sorcerers, and hypnotists. It is a dreamlike state with a marked decrease in response to environmental stimuli. In its extreme form, a state of stupor may supervene with complete unresponsiveness to environment and immobility. The duration of the trance may vary from hours to days. The onset and termination are relatively sudden and abrupt. There is complete temporary amnesia for the period of the trance.

### Highway Hypnosis

The monotony of long-distance driving and the presence of vast stretches of open country without changes in the scenery may produce a trancelike state in drivers. The driver may pass through many small country towns without recalling them and may even go beyond his destination. In its severe form, perception of the road may become distorted; a curve in the road may not be perceived, resulting in an accident.

### Automatic Writing

Sometimes a person in a trancelike state, completely out of touch with the environment, may respond with writing when a pen and paper is put in his or her hand. The writing may be meaningless and indecipherable, but certainly presents a form of communication.

### Plagiarism and Cryptomnesia

"Plagiare" in Latin means to steal. Plagiarism is usually referred to as stealing someone else's work or writing and presenting it as one's own (Meerloo, 1964).

The term cryptomnesia has been used by some people to denote an ability to become aware, while in trance, of "hidden" memories of supernatural psychic forces (Taylor, 1965). However, its use is now generally limited to the phenomenon in normal consciousness. The person expresses some thoughts verbally or in writing and believes them to be novel or original creations of his mind, but they are in fact the memories of the past. Thus in this situation, cryptomnesia becomes an unintended plagiarism.

## Ganser's Syndrome

Also known as the "syndrome of approximate answers." It was first described by Ganser in prisoners who gave approximate answers that were close to the truth but not completely true. These individuals look alert and well oriented. For a long time this was considered to be an intentional distortion of truth and malingering. It is now well recognized that it is a much more severe disorder. It may be associated with auditory and visual hallucinations, spatial and temporal disorientations, amnesias and lack of insight.

## Deja Vu

The feeling that "I have seen it before" occurs in a situation that is entirely new and unfamiliar. It is reported under conditions of fatigue, heightened sensitivity, or anxiety. It occurs more in normal young people who are inclined to daydreaming. There is some mystification of the experience implied in the phenomenon. The feeling usually lasts a few seconds, although in some pathological cases it is prolonged and may even be continuous for some time.

Several variants of this phemonenon have been described:

1. Deja entendu—the impression that what one is hearing now has been heard before.
2. Deja fait—the person is convinced that he already knew of the event that has just transpired.
3. Deja raconte—the person believes that he has already been told about an experience which in fact he is hearing for the first time.
4. Deja voulu—the person believes that something that he desires now is exactly the same thing he desired before.

Psychoanalytic theory considers deja vu to be the result of an association with past experiences that have been repressed. It has also been suggested that partial similarities between the past and present situation may promote deja vu.

## Jamais Vu

This is the converse of deja vu. The individual reports that a situation or a place well known to him seems to lack familiarity. This may occur in states of fatigue and intoxication.

## Amok and Latah

The term "amok" refers to the frenzied behavior of Malayan men who may suddenly become violent, rage through the village holding a knife or other weapon, hurting people indiscriminately, until they are overcome by force or killed. They report a complete amnesia for the whole episode. "Latah" is brief frenzied behavior among Malayan women.

Similar violent outbursts are quite common in other cultures. The common characteristics of these episodes are extremely stressful precipitating events and an amnesia for the episode.

## Confabulation

The person fills the gaps in his memory by fabrications that are considered by the person as actual occurrences. This is common among young children who may make up a long story from a few observable facts. In adults, it can occur without organic pathology as a result of dissociation or conscious lying. It is, however, quite common in the Korsakoff's syndrome.

## Hyperamnesia

Excessively pronounced memory recall may be associated with highly emotionally charged events that are registered with more than usual intensity, producing a vivid recall. It is occasionally seen in a mild state of mania and in paranoia.

## Paramnesia

This refers to distortion and falsification of memory. Deja vu, jamais vu, and confabulation are examples of paramnesia.

## Screen Memories

Some of the events recalled from early childhood may seem trivial and insignificant, but may represent a displacement of an emotionally laden event. The actual traumatic memories are thus modified through defensive operations of the ego such as repression and displacement in order to minimize the anxiety related to them. The importance of screen memories in analysis and psychotherapy is apparent since further analysis of these apparently trivial details may lead to a better understanding of early traumatic events.

## Forgetting a Name

Freud believed that forgetting a proper name is not accidental and the intrusion of false names during the process of mental effort to recall the right name follows a lawful and rational pattern that can be discovered through application of psychoanalytic technique. He showed that the substituted names had a direct relation to the lost names.

It is not uncommon that in the absence of recall of a proper name one may recall many other important aspects of the person such as his profession, his residence, and his contributions. Some attribute this difficulty to the fact that most people pay less attention to names. The name may not be heard clearly when first introduced. Most names are common and less discriminable.

## "I Can't Quite Place Him"

A face may appear familiar, but the other details about the person, including the name, may not be recalled. This happens frequently when a person is encountered out of his/her usual context. Seeing a nurse at a party in an evening gown may completely dissociate her memory from the hospital environment where she may be very familiar in a nursing uniform. The details of the context about people also become dissociated with the passage of time. A fellow worker after some years of separation may look familiar, but his context may be lost ("Where did I see him before?"), especially if the recaller has changed jobs in the meantime.

## Fleeting Thought

Fleeting thoughts of some significance may be forgotten as soon as they occur. These thoughts usually occur during intense problem-solving mental activity and are not related to the problems at hand, although they may represent the solution of another problem. Because of the preoccupation with the problem at hand, the mental activity continues and the thought is forgotten. The important fleeting thoughts are the product of the problem-solving mental activity when different solutions of a problem are tried. It is during this activity that the person hits upon a solution that is not necessarily the solution of the problem at hand, but has some importance to the other problem that the person may have been preoccupied with in the past.

## On The Tip of the Tongue

The feeling that one knows a name or a word but cannot recall it is quite common. It happens more often when a person tries to recall something out of its usual context. The subjective feeling of knowing is substantiated by quick recognition of the word if the person is presented with the word in a multiple-choice format. The person may be able to describe other characteristics of the word such as the initial letter, the length of the word, or its sound. This process frequently restores the recall of the word.

## Parapraxes

This term refers to a group of everyday minor mistakes in reading, writing, and in speech (slips of the tongue). Freud believed that they are often the consequences of a failure to repress completely some unconscious thoughts or wishes. He assigned an accessory or adjuvant role to other factors such as fatigue, inattention, haste, and excitement which may be considered by others as the primary causes of parapraxes. They are only momentary distortions of recall and do not reflect any impairment of memory.

## Amnesia of Childhood Memories

Several studies have shown that many adults can recall some memories from about 3 years of age. Henri (Henri and Henri, 1897) studied 123 adults who responded to a questionnaire about their memories. Eighty-eight percent of the adults recalled some memories from the period between the ages of 2 and 4. Dudycha and Dudycha (1933a,b) studied college students who were able to recall, on the average, memories from around 3 years of age.

Psychiatric patients between the ages of 5 and 18, comprising schizophrenics and persons with character disorder neurotics, were fairly similar to normal adults in recalling their childhood memories (Weiland and Steisel, 1958).

The number of memories recalled increases with the subject's reported age. The rate of recall increases from age 3 to 5, then decreases (Waldfogel, 1948). There are slight sex differences in the age of earliest recall. Waldfogel estimated that the average age of first recall was 3 to 23 years of age for females and 3 to 64 years of age for males.

Several theoretical explanations for infantile amnesia have been advanced. The psychoanalytic explanations center around the process of the repression of early infantile memories. It is hypothesized that since infantile desires, impulses, thoughts, and strivings are incompatible with or disturbing to the adults' consciousness and motivation, they are blocked out (repressed) from consciousness.

Other explanations include modifications of childhood memories with age, perceptual transformation of children's experiences with development (Campbell and Spear, 1972), and lack of verbal labels before the age of 2½ or 3 years.

## F. DREAM MEMORY AND DREAM AMNESIA

Neurophysiological data on sleep have established that dream sleep is one of the three principle states of human consciousness: waking, synchronized sleep (non-REM sleep), and desynchronized sleep (REM sleep). Rapid eye movement sleep is associated with dreaming and is shaped by the brain stem neuronal mechanism. It occurs on a periodic basis automatically through-out the night. It has been shown, through many replications, that when the subjects are awakened during REM sleep they report, 80 to 85% of the time, experiences that are identified by judges as dreams (Berger, 1969). Although there is some ongoing mental activity during non-REM sleep, it is more thoughtlike in character (Monroe et al., 1965). There is a shift from conceptual mental activity (or thinking) in non-REM to perceptual activity (or perceiving) in REM sleep. Hobson and McCarley (1977) suggested that the brain stem sleep mechanism also activates the forebrain which generates dreams by com-paring information generated in specific brain stem circuits with information stored in memory.

These findings negate the psychoanalytic theory thesis that proposed a wish or an impulse to be the main creator of dreams. Freud (1933) declared unequivocally that the essential part of the latent content of dreams came from a repressed wish. He believed that it is this part which contributes the major share of the psychic energy necessary for dreaming and that without its participation there can be no dream.

With regard to the content of dreams, the psychoanalytic theory pro-posed that dreams have meaning, are orderly and nonrandom, relate covertly or overtly to waking life, and they contribute to the adaptive capacity of the individual's life. Psychophysiological research in determining the meaning of dreams has lagged behind. In fact, a fair number of studies tend to support the psychoanalytic interpretation of dream content.

According to the psychoanalytic theory, the latent content of dreams is transformed into the manifest dream (dream recall) through operations called "dream work." The latent dream content usually consists of three types of information: a repressed wish or impulse, some nocturnal sensory impres-sions, and the current concerns or preoccupations of waking life. The dream work is involved in three types of processes: conversion of latent dream content into primary process thinking, disguise or distortion of the wish into acceptable form, and secondary elaboration to make the dream content more logical and more like a continuous story.

There has been some experimental support of the psychoanalytic notion that dreams reflect continuity with waking life. Foulkes et al. (1969) studied dreams of children at different age levels. They concluded that childrens' dreams are realistic representations of their waking life and when the waking life is disturbed by stresses, they are reflected in the dreams. Similarly, Hall and Domhoff (1963) concluded that dreams mirror the emotional preoccu-pations of waking life.

In adults' dreams it is frequently difficult to correlate the events of wak-ing life with the events of a dream because of the extreme variability of a day's events, any one of which may occur in the dream. This relationship is frequently tested by manipulation of the presleep situation such as promotion of sexual or aggressive feelings (Rechtschaffen and Foulkes, 1965), and var-iations in mental or physical activities. It has been shown that the contents of dreams are modified by a fairly large number of experimental as well as natural variables, such as stressful events, mood and affective states, amount of mental activity, change in occupational or study schedule, illness or injury, vacations, amount of physical activity, and hormonal changes (pregnancy, change of life).

Several studies have investigated the presence of inherent logic or continuity in several dreams of a night. The findings have been variable, showing both a continuity and a lack of it. In one study (Kramer *et al.*, 1976), judges were unable, in any significant manner, to put the several dreams of a night in a sequential order.

Cartwright and Romanek (1978) studied 87 students (46 males and 41 females, mean age 20). Sixty-four percent of the females and 54.5% of males reported one or more repetitive dreams. Most of the repetitive dreams tended to be unpleasant. They also found sex differences in the reporting of dreams. Seventy-seven percent of the repetitive dreams reported by the female students were unpleasant (compared with 48% reported by males). The females reported more total number of dreams and recalled them in greater details.

Awareness of dreaming and the affective tone of dreams vary greatly. Stressful events and blue moods are associated with greater dreaming and recall. When things are going well, we are less aware of dreaming. In acute depression, dreams are relatively bland and reflect denial and decathexis. During improvement of depression, dreams show more anxiety and hostility.

What makes us remember one dream and forget others? Why are so many dreams lost? Although with practice and increased attention one may recall many more dreams than one is generally able to, there is a recency effect in dream recall. Morning dreams are recalled better than the dreams from the early part of the night. In fact, most dreams from the early part of the night are forgotten unless the dreamer wakes up after the dream. Psychoanalytic theory suggests that the dreams dealing with unresolved issues are remembered better than the dreams dealing with resolved conflicts.

Hobson (1977) suggested a biochemical explanation of dream amnesia (reciprocal interactional model). He noted that waking and REM sleep are contrasted by opposite extremes in the ratios of aminergic (A) to cholinergic (C) activity (A/C ratios). The waking state is likely to be characterized by the highest A/C ratios. Dream sleep occurs when A/C ratios are lowest. According to this model, a shift in the state from dreaming to waking is necessary to recall the dream. Most dreams from the early part of the night are lost because no such shifts occur.

In summary, all of us dream every night, mostly during REM periods of sleep, which occur on a periodic basis in an automatic fashion. Most of the dreams from the early part of the night are forgotten in the morning unless the dreamer is awakened during REM sleep and is asked for the dream experience. Dream contents reflect concerns of waking life and are affected by many factors such as mood state and physical and mental activity during the presleep period.

## G. HYPNOSIS AND MEMORY DYSFUNCTIONS

Several memory phenomena are associated with hypnosis, including posthypnotic amnesia, hyperamnesia, and age regression.

### Posthypnotic Amnesia

Thorn (1960) introduced a distinction between two types of posthypnotic amnesia: recall amnesia and source amnesia. Recall amnesia is induced by purposeful posthypnotic suggestion. Traditionally, this type of amnesia refers to the subject's inability to recall, when asked posthypnotically, the events that occurred during hypnosis. This is a temporary forgetting of the experience that occurred under hypnosis.

Source amnesia occurs spontaneously in the hypnotic trance. This type of amnesia is said to occur when the subject subsequently remembers the hypnotic experience but has no recollection of acquiring the experience. The subject knows the information presented during hypnosis, but he does not know how and why he knows that.

Although recall amnesia depends upon suggestion, source amnesia occurs spontaneously without explicit suggestion. The source amnesia occurs spontaneously without explicit suggestion. The most salient feature of posthypnotic amnesia is that the information can be recalled at the presentation of a prearranged signal or recovered by rehypnotizing. Thus the amnesia reflects a retrieval phenomenon rather than problems with memory, encoding, or storage.

The occurrence of posthypnotic amnesia is explained on the basis of cognitive and interpersonal theories. The cognitive point of view regards the amnesia as a genuine disorder of memory retrieval analogous to ordinary forgetting. The interpersonal theories consider the amnesia as a social behavior analogous to the keeping of secrets. Orne (1966) suggested that posthypnotic amnesia results from functional separation or dissociation in different types of mental processes especially when associated with a very profound hypnotic experience.

### Hyperamnesia

Many investigators have suggested that hypnosis can improve the remembering of past events. In fact, a strong belief in this phenomenon by the public has led to its frequent use in criminal investigations to improve the recall of witnesses and victims. However, laboratory studies of hypnosis have not confirmed these claims. Controlled studies indicate no significant increase in memory span under hypnosis. Increased recall in hypnosis appears to be associated with a corresponding increase in inaccurate recollections or confabulations.

Sloan (1981) reported a study in which 44 consecutive cases were seen at the Los Angeles Police Department. Each of the victims and witnesses were first interviewed in the waking state. They were then randomly assigned to one of four groups for a second interview: (1) group 1 was investigated in a conventional format under hypnosis; (2) group 2 was investigated with special instructions for visual imagery under hypnosis; (3) group 3 was investigated in a conventional format without hypnosis; and (4) group 4 was investigated, with special emphasis on visual imagery, without hypnosis. The author concluded that there was no significant effect of hypnosis on memory (such as overall productivity, accuracy of recollection, or presence of errors) either as a main effect or in interaction with the interview technique.

## Age Regression

It has been assumed that because of the high motivational state in hypnosis, it may be possible to recall remote memories that otherwise may be difficult to retrieve in the waking state. This assumption has led several investigators to attempt to retrieve early childhood memories in adult subjects. Some studies claimed to have been successful in recalling memories as far back as early infancy and the time of birth (Hadfield, 1928). The use of hypnosis to produce a controlled return to a suggested prior age (age regression) has been studied extensively. When a subject is carried under hypnosis into the future to an age later than his current age, it is called "age progression" (Kline, 1951).

In age regression studies, the suggestion is made under hypnosis to regress and recall events occurring at a specific age or period of development. Such regression has been supported by neurophysiological data such as EEG or conditioned reflexes which have been shown to change with age regression in some studies (Schwarz *et al.*, 1955). Similarly, age regression has been validated by studies using psychological tests to monitor age-appropriate responses (Kline, 1951).

In a controlled study, Reiff and Scheerer (1959) used Piaget's Hollow Tube and Right-Left Test, an arithmetic and a word association test to monitor age regression. Five subjects were tested at the hypnotically regressed age of 4, 7, and 10 years. Fifteen control subjects were divided into three groups. Subjects in each group were asked to simulate regression (without hypnosis) to one of the three age levels. The results indicated that the performance of the hypnotically regressed subjects was consistent with their regressed age. However, a fairly good number of control subjects were also able to simulate age regression. The hypothesis tested implied that the availability of specific memories for past events is a function not only of their distance in time, but also of the mode of cognitive functioning used at the time they occurred. The authors concluded that on various tasks hypnotically regressed subjects performed more consistently with regressed age than the control subjects.

O'Connell *et al.* (1970) replicated Reiff and Scheerer's study with some design improvements. Their results indicated that the hypnotically age-regressed subjects behaved in the same manner as reported by Reiff and Scheerer. The behavior of the control subjects (role players or simulators) was similar in some respects, but there were some significant differences from the ones reported by Reiff and Scheerer. The control subjects in this study were much more capable of behaving like the regressed subjects. They did not break out of character while role playing and they did not show signs of nervousness such as defensive laughter. The authors concluded that: (1) hypnotic age regression does not involve total reinstitution of childlike mental processes and memories; (2) where activities were in some way amenable, such as through the experimentor's support and heightened motivation, hypnotically age-regressed subjects were able to perform in a childlike manner; and (3) where activities were less amenable to such influences, hypnotically age-regressed subjects performed no more successfully than the control subjects.

## H. MEMORY LOSS INDUCED BY ELECTROCONVULSIVE THERAPY

Electroconvulsive treatment (ECT) was first used in clinical practice in 1937. Soon after its introduction, it was observed that memory disturbances were common during the course as well as after a series of ECT. These early observations have been confirmed by several studies (Levy *et al.*, 1942; Wilcox, 1954).

Although there are individual variations with regard to memory disturbances, the major effects of bilateral ECT on human memory are essentially as follows (Glickman, 1961):

1. A loss of memory for experiences preceding the ECT with those closest in time to ECT being the most likely to be lost.
2. A pattern of recovery of memory in which the best-learned material is the first to be recovered.
3. The occurrence, after some delay, of an anterograde amnesia whose degree of permanence is not known.

The traditional bilateral ECT has been replaced by unilateral ECT especially of the nondominant hemisphere because of its less disruptive effect on memory functions. The results of the studies by Squire and associates (1976) indicate the following advantages of unilateral ECT over bilateral ECT:

1. Bilateral ECT produces greater retrograde amnesia than right unilateral ECT.

2. Bilateral ECT may produce retrograde amnesia for remote memories between one and three years; this effect is not observed after right unilateral ECT.

3. Significantly more patients receiving bilateral ECT than right unilateral ECT complain six to nine months after the last ECT that their memory is not as good as it was before ECT.

The nature and the mechanisms of ECT-induced memory disturbances are not well understood. Brain damage resulting from ECT has been ruled out both in human and animal studies (Wilcox, 1954). It appears that ECT affects the processes involved in memory consolidation and retrieval (Miller and Springer, 1973).

Research on the neurochemical consequences of ECT in animals has found that ECT depresses adenosine triphosphate, decreases cerebral oxygen consumption, releases and thus depletes acetylcholine, increases brain serotonin and dopamine levels, and alters the amounts of brain glutamate, gamma-aminobutyric acid, fatty acids, and RNA. With these widespread changes resulting from ECT, it may be difficult to attribute memory disturbances to a particular substance. The cholinergic system of the brain, however, has been shown to greatly influence memory processes.

## I. SUMMARY

Psychiatric disorders such as depression, schizophrenia, and dissociative disorders are often associated with memory disturbances. Most patients with mild and moderate depression complain of increasing problems with memory. Severe depression is frequently associated with short-term memory impairment which can be documented on objective tests. This deficit, however, appears to be the result of impaired registration and retention and improves with the improvement of depression. Depression is also characterized by increased recall of unpleasant memories. Differential diagnosis of depression from other causes of dementia is extremely important in the elderly patient. Several studies have indicated that as many as 20% to 50% of elderly patients with depression may be misdiagnosed as dementia.

Chronic schizophrenics have been shown to have impaired short-term and long-term memory. Young as well as older chronic schizophrenics show poor memory on various types of recall tests such as recall of words, sentences, nonsense syllables, and paired associates. Etiology of these deficits is not known. Several hypotheses relate to impaired ability in early processing of information and inability to organize the information available in the short-term memory, leading to poor consolidation in long-term memory and poor recall. It appears that multiple factors play a role in causing memory deficits in schizophrenics. For example, the presence of hallucinations and delusions would cause greater output interference during recall, narrow attention and lesser motivation may contribute to poor recall, and dysfunction in certain brain structures and the chronic use of drugs may induce some deficits in recall.

Dissociative disorders are characterized by a temporary loss of memory for a specific period of time. The loss is restored with the improvement of the disorders. The psychogenic amnesia may occur in several forms such as localized, generalized, systematized, or continuous. The localized amnesia is referred to as a loss of memory for a short period of time, whereas generalized amnesia covers a much larger segment of time or the whole of the past life. In systematized amnesia, memory loss is for a specific event such as the birth of a baby or death of a friend, whereas in continuous amnesia, anterograde memory loss continues for a specific period of time. Psychogenic fugue is characterized by an inability to recall one's past and an assumption of a new identity. At the termination of fugue, memory for the past life before the onset of fugue is restored, but the memory for the events occurring during the state of fugue is temporarily lost.

Although the major dissociative disorders are rare, several minor dissociative phenomena occur frequently in the normal population. These phenomena include highway hypnosis, deja vu, jamais vu, hyperamnesia, paramnesia, forgetting a name or a face, fleeting thoughts, and parapraxes.

The role of hypnosis in producing amnesia and hyperamnesia has been studied extensively. Posthypnotic amnesia is referred to as a temporary forgetting of the experience occurring during hypnosis. This phenomenon is further distinguished into "recall amnesia" and "source amnesia." The recall amnesia is induced by purposeful posthypnotic suggestion. The source amnesia occurs spontaneously in the hypnotic trance without a suggestion by the hypnotist. The occurrence of posthypnotic amnesia is explained on the basis of cognitive and interpersonal theories. The cognitive point of view regards the amnesia as a genuine disorder of memory retrieval, analogous to ordinary forgetting. The interpersonal theories consider amnesia as a social behavior analogous to the keeping of secrets.

Several investigators have suggested that hypnosis may improve recall of past events. Laboratory studies of hypnosis have not confirmed these claims. Controlled studies indicate that there is no significant increase in memory span under hypnosis. Increased recall in hypnosis appears to be associated with a corresponding increase in inaccurate recollections or confabulations.

## J. REFERENCES

Beck AT: *Cognitive Therapy and the Emotional Disorders*. New York, International University Press, 1976.

Berger RJ: The sleep and dream cycle, in Kales A (ed): *Sleep: Physiology and Pathology*. Philadelphia, Lippincott, 1969, pp 17–32.

Boucher J: Memory for recent events in autistic children. *J Autism Dev Dis* 1961; 11:293–301.

Calev A: Severely disturbed schizophrenics have a memory pathology distinct from mildly disturbed schizophrenics, in *Proceedings of the Annual Conference of the British Psychological Society*, London, 1981, pp 2–3.

Calev A, Venables P, Monk A: Evidence for distinct verbal memory pathologies in severely and mildly disturbed schizophrenics. *Schizophrenia Bull* 1983; 9:247–264.

Campbell B, Spear N: Ontogeny of memory. *Psychol Rev* 1972; 79:215–236.

Cartwright R, Romanek I: Nature and function of repetitive dreams of normal subjects. *Psychiatry* 1979; 42:131–137.

Dudycha G, Dudycha M: Adolescents' memories of preschool experiences. *J Gen Psychol* 1933a; 42:468–480.

Dudycha G, Dudycha M: Some factors and characteristics of childhood memories. Child Dev 1933b; 4:265–278.

Fogarty S, Hemsley D: Depression and accessibility of memories: A longitudinal study. *Br J Psychiatry* 1983; 142:232–237.

Foulkes D, Larson J, Swanson E, *et al*: Two studies of childhood dreaming. *Am J Orthopsychiatry* 1969; 39:627–643.

Freud S: *New Introductory Lectures on Psychoanalysis*, Sprott WJ (trans) New York, WW Norton and Co, Inc, 1933.

Friedman AS: Minimal effects of severe depression on cognitive functioning. *Abnorm Soc Psychol* 1964; 69:237–243.

Glickman SE: Perseverative neural processes and consolidation of the memory trace. *Physiol Bull* 1961; 58:218–233.

Hadfield J: The reliability of infantile memories. *Br J Med Psychol* 1928; 8:87–111.

Hall C, Domhaff B: A ubiquitous sex differences in dreams. *J Abnorm Soc Psychol* 1963; 66:278–280.

Henri V, Henri C: Enquete sur les premiers souvenirs de l'enfance. *L'Annee Psychol* 1897; 3:184–198.

Hobson J: Reciprocal interaction model of sleep cycle control. Implications for PGO wave generation and dream amnesia, in Colin DR, McGaugh J (eds): *Neurobiology of Sleep and Memory* New York, Academic Press, 1977, pp 159–183.

Hobson JA, McCarley R: The brain as a dream state generator: An activation-synthesis hypothesis of the dream process. *Am J Psychiatry* 1977; 134:1335–1348.

Johnson JH, Klinger D, Williams T: Recognition in episodic long-term memory in schizophrenia. *J Clin Psychol* 1977; 33:643–647.

Kahn R, Zarit S, Hilbert N, *et al*: Memory complaints and impairment in the aged: The effects of depression and altered brain functions. *Arch Gen Psychiatry* 1975; 32:1569–1573.

Kanner L: Early infantile autism. *J Pediatr* 1944; 25:211–217.

Kline M: Hypnotic age regression and intelligence. *J Genet Psychol* 1950; 77:129–132.

Kline M: Hypnosis and diagnostic psychological testing. *Personality* 1951; 1:243–251.

Koh S, Kayton L, Berry R: Mnemonic in young non-psychotic schizophrenics. *J Abnorm Psychol* 1973; 81:299–310.

Koh S, Grinker R, Marusarz T, *et al*: Affective memory and schizophrenic anhedonia. *Schizophr Bull* 1981; 7:292–307.

Korboot P, Yates A: Speed of perceptual functioning in chronic nonparanoid schizophrenics: A partial replication and extension. *J Abnorm Psychol* 1973; 81:296–310.

Kramer M, Hlasny R, Jacobs G, *et al*: Do dreams have meaning? An empirical study. *Am J Psychiatry* 1976; 133:778–781.

Levy N, Serota N, Grinker R: Disturbances in brain function following convulsive shock therapy: Electroencephalographic and clinical studies. *Arch Neurol Psychiatry* 1942; 47:1009–1029.

McGhie A: Attention and perception in schizophrenia, in Mahr BA (ed): *Progress in Experimental Personality Research*. New York, Academic Press, 1970. vol 5.

Meerloo J: Plagiarism and identification. *Arch Gen Psychiatry* 1964; 11:421–424.

Miller RR, Springer AS: Amnesia: Consolidation and retrieval. *Psychol Res* 1973; 80:69–70.

Monroe L, Rechtschaffen A, Foulkes D, *et al*: Discriminability of REM and NREM reports. *J Pers Soc Psychol* 1965; 2:456–460.

Nott P, Fleminger J: Presenile dementia: The difficulties of early diagnosis. *ACTA Psychiatr Scand* 1975; 51:210–217.

O'Connell D, Shor R, Orne M: Hypnotic age regression: An empirical and methodological analysis. *J Abnorm Psychol Monogr* 1970; 76:1–32.

Orne MT: On the mechanisms of post-hypnotic amnesia. *Int J Clin Exp Hypn* 1966; 14:131–134.

Popkin S, Gallagher D, Thompson L, *et al*: Memory complaints and performance in normal and depressed older adults. *Exp Aging Res* 1982; 8:141–145.

Rado S: *Psychoanalysis of Behavior: Collected Papers*. New York, Grune and Stratten, 1956.

Rechtschaffen A, Foulkes D: Effects of visual stimuli on dream content. *Percept Mot Skills* 1965; 22:1149–1160.

Reiff R, Scheerer M: *Memory and Hypnotic Age Regression*. New York, International University Press, 1959.

Ron M, Toone B, Garralda M, *et al*: Diagnostic accuracy in presenile dementia. *Br J Psychiatry* 1979; 134:161–168.

Russell P, Beekhuis M: Organization in memory: A comparison of psychotics and normals. *J Abnorm Psychol* 1976; 85:527–534.

Schwarz B, Bickford R, Rasmussen W: Hypnotic phenomenon including hypnotically activated seizures, studied with electroencephalogram. *J Nerv Ment Dis* 1955; 122:564–574.

Sloane MC: *A Comparison of Hypnosis vs Waking State vs Nonvisual Recall Instructions for Witness/ Victim Memory Retrieval in Actual Major Crimes*, PhD thesis. Florida State University, Tallahassee, 1981.

Squire L: Retrograde amnesia following electroconvulsive therapy. *Nature* 1976; 260:775–777.

Sternberg D, Jarvik M: Memory functions in depression. *Arch Gen Psychiatry* 1976; 33:219–224.

Taylor F: Cryptomnesia and plagiarism. *Br J Psychiatry* 1965; 111:1111–1118.

Teasdale J, Russell M: Differential effects of induced mood on the recall of positive, negative and neutral words. *Br J Clin Psychol* 1983; 22:163–171.

Thorn WA: *A Study of the Correlates of Dissociation as Measured by Post-hypnotic Amnesia*, unpublished bachelor's (Hans) thesis. University of Sydney, 1960.

Velten E: A laboratory task for the induction of mood states. *Behav Res Ther* 1968; 6:473–482.

Waldfogel S: The frequency and affective character of childhood memories. *Psychol Monogr* 1948; 62(whole No. 291).

Walton D: The diagnostic and predictive accuracy of the Wechsler Memory Scale in psychiatric patients over sixty-five. *J Ment Sci* 1958; 104:1111–1116.

Weiland I, Steisel Z: An analysis of manifest content of the earliest memories of children. *J Gen Psychol* 1958; 92:41–52.

Wilcox KW: *Intellectual Functioning as Related to Electroconvulsive Therapy*, PhD thesis. University of Michigan, 1954.

Yates AT: Psychological deficit. *Annu Rev Psychol* 1966; 17:111–144.

CHAPTER 12

# Memory Changes with Aging

Almost every elderly person can attest to his or her diminishing memory. Similarly, younger persons coming in contact with the elderly can verify a decline in the memory capacity of the elderly. However, a scientific approach to determine the amount or the type of memory deficits in the elderly has not produced definitive results. Contradictory findings abound in the literature.

This state of knowledge may be the result of poor techniques, unsophisticated tests, and/or the presence of other factors directly or indirectly related to poor memory performance. In this chapter, we have reviewed the psychological studies of memory processes in the elderly. Although a brief summary of the biological changes in the central nervous system of the elderly has been added, only a few of these changes have been related directly to the memory impairment.

## A. PSYCHOLOGICAL ASPECTS OF MEMORY CHANGES WITH AGING

Memory evaluations in the elderly have utilized the usual tests based on common models of memory (refer to Chapter 1 for further details). Most of the studies in this area are based on the dual-process and the level of processing models. According to the dual-process model, memory is broken down into short-term and long-term components. The level of processing model implies depth of processing of incoming material.

### Sensory Memory in the Elderly

The first impression that an external stimulus makes on our senses is called sensory memory. The impression is very brief and is either lost or transferred to the short- and long-term memories.

Schonfield and Wenger (1975) studied age differences in visual sensory memory. They found a dramatic increase in the time required to identify a visually presented (tachistoscopically) letter string in an older age group, when the string was increased from four to five letters. No such increase in time was found for young subjects until the string was increased to six or seven letters. This study suggested some decrement in perceptual span in the elderly.

Walsh and Thompson (1978) presented the letter "O" in two brief flashes. The interval between the two flashes was adjusted to find the longest interval in which the subjects would report seeing a continuous stimulus. This interval was found to be longer for younger subjects, suggesting a more rapid decay of sensory memory in older subjects.

Evidence for age differences with regard to auditory sensory memory is much less direct than for visual sensory memory. Dichotic listening experiments indicate that older subjects are somewhat impaired in the initial perception or registration of auditory information (Clark and Knowles, 1973).

### Short-term Memory in the Elderly

Short-term memory (STM) is different from the sensory memory or the afterimage since it lasts a little longer (for a period of a few seconds) and makes one aware of the "just past." Short-term memory is a temporary store of limited capacity, but not as temporary as the sensory memory. The study of STM involves a broad range of techniques organized on the basis of theoretical issues concerning the nature of the memory. Commonly used tests include free recall, serial recall, probe tasks, distractor tasks, and recognition tests.

*Memory span* tests require recall of previously learned material and learning of new material such as a series of digits, letters, or words. The tasks are varied in length, stimulus repetition, timing, and the use of interference techniques. Several studies have reported age differences in these test indicating a shorter memory span for the elderly, while other studies have found no significant difference between the young and the elderly.

In the number span techniques (Barbizet and Cany, 1968), the subject is given increasingly longer number sequences. However, each succeeding sequence differs from the one before it in its last number. The young adults are able to recall on the average 9.06 numbers while older persons (> 65 years) can retain only 5.87 numbers.

In the digit sequence learning task, the subject learns varying lengths of digit sequences. The task is continued until the subject has repeated the digit sequence correctly for two consecutive trials or until the 12th trial. Young adults perform significantly better on this test than the elderly.

*Letter span* tests are similar to the digit span tests except that letters are substituted for the digits. The norms for letter span are 6.7 letters for people in their 20s and 6.5 letters for people in their 50s.

Several studies have found no age differences in digit span (Craik, 1968a; Bromley, 1958) while others have reported slight but reliable age decrements in digit span and letter span (Botwinick and Storandt, 1974; Taub, 1973). Talland (1968) found no age differences for word span. Backward span of letters and words appears to be shorter for elderly than for young adults. Bromley (1958) found that backward span scores declined more rapidly than forward span with increasing age.

In the *Running Memory Span* test, subjects are given a relatively long string of items of unknown and variable length. When the string ends, the subject's task is to reproduce as many items as possible from the end of the string. The items must be reproduced in their correct serial order. Talland (1968), in a series of studies, found that older subjects showed a relatively slight but reliable decrement on these tasks.

In the *dichotic listening* tasks, two short series of digits, letters, or words are presented simultaneously, one series to each ear. In free recall, subjects typically recall all available items from one ear before recalling the other series. As a rule more words are recalled from the first "half-set" which is held in the STM. The items in the second series are likely to be held in sensory memory which are subject to rapid decay. Fewer items are recalled from the second half-set. A decrement in the recall of the items in the second half-set is frequently attributed to a deficit in sensory memory or a decreased capacity of perceptual store. Inglis and Caird (1963) demonstrated through a series of dichotic listening experiments that normal aging was associated with no decrement in the recall of the first half-set, indicating normal STM. However, they also found that the performance on the second half-set drops progressively with age, suggesting a decrement in sensory memory with age. In similar experiments, when the ear is specified for the first recall, all subjects tend to show right-ear superiority in first recall and do less well in recalling from the left ear. However, elderly subjects perform poorly in recalling digits presented to the left ear.

Retention of *supra span* material was tested by Friedman (1966) who presented letter strings, 4 to 12 items in length, to a group of young subjects (20–34 years old) and to a group of older subjects (60–81 years). The groups were matched on letter span. The subjects were asked to recall the items in serial order. Decrement in performance with age was found on serial recall, but there was no age difference when the data were scored without regard to the order. The results were interpreted to suggest that when the subjects are required to organize the material before recall, older subjects do less well than the younger subjects.

## Conditions of Divided Attention

Older subjects tend to perform poorly on tasks that require division of attention between two input sources. In one study subjects watched a display of 12 light bulbs; a morse key was positioned under each bulb and the subject was asked to press the key when its corresponding light came on. Pressing the key extinguished the light but caused another light to come on. Older subjects could perform this task well. However, when the task was complicated by asking subjects to press the key corresponding to the previous light, older subjects performed less well than the younger subjects. When the memory load was increased by making subjects work "two back" or "three back," the performance of older subjects became progressively worse.

In other distraction studies, subjects are given stimuli (e.g., 3 letters or words) to remember, which are immediately followed by a counting task in which the subjects participate actively. After a brief period of counting, subjects are asked to recall the initial stimuli. In this situation efficiency of recall declines as a function of time interval between the stimulus and recall. The older subjects do as well as the young subjects (Kriauchiunas, 1968).

Older subjects do poorly when they are required to perform two tasks simultaneously. Broadbent and Heron (1962) required subjects to perform on a visual letter cancellation task while monitoring a series of auditory letters for a repeated letter. The older subjects tended to concentrate on one task at a time resulting in a deterioration of performance on the other task.

In another study, Broadbent and Gregory (1965) presented three visual and three auditory stimuli simultaneously. The visual items were lights while the auditory items were a letter, a digit, and a letter. Subjects were asked to recall the visual items and then the auditory items. The performance remained at a constant level with age up to 45 years of age, then it dropped significantly.

McGhie et al. (1965) presented five numbers visually and another five numbers auditorily simultaneously at a rate of 2 sec each. The task was to detect and write down repeated numbers. No age differences were found when the repeated numbers occurred first on the auditory channel, but there were substantial age differences in performance when the number occurred first on the visual channel.

## Rate of Processing Short-term Memory

It has been suggested that normal aging is associated with slowing of all biological activity including the activities of the central nervous system which leads to generalized decline in the rate of cognitive processing and slowing of reaction time. In general, past research has been consistent with this position. Sternberg (1966) presented subjects with a short set of digits or letters. Immediately after the presentation, a test item was given. The subject was to decide as quickly as possible whether the test item was a member of the memory set presented before. The decision latency increased for all subjects as the size of the memory set increased. However, the reaction time became much longer for the older age subjects than the young adults. Similar results have been reported by subsequent studies (Anders et al., 1972; Erikson et al., 1973) that show that older persons normally perform slower than younger persons on a variety of cognitive tasks.

Craik (1977) suggested that the difficulty or the slowing of mental operations may be the result of the use of different and less optimal processing strategies by the elderly as compared with younger adults. In order to determine whether cognitive processes are inherently slower in the aged or whether the slowness is due to strategy differences between the young and the old, Macht (1984) investigated age differences in the speed of recall under conditions that induced both the aged and the young to carry out the same kind of processes during learning and recall. All subjects learned a set of items by a procedure that required them to search a list to identify instances of common conceptual categories. This search procedure was used to control for age differences in initial processing. Memory for target items was tested by free recall and cued recall in which each item was cued by the category label. No age differences were found in either the rate of free recall or the speed of cued recall under these conditions.

Lorsbach and Simpson (1984) used a probe recognition task to determine the rate of processing in short-term memory. Subjects were presented lists of words at the exposure rate of either 350, 700, or 1400 msec/word. An instructional cue (letters I, H, or S) followed by a probe word was then presented. When given the letter I, the subject was expected to judge whether or not the forthcoming probe word was identical to any word in the preceding study list. When given the letter H, the subject was to determine whether the probe word was a homonym of any word in the previous study list. The letter S indicated that the subject was to determine if the probe word was a synonym of any word in the study list. This technique was used to test the efficiency of visual, phonemic, and semantic encoding in the STM. The dependent variables were speed and accuracy of recognition. The results indicated that the two age groups were equivalent in their ability to identify recently presented identical words, homonyms and synonyms. Age differences, however, were observed in the speed of access to information and these differences were greatest on tasks requiring retrieval of semantic information from the secondary component of STM. The authors concluded that the information held in STM is equally available to young and older subjects, regardless of the presentation rate, complexity of the information, or input position. The older individuals, however, require a somewhat greater amount of time to gain access to the information, particularly semantic types of information. Age-related slowing thus appeared to manifest itself more clearly with tasks requiring the retrieval of semantic information from secondary memory and has no clear effect upon the initial encoding of information in STM.

The rate of learning for certain types of material appears to be faster for young adults than for the elderly. Drachman and Leavitt (1972) made repeated presentations of a 15-digit string for serial recall. The young adults learned the string faster than the elderly.

### Short-term Forgetting

Loss from the STM may depend on the process of decay with time and the interferences occurring after the learning. Conrad and Hille (1958) showed that fast presentation coupled with fast recall led to higher performance levels than slow presentation and recall. Frazer (1958) found no difference between young and old subjects' performance on an immediate recall test at fast rates, but found that the old group's recall level dropped more than the young group's performance at slow rates.

Kinsbourne (1973) showed the opposite result. Older subjects were generally poorer than the young group at recalling an eight-letter sequence, but while the young group was unaffected by variations in presentation rate (from one letter per 2 seconds to four per second), the older group performed disproportionately worse at a faster rate. The author concluded that the performance of older subjects is disrupted somewhat with fast presentation, although a presentation through the auditory channel is less affected than a visual presentation.

## Long-term Memory in the Elderly

The long-term memory (LTM) holds the stable behavioral repertoire for lifetime experience. Since all performances have to be obtained under controlled conditions, the methods of studying LTM are limited to those that can be accommodated within the time constraints of longitudinal laboratory work. Standard memory terminology reflects this constraint. Psychological literature refers to memories as "long term" if the retention interval exceeds 30 sec and the bulk of the articles on memory deals with intervals of a few seconds or minutes.

It was generally believed that the older individual could recall past memories easily and that they suffered no impairment in LTM. These impressions, however, are based on anecdotal descriptions and have not been validated by scientific investigations. In fact, most studies find that elderly subjects do less well than the younger subjects on LTM tasks.

In a typical experiment of free recall, a list of 12 to 30 words is presented to the subjects who are instructed that following the presentation they will be asked to reproduce the items in any order they choose. It is hypothesized that the items in the initial portion of the list have to be stored in the secondary or LTM before they are recalled at the end of the presentation. The items from the last portion of the list are retained in the sensory and STM. No age differences are found in the recall of the last few items (the recency effect), but the older subjects recall fewer words from the beginning and the middle of the lists; that is, from the LTM portion (Craik, 1968b).

### Recall versus Recognition

Schonfield and Robertson (1966) compared performance of various age groups on tasks of recall and recognition. The subjects were presented with a list of 24 words to learn. The acquisition phase was followed by free recall or recognition. The recognition test was a forced choice task in which each word in the list was presented in a group with four distractor items. There was a large and systematic drop in the recall performance with increasing age, but no age decrement was found in the recognition task. The data suggest that retrieval from memory storage is one major cause of decreased memory performance in older people.

Subsequent studies have confirmed these results except that some studies have also shown an age-related decrement in recognition tasks (Crenshaw, 1969; Gordon and Clark, 1974). Harwood and Naylor (1969) presented 20 line drawings of items until subjects could recall at least 16 of the item names. Four weeks later, subjects were asked to recall the names again and then to recognize the 20 drawings from a set of 60. The mean recall of the older subjects was 74% of the young group while the mean recognition was 87% of the scores obtained by the young adults. Erber (1974) has also shown a decline with age in both recall and recognition tasks.

Robinowitz (1984) studied recognition failure with increasing age. Subjects were tested on four lists of weakly related paired associates (A-B). Following the first two practice lists, they were given a standard cued recall test (A-?). Following the third critical list, they were first given a surprise recognition test of the B items in the presence of other single words. Following this recognition test, the expected cued recall test was administered. In this paradigm, people often fail to recognize many words that can be recalled subsequently. This is termed the recognition failure phenomenon. Participants also studied a fourth list which was followed by a recognition test for the items. The participants were then given an unexpected backward recall test in which recall of the A items was requested while B items were given as cues. The results indicated significant age deficits for both recall and recognition. The age deficit in recognition was attributed to differences in the effectiveness of the retrieval process in recognition. The phenomenon of recognition failure (the failure to recognize items that are subsequently recalled) was observed in all subjects. However, the older subjects showed a higher recognition failure rate than the younger subjects.

## Aging and Category-Recall Relationship

When appropriate cues are provided, the performance of the elderly on free recall is improved greatly. Laurence (1967) presented a list of 36 words, broken down into six categories (e.g., birds, flowers, etc.). Giving subjects the names of the category at the time of recall benefited the older subjects but not the younger group. The performance of the older subjects was enhanced to equal that of the younger group. Mandler (1968) documented the categorical-recall functions, showing that young adults will remember an average of roughly four items from every additional category into which they chunk the items, up to seven categories.

Worden and Meggison (1984) used a sorting-recall procedure to investigate how LTM in the elderly is affected by categorical organization. The study was designed to estimate chunk size in the young versus the elderly by directly manipulating the number of categories into which words could be organized. Sixty-four young adults and retirees (67 years) sorted 48 unrelated words into two, four, six, or eight categories prior to recall. High- and low-frequency lists were tested, a manipulation that only affected the young adults. Surprisingly, overall initial recall was equally high for both groups, but the effect of increasing the number of categories on recall differed dramatically for young and old groups. Subsequent assessment of long-term recall showed greater memory loss for the older group.

## *Retrieval of Information from Long-term Memory*

Madden (1985) investigated age differences in the retrieval of information from LTM. Each trial required a decision regarding the synonym of two visually presented words. On the yes-response trials, the two words were either identical, differed only in case, or were synonyms that differed in case. Age differences in absolute decision time were greater for the synonyms than for the other word pairs. The author concluded that a generalized age-related slowing in the speed of information processing can account for age differences in the retrieval of letter identity and semantic information from LTM.

Warrington and Silberstein (1970) devised a questionnaire to study the relation of news items that had been current for one month to two years previously. They found a decline on recall of the events, both with increasing retention interval and with increasing age of the subjects; however, there was much less decline in recognition performance with either variable. It is generally very difficult to determine the loss of retention for social and political events because of the great variation in the individual interest in such events. Several other studies that have attempted to determine retention loss from past events find that memory is frequently inversely related to the remoteness of events in the older subjects. Other factors contributing to forgetting in LTM include (1) acquisition problems due to sensory deficits, poor use of mediators, and poor organization of material, and (2) interference arising either from previously learned material (proactive inhibition) or from subsequent material (retroactive inhibition).

## Nonverbal Memory

Age-related differences in memory for pictures, tones, touch, and smell have been reviewed by Neisser (1967). In general, the ability to reproduce or recognize geometric designs declines with age, but the loss is gradual until the 60s or 70s when the loss becomes much greater. Harwood and Naylor (1969) had subjects learn a series of 20 line drawings. Four weeks later, young subjects recognized 19.0 of the drawings on the average while the older subjects recognized an average of 16.6 drawings. Although the difference was significant, the loss in absolute terms does not appear to be too great. Reige and Inman (1981) found an age-related decline on six different memory tests using visual, auditory, and tactile items that defied verbal labeling.

Howell (1972) documented age-related changes in memory for different classes of pictorial stimuli. Elderly persons seemed to have better recall of pictorial materials compared with verbal material. Park and Puglis (1984) examined how the addition and deletion of various pictorial components affected the memory. They presented slide photographs of cartoons, intact or with much of the background obliterated, to a group of young and elderly subjects (>60 years old). During recognition, 120 items were presented for 8 sec each. Half of the items were distractors, 30 with context and 30 without. The participants indicated if they recognized the central figures in the picture with a written "yes" or "no" response. The young subjects recognized pictures with contextual details better than without the details, whereas the reverse appeared to be true for older individuals. The authors concluded that the elderly individuals encode events in a less context-specific manner than young adults.

## Aging and Level of Processing Model

According to the level of processing model, the durability of the memory trace is simply a function of the depth of processing carried out on the stimulus. Greater depth implies more elaborate, semantic analysis. Studies indicate that, in general, when the subjects carry out more elaborate analysis of words, they remember them better (Craik and Tulving, 1975).

It was suggested that perhaps older subjects perform poorly on free recall because they do not carry out sufficient depth analysis of the presented stimuli. This notion was further elaborated by Bromley (1958) who observed that older subjects did not process irrelevant details to the same extent as the younger adults did. This reduction in attention to incidental details may be the result of increased accumulated knowledge of the elderly about their environment which reduces their need to attend to the irrelevant and incidental stimuli.

Several studies of memory functions in the elderly based on the level of processing model have been carried out, but the results are inconclusive and sometimes contradictory. Eysenck (1974) presented words to his subjects and asked them to carry out various processes with the words. Some involved shallower levels of processing (counting the number of letters in the words). Others allegedly involved deeper processing by generating appropriate adjectives or images for each word. The subjects were led to believe that this was all that they had to do. However, later instruction asked them to recall the words. All the subjects recalled the words that were subjected to deeper levels of processing better than the rest. However, when compared with the young adults, the older subjects had an especially difficult time in recalling words that were allegedly processed at a deeper level. Eysenck concluded that these results indicated that the elderly had a deficit in semantic processing.

White (quoted by Craik, 1977) presented a series of single words to subjects under one of four instructional conditions: (1) Is the word in capital letters? (2) Does the word rhyme with _____? (3) Does the word belong to the _____category? (4) Just learn the word. The subjects expected that they were supposed to remember only one quarter of the words while they were making judgments about the rest of the words as instructed. After all the words were presented, the subjects were asked to recall as many words as they could from all the words presented. They were then given a recognition list from which to recognize the presented words. It was hypothesized that the depth of processing increased from condition 1 to condition 3, thus increasing the recall of words—least under condition 1 and most under condition 3. The results supported the hypothesis that more words were recalled from condition 3 than from condition 1 by all subjects. The words given under condition 4 yielded the same level of recall as in condition 3. Younger adults recalled significantly more words than the older subjects in the last three conditions. These results may be interpreted in a similar manner as in Eysenck's study, showing a deficit of semantic processing in the elderly, or they may simply indicate a deficit in the retrieval process. The latter interpretation was further supported by a recognition test that was administered to all subjects after the recall test. On recognition, elderly subjects did as well as the young adults on the first three conditions.

## B. OTHER FACTORS AFFECTING MEMORY IN THE ELDERLY

A general decline in the level of interest in the surrounding environment is common in the elderly. There are increasing inhibitions, cautions, and diminishing motivation to do new and exciting things. It has been suggested that the poor performance of the elderly in some of the memory experiments may be the result of poor motivation. The studies that have tried to manipulate motivation during cognitive and memory tests have failed to find the age-related decline to be an artifact of poor motivation (Ganzler, 1964). These studies, however, barely scratch the surface of the complex nature of human motivation.

A decline in overall intellectual functions with increasing age has been taken as an indicator for a parallel decline in memory functions. Intellectual ability (such as tested with the Wechsler Adult Intelligence Scale) in cross sectional studies typically increases through childhood but levels off by about the age of 20 years. It then remains static for only a decade or so before it starts to decline. The decline is slow at first but starts to accelerate as the individual reaches the end of middle age. These trends are not confirmed by longitudinal studies in which the same individuals are retested at later ages. Owens (1966) reported the results of intelligence tests on a sample of males who were first tested on the Army Alpha Test at around the age of 50 years.

The sample was retested 11 years later. The subjects showed only the slightest but nonsignificant trend toward lower scores on retesting.

Similar results are obtained by other investigators who have employed longitudinal testing (Schaie and Strother, 1968). They indicate that cross sectional data exaggerate the amount of intellectual decline with old age. Speed of performance seems to play an important role in decreasing the performance. Since most of the data on memory in the elderly are derived from cross sectional studies, it is inferred that the real memory decline may not be as great as reported.

## C. BIOLOGICAL ASPECTS OF AGING AND MEMORY

Biological theories of memory postulate formation of new proteins, development of new dendritic spines, activation of new enzymes, and participation of neurotransmitters. Although aging influences all these biological processes, there is as yet no direct evidence that the slowing down or decrease in these biological activities are directly related to memory impairment in the elderly.

Biological aging is believed to originate in molecular changes, presumably in DNA or DNA-associated enzymes, which progress with varying speed through systems of cells, tissues, and organs until vital functions are affected. It is believed that the maximum lifespan is probably determined by genetically regulated metabolic and enzymatic functions and the morphologic integrity of vital organs such as the lungs, the liver, the brain, and the cardiovascular system. The rate of aging and how long we live are the result of an interaction at the cellular level between genetic programs and environmental influences, some of which may be controllable.

Studies investigating the effects of aging on brain functions have focused on the following three major areas:

1. Aging related to cell death, particularly of neurons for reasons not understood, and an increase in the signs of cellular aging in the brain, including the formation of lipofuscin, neuritic plaques, and neurofibrillary tangles.
2. Aging related to metabolism and a lack of oxygen supply to the brain including atherosclerotic or cardiovascular problems due to the weakening of the heart or difficulties in the flow of blood through capillaries in the brain.
3. Aging due to impaired neuronal communication, ranging from changes in transmitter levels and turnover, synthesizing and catabolizing enzymes, as well as changes in receptors and in the structure and functioning of neuronal membranes.

## Brain Growth and Neuronal Loss

There is an early period of brain growth in childhood that reaches its peak by the end of the first decade and remains relatively stable through adulthood until there is a decline into senescence. The aging process in most organs (except the brain) involves a diminishing potential for cell division and consequently gradual replacement of parenchymal cells with connective tissue. The brain has no connective tissue except that in the vascular system. The death of neurons is associated with the proliferation of glial cells (gliosis).

In 1958, Burns calculated from Brody's data that during every day of adult life more than 100,000 neurons die. How were these figures arrived at? It is not clear. Brody's (1955) estimation of neuronal loss in the human cortex between 20 and 80 years of age was 30% while Leboucq's (1929) data showed a decrease of the surface of the brain, between 20 and 76 years of age, of 10%. Brody's recent comments indicate that he considered Burns' calculations to be unscientific.

Earlier studies provided support for progressive loss of neurons with age (Shefer, 1973). In these studies the decreased packing density of neurons was interpreted as neuronal loss. In contrast, studies of neurons in the nuclei of the medulla and the pons showed no loss with age. Recent studies (Terry et al., 1981) have raised serious questions as to the extent of neuronal loss with age. These studies show some loss of small cell components (soma size below 40 $\mu m^2$), but apparently no significant losses of cellular elements above that size. It has been suggested that the small elements may be largely glial and there may be only a slight decrease of neurons with age.

## Changes in Dendritic Spines

Dendritic spines in the cerebral cortex are small appendages that extend from the dendrites of most, but not all, types of neurons. Spines form a variety of shapes and lengths. They are common sites of synaptic contact. Thus a change in their density or structure could result in a reduction or loss of input to the neuron. Spine density and structure are influenced by both age and environment. An enriched environment has been shown to cause an increase in dendrites and spine density in an aged rat brain (Diamond, 1978).

Old rats show a patchy loss of dendritic spines at various stations along the dendrite shafts. In the cerebral cortex, changes are most obvious in the pyramidal cells of layers 3 and 5 in the prefrontal, temporal, and parieto-occipital association areas. The most distal portion of the dendrite arbor and the most proximal portions near the soma seem to suffer early. The spine-bare areas often become modulated, especially peripherally, whereas more proximally affected segments, zones of irregular swellings, become increasingly obvious. Horizontally oriented dendrites appear to undergo selective degenerative changes, fragmenting and dying back upon the central axis of the neuron. The basilar dendrite system is the most severely affected as the aging process continues. An increasing number of pyramidal cells are found to be totally deprived of basilar shafts. Oblique branches of the apical element and the terminal dendritic bouquet show progressive loss until they approximate in general configuration the primitive pyramidal neuron of the embryonic cortex.

The potential to develop new spines is not lost with age. Possibly a small loss of neurons may be compensated by an increase in dendrites and spines. Buell (1979) have shown that some dendrite systems respond to the challenge of aging with increased dendrite growth and spines.

## Glial Cell

It has been reported that an increased neuronal loss with age is replaced by glial cells, producing an increased gliosis in the aged brain. Brizzee *et al.* (1981) for example found an increased number of glial cells in several brain regions with age, while others have reported that the number of glial cells in the anterior commissure decreased with age in the mouse and no increase was found in the cerebral cortex of a 650-day-old rat. It appears that an increase in the number of glial cells with age may not be a uniform phenomenon, but may vary considerably across brain regions and perhaps life span environmental conditions.

## Intracellular Changes

In most organs the lipid content increases with age while intracellular water, carbohydrate, proteins, and minerals are lost. In the brain, the content of lipid, carbohydrate, proteins, and minerals remains the same or declines with age, but the water content increases slightly.

The appearance of lipofuscin is the most characteristic phenomenon in the aging of the cells of various organs—the myocardium, the spleen, the liver, and the neurons. The accumulation increases with age. Twenty-five percent of the intracellular perinuclease volume of neurons in rodents is occupied by age pigment in 28-month-old rats and mice.

Hannover (1842) was the first to describe a pigment in the nervous system that probably corresponds to lipofuscin. Subsequently, several other investigators reported pigment accumulation in the CNS. Borst (1922) introduced the term lipofuscin, which means dark, dusky pigmented lipid.

Lipofuscin has a very heterogeneous chemical structure so that it cannot be identified by a single histochemical process. The origin of the pigment is not definitely known. It has been suggested that it may originate in the golgi apparatus and the lysosomes. Similarly, the functional relationship of the pigment to the aging process is also not clear.

Pathological changes such as senile plaques, amyloidosis, neurofibrillary tangles, and granulovascular degeneration, some of which occur in the brain of normal man during senescence, appear frequently in selected brain regions of individuals with Alzheimer's disease.

Some changes in the molecular and physical properties of the neuronal membrane have been demonstrated with aging. The increased stiffness of the membrane phospholipids appears to be caused by an augmented cholesterol content and a decreased unsaturated fatty acid content. Similarly, changes in the phospholipid methylation can lead to an increased rigidity of the entire structure of the membrane. The increased rigidity of the membrane is reflected in decreased permeability and in changes in bioelectrical characteristics.

## Neurotransmitters

Brain neurotransmitters undergo progressive changes in their concentration as animals age. These changes lead to quantitative differences between various transmitter systems, causing an altered relationship among interacting neuronal circuits whose activities regulate common physiological functions. A deficit in one metabolic system could lead to overactivity in another system or vice versa as animals grow old. Alterations in hypothalamic catecholamines and serotonin are associated with a decline in gonadotropin release in aging rats.

Monkeys tested at 4, 10, and 20 years of age consistently show a gradual downward shift in monoamine histofluorescence intensities in the locus coeruleus, the substantia nigra, and the dorsal raphe nucleus.

Depressed levels of monoamines in the human brain with aging are well established as are correlative declines in the catecholamine synthetic enzymes along with an elevation in degenerative enzyme activity (McGeer and McGeer, 1976).

Impairment of neurotransmission during aging may result from a decreased synthesizing of enzymes, a slower uptake mechanism, increased activity of catabolic enzymes, and a decrease in the number of receptors.

## Enzymes

Age-related reduction occurs in choline acetyltransferase (ChAT) and glutamic acid decarboxylase (GAD). The cerebral cortex is very vulnerable to the changes in ChAT activity, in both 18- and 26-month-old rats compared with a 10-month-old age group. No significant changes in ChAT activity were found in the hippocampus.

Glutamic acid decarboxylase activity was also reduced in the cerebral cortex of older rats—a 50% reduction at 26 months of age compared with 10 months of age.

In a study of neurologically normal humans 5 to 87 years old (McGeer and McGeer, 1976), almost one third of the brain areas examined showed a significant negative correlation between ChAT activity and age. The decline in ChAT activity is particularly notable in the cortical areas. Perry et al. (1977) found a significant linear correlation in both area 21 of the cortex and the hippocampus in a series of 60 normal brains from humans 60 to 90 years of age. No statistically significant correlation between age and ChAT activity was noted in the normal human frontal cortex by White *et al.* (1977), in the temperal lobe, or in any of the 20 areas of the brain studied by McKay *et al.* (1978) in neurologically and psychiatrically normal humans ranging between the ages of 46 and 74 years.

Loss of ChAT and GAD activity appears to be somewhat species specific with fewer changes noted in the mouse than in the rat brain. They are virtually unchanged in the mouse cerebral cortex.

Studies of the dopaminergic and the norepinephrine systems indicate a sharp decline with age in the activities of tyrosine hydroxylase and dopadecarboxylase in some areas of the brain. The most significant decline has been noted in the basal ganglia and the nucleus accumbens.

## Receptors

Binding assays for receptors show a decrease in old rodents and humans. The decrease is more pronounced in some areas than in others and is generally the result of fewer receptors, not changes in the receptor affinity. The old rodents also show a reduced ability to increase the number of receptors (supersensitivity) to diminished presynaptic stimulation. This may reflect lowered responsiveness of the old nervous system. A decrease in the number of receptors may be due to a decrease in the receptor-binding sites at the membrane level, dendritic degeneration, and cell loss.

There are significant age-related changes in β-adrenergic and cholinergic muscarinic receptor binding in selected regions of the rat brain. The cholinergic receptor binding was shown to be 20% lower in the cerebral cortex and the corpus striatum of the oldest animals (26 months) compared with the youngest age group (10 months). Binding in the hippocampus was identical in all three age groups. β-Adrenergic receptor binding was also reduced in two of the brain regions of older animals: 30% down in the cerebellum and greater than 50% reduction in the brain stem. Similarly, 50% fewer β-adrenergic receptor sites were found in the cerebellar tissue obtained from human subjects aged 62 to 80 years compared with the number found in samples from individuals up to 2 years of age.

Gamma-aminobutyric acid receptors also decrease in the rat brain with aging. The regional distribution of such a decrease reveals a rather specific localization such as the substantia nigra, the hypothalamus, the striatum, the cerebral cortex, the hippocampus, the pons, and the medulla oblongata.

## Blood Flow and Metabolism

Cerebral blood flow is regulated to meet the requirements of cerebral metabolism and functions. Because glucose is the major substrate for oxidation metabolism in the adult brain, the cerebral metabolic rate for glucose reflects the local metabolic rate and functional activity. There are age-related changes in the metabolic rate. The regional cerebral metabolic rate for glucose falls in the awake rat between the age of 3 to 12 months while the regional cerebral blood flow remains unchanged. There is no further decline in this metabolic rate in the rat between 12 to 34 months of age (Smith *et al.*, 1980).

Rapoport *et al.* (1984) studied 21 healthy male volunteers between the ages of 21 and 83 years. They were carefully selected to rule out subclinical cerebrovascular disease. They were studied for brain metabolism with the help of a positron emission tomography scan. The results indicated that the cerebral metabolic rate for oxygen, cerebral blood flow, and cerebral metabolic rate for glucose were not reduced in the healthy elderly.

A few studies have shown that an aging brain possesses a reduced ability to utilize water-soluble precursors for phospholipid synthesis.

Degrell *et al.* (1983) studied the effects of profound arterial hypoxemia on the metabolism of carbohydrates, energy pool, and neurotransmitters of brains of 1- and 2-year-old male rats. No significant decrease in carbohydrate and energy metabolism was found in hypoxemic conditions. However, in hypoxemic conditions, older rats showed a significant decrease in the levels of dopamine by 25%.

Cyclic adenosine monophosphate (cAMP) and cyclic guanosine monophosphate (cGMP) are considered to be the intracellular messengers for several neurotransmitters in the central nervous system. Norepinephrine increases cAMP and acetylcholine increases cGMP in some regions of the brain. Dopamine also stimulates cAMP. Both cAMP and cGMP can be rapidly catabolized to 5-AMP and 5-GMP by specific phosphodiesterases. Alternatively, they can attach themselves to certain protein-phosphorylating enzymes (collectively referred as protein kinases) that are intracellular "effectors" for the most physiologically important effects of cAMP. Animal studies indicate that steady-state levels of cAMP and cGMP do not change in most brain areas with age. Similarly, adenyl cyclase, the enzyme responsible for the production of cAMP, is unaffected by aging.

## Neurophysiology

There is progressive deterioration of sensory functions with age. Hearing abnormalities and diminished olfaction are common. Sense of smell is impaired in four out of five individuals over the age of 65 and the sense of taste, which is closely allied, diminishes in about the same proportion. In part, this is due to a profound loss in the density of taste buds in the tongue of old people: as many as two thirds of the taste buds become atrophic in old age. The loss of peripheral receptors, however, is not the only explanation for the impairment of taste in the aged individual. It is presumed that there is an accompanying loss of cells in the cerebral cortex.

Vibration threshold rises progressively with age. A similar increase in the touch-pressure threshold has been found for the index finger and great toe of older individuals (Dyck *et al.*, 1972).

Nerve conduction velocity in the peripheral system in man undergoes a continuous gradual reduction with age. A 16% slowing between the third and ninth decade of life has been reported. The slowing of conduction is accompanied by a decrease in amplitude and a prolongation of the compound action potential with advancing age. Lehmann (1977) reported no significant change in the refractory period up to 70 years of age.

Roger *et al.* (1981) have reported electrophysiological changes in cerebellar function with age. They found that the firing patterns of primary output neurons of the cerebellum, the Purkinje's cells, are disrupted in senescence and the firing rate declines.

## D. SUMMARY

At the psychological-phenomenological level, the major changes in human memory with age that have been scientifically documented to date include the following (1) There seems to be only minimal differences between old and young persons—and thus only slight age decrements—in what has been called "primary memory" which "is involved when the retained material is still in mind, still being rehearsed, still at the focus of conscious attention" (Waugh and Norman, 1965), and whose capacity has been estimated to range from 2.6 words to 3.4 words. (2) When memory tasks and information exceed the capacity of the primary memory so that only secondary or LTM processes are involved, older persons are less able to form long-term memories and less able to retrieve them than young persons. (3) Memory tasks requiring the manipulation or reorganization of recently stored information and tasks in which attention must be divided involve secondary rather than primary memory processes and are thus tasks on which older persons perform significantly more poorly than young persons. (4) When divided attention memory tasks are presented auditorily, older subjects show small decrements in short-term retention, but not when such tasks are presented visually. (5) Older persons perform more poorly on tasks requiring recall than on tasks requiring recognition. This may be due in part to a failure of older persons to organize or reorganize the material to be remembered, to a failure to use mnemonic devices, and to a tendency to use verbal rather than visual mediators to make material more memorable. Since these activities are carried out during acquisition, they can be referred to as encoding operations and it can be hypothesized that older persons do not carry out as many encoding procedures as young persons (or carry them out less deeply and less thoroughly) with the result that the material to be remembered is processed less, encoded less, and thus more poorly recalled. It has also been hypothesized that older persons are less likely to recall information because retrieval cues used in recall have become attached to so many items that they are "overloaded" and thus ineffective. (6) There are very few studies of the effect of age on nonverbal memory such as for pictures, tones, or smell, but the few studies that have been conducted show gradual memory deficits with increasing age (Botwinick and Storandt, 1974). (7) Contrary to popular belief, older persons do *not* recall or recognize information from the distant past (such as the names and faces of high school classmates) as well as young persons, although they do show high levels of retention. (8) There is evidence that giving older persons special instructions before learning, instructions that force them to carry out a greater number of more elaborate, or deeper encoding/processing operations, significantly decreases or entirely abolishes the difference usually found between older and younger persons in recall and recognition. Under these conditions, older persons perform almost as well in recall and recognition tasks as young persons. The failure to engage in elaborate or deep encoding may also explain the poorer performance of young children on certain memory tasks.

## E. REFERENCES

Anders T, Fozard J, Lilliquist T: Effects of age upon retrieval from short-term memory. *Dev Psychol* 1972; 6:214–217.

Barbizet J, Cany E: Clinical and psychometric study of a patient with memory disturbances. *Int J Neurol* 1968; 7:44–45.

Borst M (ed): *Pathologische Histologie*, Vogel, Leipzig, 1922.

Botwinik J, Storandt M: *Memory Related Functions and Age*. Springfield, Ill, Charles C Thomas, 1974.

Brizzee KR: Structural correlates of the aging process in the brain. *Psychopharmacol Bull* 1981; 17:43–52.

Broadbent D, Gregory M: Some confirmatory results on age differences in memory for simultaneous stimulation. *Br J Psychol* 1965; 56:77–80.

Broadbent D, Heron A: Effects of a subsidiary task on performance involving immediate memory in younger and older men. *Br J Psychol* 1962; 53:189–198.

Brody H: Organization of the cerebral cortex. III. A study of aging in human cerebral cortex. *J Comp Neurol* 1955; 102:511–556.

Bromley DB: Some effects of age on short-term learning and memory. *J Gerontal* 1958; 13:398–406.

Buell SJ, Coleman PD: Dendritic growth in the aged human brain and failure of growth in senile dementia. *Science* 1979; 206:854–855.

Burns BD: *The Mammalian Cerebral Cortex*. London, Edward Arnold, 1958, p 90.

Clark L, Knowles J: Age differences in dichotic listening performance. *J Gerontal* 1973; 28:173–178.

Conrad R, Hille B: The decay theory of immediate memory paced recall. *Can J Psychol* 1958; 12:1–6.

Craik FI: Short-term memory and the aging process, in Talland GA (ed): *Human Aging and Behavior*. New York, Academic Press, 1968a, pp 131–168.

Craik FI: Two components in free recall. *J Verb Learn Verb Behav* 1968b; 7:996–1004.

Craik FI: Age differences in human memory, in Birren JE, Schaie KW (eds): *Human Aging and Behavior*. New York, Van Nostrand Reinhold, 1977.

Craik FI, Tulving E: Depth of processing and the retention of words in episodic memory. *J Exp Psychol Gen* 1975; 104:268–294.

Crenshaw DA: *Retrieval Processes in Memory and Aging*, PhD thesis. Washington University, 1969.

Degrell I, Zenner K, Kummer P, *et al.*: Monoamine metabolites in the CSF of conscious unrestrained rats. *Brain Res* 1983; 277:283–287.

Diamond MC: The aging brain: Some enlightening and optimistic results. *Am Sci* 1978; 66:66–71.

Dyck PJ, Schultz P, O'Brien P: Quantification of touch-pressure sensation. *Arch Neurol* 1972; 26:465–473.

Drachman D, Leavitt J: Memory impairment in the aged: Storage versus retrieval deficit. *J Exp Psychol* 1972; 93:302–308.

Erber J: Age differences in recognition memory. *J Gerontal* 1974; 29:177–181.

Eriksen C, Hamlin R, Daye C: Aging adults and rate of memory scan. *Bull Psychol Soc* 1973; 1:259–260.

Eysenck MW: Age differences in incidental learning. *Dev Psychol* 1974; 10:936–941.

Frazer DC: Decay of immediate memory with age. *Nature* 1958; 182:1163.

Friedman H: Memory organization in the aged. *J Genet Psychol* 1966; 109:3–8.

Ganzler H: Motivation as a factor in the psychological deficit of aging. *J Gerontol* 1964; 19:425–429.

Gordon S, Clark W: Application of signal detection theory to prose recall and recognition in elderly and young adults. *J Gerontol* 1974; 29:64–72.

Hannover A: Mikorskopiske undersogelser af nervesystemet, in *Danske Videnskabernes Selskab, Copenhagen.2. Naturvidenskapsselsk*. Og Mathe, Matisk, Afdeling, Ser 4, vol 10, 1942, pp 1–112.

Harwood E, Naylor G: Recall and recognition in elderly and young subjects. *Aust J Psychol* 1969; 21:251–257.

Howell S: Familiarity and complexity in perceptual recognition. *J Gerontol* 1972; 27:364–371.

Inglis J, Caird W: Age differences in successive responses to simultaneous stimulation. *Can J Psychol* 1963; 17:98–105.

Kinsbourne M: Age effects on letter span related to rate and sequential dependency. *J Gerontol* 1973; 28:317–319.

Kriauchiunas R: The relationship of age and retention interval activity in short-term memory. *J Gerontol* 1968; 23:169–173.

Laurence MW: Memory loss with age: A test of two strategies for its retardation. *Psychonom Sci* 1967; 9:209–210.

Leboucq G: Le rapport entre lipoids et la surface de l'hemisphere cérèbrale chez l'homme et les singes. *Mem Acad R Med Belg* 1929; 10:55.

Lehmann D: Pattern evoked average EEG potentials and dichotic visual receptors. *Perception* 1977; 6:77–84.

Lorsbach TC, Simpson GB: Age differences in the rate of processing in short-term memory. *J Gerontol* 1984; 39:315–321.

Macht ML: Speed of recall in aging. *J Gerontol* 1984; 39:439–443.

Madden DJ: Age-related slowing in the retrieval of information from long-term memory. *J Gerontol* 1985; 40:208–210.

Mandler G: Organized recall: Individual functions. *Psychonom Sci* 1968; 13:235–236.

McGeer E, McGeer P: Neurotransmitter metabolism in the aging brain, in Terry RD, Gerson S (eds): *Neurobiology of Aging*. New York, Raven Press, 1976, pp 389–403.

McGhie A, Chapman J, Lawson J: Changes in immediate memory with age. *Br J Psychol* 1965; 56:69–75.

McKay A, Davies P, Dewar A, et al.: Regional distribution of enzymes associated with neurotransmission by monoamines, acetylcholine, and GABA in the human brain. *J Neurochem* 1978; 30:827–839.

Neisser U: Cognitive Psychology. New York, Appleton-Century-Crofts, 1967.

Owens WA: Age and mental abilities: A second adult follow-up. *J Educ Psychol* 1966; 57:311–325.

Park DC, Puglis J: Picture memory in older adults: Effects of contextual details at encoding and retrieval. *J Gerontol* 1984; 39:213–215.

Perry E, Perry R, Blessed G, et al.: Necropsy evidence of central cholinergic deficits in senile dementia. *Lancet* 1977; 1:189–190.

Rapoport SI, Duara R, Haxby J: Positron emission tomography in normal aging and Alzheimer's disease. *Psychopharmacol Bull* 1984; 20:466–471.

Reige W, Inman V: Age-differences in nonverbal memory tasks. *J Gerontol* 1981; 36:51–58.

Rogers J, Zornetzer S, Bloom F: Senescent pathology of cerebellum: Purkinje neurons and their parallel fiber afferents. *Neurobiol Aging* 1981; 2:15–26.

Robinowitz JC: Aging and recognition failure. *J Gerontol* 1984; 39:65–71.

Schaie K, Strother C: The effect of time and cohort differences upon age changes in cognitive behavior. *Multivar Behav Res* 1968; 3:259–294.

Schonfield D, Robertson B: Memory storage and aging. *Can J Psychol* 1966; 20:228–236.

Schonfield D, Wenger L: Age limitation of perceptual span. *Nature* 1975; 253:377–378.

Shefer VF: Absolute number of neurons and thickness of the cerebral cortex during aging, senile, and vascular dementia, and Pick's and Alzheimer's. *Neurosci Behav Physiol* 1973; 6:319–324.

Smith CB, Goochee C, Rapoport S, *et al.*: Effects of aging on local rates of cerebral glucose utilization in the rat. *Brain* 1980; 103:351–365.

Sternberg S: High-speed scanning in human memory. *Science* 1966; 153:652–654.

Talland G: *Disorders of Memory and Learning*. Middlesex, England, Penguin Books, 1968.

Taub HA: Memory span, practice and aging. *J Gerontol* 1973; 28:335–338.

Terry RD, Peck A, Deteresa R, *et al.*: Some morphometric aspects of the brain in senile dementia of the Alzheimer type. *Ann Neurol* 1981; 10:184–192.

Walsh S, Thompson L: Age differences in visual sensory memory. *J Gerontol* 1978; 33:282–287.

Warrington E, Silberstein M: A questionnaire technique for investigating very long-term memory. *Q J Exp Psychol* 1970; 22:508–512.

White P, Goodhardt M, Keet J, *et al*: Neocortical cholinergic neurons in elderly people. *Lancet* 1977; 1:668–670.

Worden PE, Meggison DL: Aging and category recall relationship. *J Gerontol* 1984; 39:322–324.

# Treatment Strategies for Memory Disorders

Establishment of etiology is an essential prerequisite for the treatment of memory disorders. It is estimated that 20% to 40% of the patients may have treatable disorders resulting from metabolic disturbances, alcohol abuse, intracranial pathology such as hematoma, tumor, and abcess, and psychiatric disorders such as dissociative disorders and depression. The remaining 50–60% of the cases of dementia are likely to suffer from primary degenerative diseases, including Alzheimer's disease. This group of patients should be differentiated from the rapidly growing population of aged individuals in their 60s and 70s who suffer from progressive deterioration of cognitive and memory functions.

In the absence of an effective treatment for memory impairment in the aged and in Alzheimer's disease, multiple therapies have become the main mode of treatment. The goal of these therapies at present is not to cure, but merely to improve the quality of life for the sufferers who progressively deteriorate in their cognitive and physical functions.

The currently available therapies may be divided into the following categories:

1. Pharmacological treatment
2. Memory skill training
3. Psychiatric treatments
4. Environmental management
5. Reality orientation program
6. Other therapies

## A. PHARMACOLOGICAL TREATMENT

A fairly large number of drugs have been tried in the treatment of senile dementia and in the improvement of memory deficits suffered by the elderly. Most of these drugs can be categorized under the following classes of drugs:

1. Cholinergic drugs
2. Central nervous system stimulants
3. Nootropic drugs
4. Vasodilators
5. Convulsant stimulants
6. Anabolic agents
7. GABA-ergic drugs
8. Neuropeptides

A detailed discussion of these drugs can be found in the Chapters 3 and 5. Only a few of the drugs that have shown promising results in human studies will be discussed here.

### Cholinergic Drugs

Neurochemical changes in normal aging and dementia indicate that the cholinergic system may be involved with characteristic memory changes. For example, it has been found that the enzyme choline acetyltransferase (ChAT), which catalyzes the synthesis of the neurotransmitter acetylcholine (ACh), decreases after age 20. There is also an increase in the activity of acetylcholinesterase (which breaks down ACh) in old age and Alzheimer's disease. The drugs utilized in enhancing the cholinergic activity of the brain may be classified in the following categories:

1. Direct precursors of ACh
   a. Choline
   b. Phosphorylcholine
2. Indirect precursors of ACh
   a. Lecithin
   b. Dimethylaminoethanol
3. ACh releasers
   a. Phosphatidylserine
4. Cholinesterase inhibitors
   a. Physostigmine
5. ACh agonists
   a. Arecoline

*Physostigmine*

Physostigmine enhances cholinergic activity by delaying hydrolysis of liberated ACh by cholinesterase. It has been tried in young adults, healthy elderlies, and patients with Alzheimer's disease with variable results.

Davis *et al.* (1978) gave intravenous infusion of 1.0 mg of physostigmine or saline to 19 normal young volunteers (18 to 35 years) over a period of 1 hr. Approximately 20 min prior to the start of infusion, each subject received 0.5 mg of methscopolamine bromide subcutaneously in order to block the peripheral effects of physostigmine. The memory tests included two tests of short-term memory (STM; digit span and memory scanning) and two tests of long-term memory (LTM) for retrieval of information from LTM and the storage of information in LTM. Physostigmine, compared with saline, had no quantifiable effect on any aspect of STM. However, the retrieval of words was enhanced significantly more on the day that subjects received physostigmine than the day they received saline. Similarly, storage of words was enhanced with physostigmine.

Davis *et al.* (1979b) also carried out a study of physostigmine in Alzheimer's disease patients in two phases: an initial dose-finding phase with different doses of intravenous infusion because of a fairly narrow dose range of effectiveness, and then a replication phase in which the dose that was associated with the best memory performance was compared with a placebo in a double-blind crossover study design. The authors concluded that for nearly every patient, at least one dose of physostigmine enhanced memory performance in a way that can be reproduced reliably during the replication phase.

Christie *et al.* (1981) gave 11 patients with a clinical diagnosis of Alzheimer's disease an intravenous infusion of physostigmine (0.25–1 mg), arecoline (2 and 4 mg), and a saline in a randomized double-blind design. A significant improvement was seen on a picture recognition test with physostigmine 0.375 mg and arecoline 4 mg. For the majority of the patients improvement was only slight, but in two patients it was clear-cut and consistent.

Sullivan *et al.* (1982) studied five men and seven women with a clinical diagnosis of Alzheimer's disease (mild = 6, moderate = 5, severe = 1). Physostigmine (0.25 and 0.5 mg) and a saline placebo were infused intravenously over 30 min on three separate days according to a double-blind protocol. A 1-hr-long memory assessment began 15 min after the start of the infusion. Patients received 2.5 to 5 mg methscopolamine 1 hr before each infusion to minimize systemic cholinergic toxicity. The memory tests included paired-associate and recognition tasks. Physostigmine did not produce any reliable change in performance in the whole group. Four of eight patients performed better on verbal paired-associate learning tests whereas three did worse than their baseline and the rest did not show any change at all. The authors concluded that patients with mild dementia are more likely to show improvement in memory functions during physostigmine treatment than those with greater cognitive disability.

Caltagirone *et al.* (1983) showed no memory improvement in Alzheimer's disease patients both with acute and chronic administration of physostigmine. In one study, eight patients received acute administration of physostigmine in an idividual optimal dose orally or subcutaneously. The individual optimal dose was assessed by monitoring serum cholinesterase activity. Memory performance was assessed by two tests: the Rey's 15 Words Test and the digit span subtests from the Wechsler Memory Scale. Although a slight behavioral activation was noted in all patients after the treatment, the comparison between the mean scores obtained by Alzheimer's disease patients on memory tests before and after the acute physostigmine administration failed to reach the level of statistical significance.

In their second study, Caltagirone *et al.* (1982) administered orally 1 mg of physostigmine four times a day for one month to eight patients with a clinical diagnosis of Alzheimer's disease. The possible beneficial effect of the drug was evaluated by means of a neuropsychological battery administered to all patients before and after the treatment. The performances of demented patients on retest did not show any difference in comparison with performances obtained on the first assessment.

Mohs *et al.* (1985) reported the effects of oral physostigmine in ten patients with Alzheimer's disease (ages 52–76 years). After an initial optimal dose-finding phase, physostigmine was administered every 2 hr from 7 AM to 9 PM in doses of 0.0, 0.5, 1.0, 1.5, and 2.0 mg for three to five days. Improvement was assessed with the Alzheimer's Disease Assessment Scale and compared with a placebo condition. Three of the patients showed a significant improvement (41.7%, 43.4%, and 17.3%). Four other patients showed marginal improvement while the remaining three had inconsistent responses. Serum cortisol measures obtained during sleep suggested that the patients whose symptoms improved with physostigmine were those in whom oral physostigmine enhanced central cholinergic activity.

Most studies of acute administration of physostigmine tend to show some improvement in memory performance, but the improvement is generally small and short-lasting. The improvement in memory functions may also depend upon the severity of Alzheimer's disease. It has been suggested that severe neuronal loss is unlikely to respond to treatment with physostigmine. Glen and Whalley (1979) claimed that only patients at the onset of mental deterioration could obtain some improvement by treatment with cholinergic agents. Most investigators agree that physostigmine exerts its maximal beneficial effect on memory functions in a narrow range of doses and it is important to determine each subject's optimal dose for maximum improvement. For a given patient, doses lower than the optimal dose have no effect, but doses higher than the optimal dose actually impair cognition. The individual dose may be assessed by monitoring serum cholinesterase and an initial trial of several doses with the optimal dose producing the maximal improvement on memory performance tests.

### Arecoline

This drug acts directly on postganglionic neurons and on the effector tissue. Like physostigmine, arecoline has been studied for its memory-enhancing effect in young, healthy volunteers as well as in patients with Alzheimer's disease. Sitaram *et al.* (1978) found that intravenous arecoline in small doses improved memory functions in normal young volunteers. The subjects were first given scopolamine (0.5 mg), which impaired learning recall. This effect was reversed by subsequent subcutaneous injection of arecoline in different doses (4 and 6 mg). Memory functions were assessed with a categorized serial-learning task of a fixed sequence of ten words belonging to a familiar category (e.g., vegetables, fruits).

Christie (1982) studied eleven patients with Alzheimer's disease. Arecoline was given in 2- and 4-mg intravenous infusion for 30 min. Improvement in memory functions as assessed by a picture recognition test was small and many functions remained grossly impaired compared with normal subjects.

### Choline and Lecithin

The observation that oral or parenteral choline administration could raise brain ACh was first reported in 1975 by two independent laboratories (Cohan and Wurtman, 1975; Haubrick *et al.*, 1975). Sitaram *et al.* (1978) also reported enhancement of serial learning in normal volunteers 90 min after oral administration of 10 g of choline chloride. Subsequent studies have not confirmed the earlier optimism. Davis *et al.* (1979a) and Mohs and Davis (1980) showed that normal young volunteers as well as the healthy elderly did not show any significant improvement in their memory functions with choline. The young volunteers were given 8 g and 16 g of choline for three days. Neither dose had any significant effect on memory. A few subjects who were very responsive to physostigmine in an earlier study showed a slight memory improvement with choline. In a second study, healthy adults over the age of 55 years were given 16 g of choline for seven days and 8 g of choline for 21 days. They also showed no significant improvement of memory functions.

Mohs *et al.* (1980) suggested that although many clinical studies show that choline does not improve memory in normal young adults, it does enhance memory in certain conditions, such as in cholinergic blockade produced by scopolamine. They administered choline, scopolamine, and a placebo to 20 young volunteers in three experimental conditions: choline-scopolamine, placebo-scopolamine, and placebo-placebo. Memory performance was found best in the placebo-placebo condition, poorest in the placebo-scopolamine condition, and slightly but significantly better in the choline-scopolamine condition than in the placebo-scopolamine condition.

Choline is normally present in choline-rich foods such as cauliflower and cabbage. Large doses of pure choline chloride are not well tolerated by most patients. Therefore, a more palatable substitution is made with lecithin. Lecithin-rich foods include eggs, soybeans, and liver. The amount of choline present in lecithin varies in different commercial preparations.

Vroulis and Smith (1981) administered lecithin and a placebo to 18 Alzheimer's disease patients in a double-blind crossover design for a period of two to eight weeks. Although there was no statistically significant improvement in memory, some patients showed significant improvements in specific memory functions. The data indicated that lecithin took at least two to three weeks to show a therapeutic effect and the effect persisted for about three to four weeks after the cessation of lecithin therapy. The authors suggested that short-term treatment periods may not provide an accurate picture of lecithin effect.

Etienne *et al.* (1982) studied 11 patients with Alzheimer's disease with 30 g of lecithin (55% phosphatidylcholine) and wheat germ for three months each. Memory functions were assessed with a digit span test, a paired-associate learning test, a Benton Visual Retention Test, the Logical Memory Test, and facial recognition tasks. There was no substantial difference between the test scores obtained during placebo and those during lecithin administration. Similarly, several other studies of lecithin treatment with healthy geriatric volunteers (Domino *et al.*, 1982) have shown no significant change in memory performance in spite of the elevated blood choline levels.

Several studies that have combined lecithin preloading with physostigmine treatment show variable results. Peters and Levin (1982) gave lecithin to a group of Alzheimer's disease patients for 18 months. Memory assessments were made at intervals 1 hr after taking physostigmine or placebo. The physostigmine treatment with lecithin preloading appeared to augment retrieval from LTM in some patients. In two patients, a progressive continued cognitive decline characteristic of Alzheimer's disease was observed with failure to respond to physostigmine in spite of 10 to 18 months of lecithin treatment. One patient with benign memory impairment showed consistent memory augmentation and no apparent cognitive decline after 15 months of treatment. Bajada (1982) found no extra beneficial effect from a combined treatment with choline and physostigmine in six moderate to severe Alzheimer's disease patients when compared with placebo and to each drug given alone.

Choline and lecithin administration increases the serum and brain levels of choline. Choline shares this property with tyrosine, trytophan, histidine, and threonine which affect the synthesis of neuronal catecholamine, serotonin, histidine, and glycine, respectively. However, an increase in ACh synthesis caused by providing neurons with more choline may or may not be associated with an increase in the amount of ACh actually released into synapses during a given unit of time.

## Central Nervous System Stimulants

The most commonly used CNS stimulants are dextroamphetamine (Dexedrine), methylphenidate (Ritalin), and magnesium pemoline (Cylert). Dexedrine crosses the blood–brain barrier and appears to have a stimulating effect on the reticular activating system, the respiratory and vasomotor centers, and the cerebral cortex. The exact mechanism of magnesium pemoline is not clear since it has several actions on the CNS. Its stimulating property may be related to its ability to increase the rate of dopamine synthesis and dopamine levels in certain areas of the brain such as the basal ganglia and the brain stem.

### Methylphenidate (Ritalin)

This is a CNS stimulant and produces activation of EEG responses and enhances sympathetic activity in the hypothalamic area. After several open trials indicated beneficial results in the treatment of geriatric patients, several controlled studies have been carried out. Kaplitz (1975) studied Ritalin in 44 withdrawn, apathetic geriatric patients whose characteristic symptoms were lack of interest and motivation, lowered self-esteem, restricted activity, listlessness, and general inattention to personal appearance. Excluded from the study were agitated, psychotic, and severely mentally deteriorated patients. Ritalin was given in a dosage of 10 mg twice daily for six weeks in a randomized double-blind design. The drug effect was measured by the changes in mental status, ward behavior and target symptoms, and by global ratings. The results indicated a significant improvement in several areas such as interest, attention, self-esteem, and involvement.

There are several studies of Ritalin that have shown no significant improvement in geriatric patients (Holliday and Joffe, 1965; Darvill, 1959). Crook et al. (1977) evaluated the cognitive performance of 12 elderly subjects (ages 65–80 years) who were residing in the community and complaining of diminishing cognitive and memory functions. This study was a single-dose trial of Ritalin using 10 mg and 30 mg dosages. The changes were assessed with tests for motor speed, perceptual speed, memory for faces, digit span, and paragraph recall. The results showed no significant differences between performance after Ritalin or placebo.

Dextroamphetamines and Ritalin are generally considered mood elevators and attention enhancers. They frequently reduce fatigue and improve motivation. They may not have any direct beneficial effects on cognitive functions especially in severely deteriorated patients. However, patients with mild to moderate dementia may benefit from Ritalin, especially from its attention-enhancing and fatigue-reducing effects. Several investigators have been concerned about the side effects of large doses of amphetamines and Ritalin which may produce cardiac acceleration, high blood pressure, insomnia, anorexia, and agitation. Treatment of elderly demented patients currently requires multiple approaches. When attention and motivation are poor, small doses of Ritalin may be helpful.

## Magnesium Pemoline

Eisdorfer (1968) studied 29 male patients (ages 55 to 79 years) in a Veterans Administration hospital with a clinical diagnosis of mild to moderate chronic brain syndrome. The patients were well oriented and were not psychotic. A placebo or magnesium pemoline in a single dose of 25 mg each morning were administered for 28 days in a randomized double-blind schedule. A battery of psychological tests was given to assess cognitive and memory functions and included subtests of the Wechsler Adult Intelligence Scale, the Gottschaldt Embedded Figures Test, and the Proteus Maze Test. The drug group showed significant improvement on two of the nine tests administered: the Embedded Figures Test and a nurses' rating on the Stockton Geriatric Rating Scale reflecting day-to-day ward behavior (apathy, socially irritating behavior, communication, and physical disability). The drug group also showed better performance on a vigilance task. The authors concluded that the changes in the behavior and the cognitive functions were quite small and the two groups differed little in their overall functions.

Several other studies of pemoline in geriatric patients have shown negative results or minor improvement. Gilbert et al. (1973) studied methylphenidate and pemoline in a group of normal elderly. The drugs did not produce any significant improvement in cognitive and memory functions. In fact, pemoline seemed to cause some depression and worry in the elderly and did not reduce fatigue, while methylphenidate decreased fatigue.

## Nootropic Drugs

These drugs generated a great deal of research interest in the 1970s. Giurgea (1982) designated these drugs as "nootropic," implying that these drugs influenced only the higher integrative mechanisms of the mind. Several members of this group such as piracetam, oxiracetam, paramiracetam, and aniracetam have shown promising results in animal studies. Human studies are just beginning to appear in the United States. These drugs seem to enhance cerebral energy metabolism via an increase in ATP formation and protein synthesis. They also produce alertness without the side effects of CNS stimulants.

The initial optimism derived from animal studies has not, however, been sustained after human trials. One of the two placebo-controlled studies of piracetam (Abuzzahab *et al.*, 1978; Minduse *et al.*, 1976) in the normal healthy elderly found a significant improvement in both a conventional and a computerized perceptual motor task. With respect to the treatment of primary degenerative disease with piracetam, there are several positive and negative studies. Ferris' (1981) review of piracetam studies concluded that the therapeutic efficacy of piracetam was equivocal.

Ferris *et al.* (1982) studied 20 patients with mild to moderate Alzheimer's disease who were living in the community. Piracetam in dosage of 7.2 g/day was given in a double-blind crossover schedule for two four-week treatment periods. Each treatment period was preceded by a one-week placebo period. Cognitive assessment was carried out with an extensive psychological battery. The result showed no consistent pattern of drug effects.

Some authors tried a combination treatment of piracetam and choline in ten patients with mild to moderate Alzheimer's disease. The dosages were 9 g of choline and 4.8 g of piracetam per day for seven days. Three of the patients who showed marked clinical improvement also showed significant improvement in their cognitive and memory functions.

Although piracetam appears devoid of the common side effects of CNS drugs such as sedatives, tranquilizers, analgesics, analeptics or autonomics, several studies (Chouinard *et al.*, 1983) have indicated that piracetam in higher dosages may produce overstimulation, sleep disturbances, and dizziness. Several analogues of piracetam appear to be more potent than piracetam. Itil *et al.* (1982) compared oxiracetam and piracetam (up to 2.4 g/day) in a sample of patients with Alzheimer's disease. The results indicated that oxiracetam had a greater effect in improving memory functions than piracetam. Similarly, pramiracetam has been found more effective than piracetam in the treatment of primary degenerative disease (Branconnier 1983).

## Vasodilators

In general, vasodilating drugs have not been successful in improving brain blood flow in cerebral arteriosclerosis. There is, however, no reason to believe that the occlusion caused by arteriosclerosis can be modified by vasodilator drugs any more than in the vessels of the heart or the extremities. However, some of these drugs may relieve the vasospasm that is present in some cases.

Among the large number of vasodilators (such as papaverine, isoxsuprine, cyclandelate, nylidrin, nicotinic acid), the most extensively studied drug is ergoloid mesylate (Hydergine). Hydergine is an ergot alkaloid and is one of the most popular cognitive adjutants used in elderly patients. It has several well-documented pharmacological effects such as being a dopamine agonist, a phosphodiesterase inhibitor, a stimulator of cerebral metabolism, and a mild vasodilator. The original inference that it modified dementia by vasodilation has been abandoned in favor of its other effects on the CNS.

Hydergine was first introduced in Europe in 1949 and in the United States in 1954. It was initially used for the treatment of hypertension and peripheral vascular disorders. It was several years later that its use in dementia was discovered. There have been several reviews of Hydergine studies published in the last decade. Hughes *et al.* (1976) published the first critical review of 12 clinical trials of Hydergine in the treatment of dementia. Although there were differences in the study designs, all studies had used double-blind, placebo-controlled protocols. The diagnostic criteria of the subjects, however, varied greatly among the studies. Although Hydergine was shown to produce significant improvement in the symptoms of dementia in most studies, the overall change was quite small. The authors also failed to find indications for long-term use of Hydergine.

Venn (1980) criticized the conclusions of Hughes' review. He noted that Hughes *et al.* arrived at their conclusion by averaging the results of the studies. He pointed out that Hydergine afforded a one- to two-point improvement on the global impression scale in more than 50% of the cases, with fewer patients exhibiting worsening or no change than the other treatment categories. More than 23% of the patients improved in excess of three points or greater on a seven-point scale in overall clinical status. Venn emphasized that in the present state of pharmacotherapy of senile dementia, these results may be considered fairly good.

Yesavage *et al.* (1979) reviewed 102 studies of vasodilators used in the treatment of dementia. Only 22 of the studies were considered well-controlled trials of Hydergine. In 8 of the 22 studies, Hydergine produced significant improvement in behavioral and psychological measures.

Several long-term studies (24 to 60 weeks) carried out in Europe and in the United States show significant improvement in demented patients after 6 to 12 weeks of treatment. These gains are sustained by most patients for the duration of the studies (Arrigo, 1973; Gaitz *et al.*, 1977; Eisdorfer, 1975).

The safety of the drug is well established in the elderly with a dosage of 3.0 to 4.5 mg/day. A minimum period of 6 to 12 weeks of treatment is necessary before symptomatic improvement becomes apparent.

## Neuropeptides

Neuropeptides are thought to function in the brain as neurotransmitters or as modulators of neurotransmitters. Naturally produced neuropeptides such as adrenocorticotropic hormone and vasopressin have been related to processes involved in memory functions. It has been suggested that the process of aging and senile dementia may include some dysfunction of neuropeptides.

De Wied (1980) initially observed that neurophysectomy accelerated the extinction of a conditioned avoidance response and that the administration of Pitressin, an extract of the posterior pituitry, corrected the deficit. Subsequent studies have indicated more clearly that vasopressin plays a role in the consolidation of memory processes. Clinical studies in humans have produced variable results. Chase *et al.* (1982) found a significant improvement in memory and cognitive functions in a group of Alzheimer's disease patients treated with lysine-8-vasopressin. Because of the classical endocrine activities displayed by the whole molecule of vasopressin, several analogues that are practically devoid of endocrine effects are now being tested. Tinklenberg *et al.* (1982) found that 1-desamino-*D*-arginine-vasopressin (DDAVP) and desglycinamide-9-arginine-8-vasopressin (DGALP) were helpful in improving memory functions in a small sample of dementia patients. There are, however, several studies with negative results.

### Opioid Antagonists

Recent theories link endogenous opiate systems to memory storage processes. It has been suggested that endorphins and enkephalins may control the memory process through their activity on opiate receptors (Reisberg *et al.*, 1983). Rigter *et al.* (1980) showed that the impairment of an active avoidance learning response caused by enkephalins was blocked by naloxone.

### Naloxone

Naloxone is an opioid antagonist. Several mechanisms of action have been suggested by animal studies. It may influence the cholinergic and gamma-aminobutyric acid neurotransmitter systems. It may also release the dopaminergic and β-adrenergic systems from the tonic inhibition of opiate peptide systems.

Reisberg *et al.* (1983) first conducted an open preliminary trial of 1 mg of naloxone given intravenously to five patients with Alzheimer's disease. Clinical and psychometric assessments showed notable improvement in three patients. Then a double-blind, placebo-controlled study was carried out in seven patients with moderate to severe Alzheimer's disease. Naloxone was given intravenously in dosages of 1, 5, and 10 mg alternating with a placebo. Single injections were given at intervals of seven days over a six-week period. Psychometric assessment was carried out before and 15 to 60 min after the injections. The only side effect noted was anxiety in two patients with 10 mg doses. There was a significant improvement in psychometric tests including digit symbol, digit span, substitution test, perceptual speed, and category retrieval. The authors suggested that naloxone appears to have at least a temporary beneficial effect in Alzheimer's disease.

## B. MEMORY SKILL TRAINING

Several training programs have been designed to improve the cognitive skills involved in learning and memory. These programs vary in degree of complexity and are claimed to be effective for the normal elderly as well as for demented individuals.

These training programs focus on learning attitude, interest, motivation, better organization of the material, enhancement of visual imagery, use of mnemonics, and deeper levels of processing.

## Improving Attitude

Most of the elderly believe in the age stereotype of a failing memory which leads to a self-fulfilling prophesy. Subjective complaints of memory impairment are common in the normal elderly. These complaints are frequently related to poor recall of recent events while the remote memory is perceived as adequate. Several studies have shown that there are significant differences between the subjective evaluation of memory and the actual performance on memory tests. Most of the elderly tend to perform better on memory tests than their self-evaluations about their memory would predict (Gurland et al., 1976; Kahn et al., 1975). It has been suggested that age stereotypes and depression may contribute heavily to this disparity (Kahn, 1971). The elderly are more likely to interpret their occasional memory lapses and absent-mindedness as due to their old age. The depression is most frequently associated with subjective complaints of memory impairment. Zarit et al. (1981) showed that in a group of healthy elderly living in the community, subjective complaints about memory decreased after memory training or with increased participation in a discussion group to improve attitude and motivation toward learning.

## Improving Visual Imagery

Several studies have indicated that the elderly appear to have difficulty in generating and remembering visual images and in making visual imagery associations (Winograd and Simon, 1980). A series of techniques have been imployed to improve imagery ability (Yesavage, 1983): (1) imagining various vivid scenes from poems or literature; (2) studying pictures, paintings, or line drawings and then reviewing them in detail from memory; (3) mental rotation of three-dimensional objects; and (4) exercises based on "find the mistakes" in pictures which were slightly altered from their original scenes.

Yesavage showed that pretraining in visual imagery improved the ability of a group of elderly subjects to recall names and faces. Imagery training has been criticized (Cermak, 1980) as being applicable only to a small range of tasks such as memory for lists or pairs of words. Performance decreases over time and shows little transfer to other tasks.

## Improving Organization and Use of Mnemonics

The elderly have also been shown to have difficulty in learning due to poor organization of the material (Craik, 1977). Several studies have indicated that organizational ability decreases with age (Denney, 1974). The use of categorization, cues, mnemonics, and active rehearsal is deficient in the elderly.

Schmitt *et al.* (1981) compared three groups of older adults (mean age 72.1 years) on a free recall task with categorizable lists. One of the groups was instructed to rehearse overtly while studying. The second group was instructed to rehearse by category. The third group, a control, was asked only to remember. The second group showed higher levels of recall than the other two groups. The authors concluded that the memory performance of older adults is modifiable and that efficient performance is obtained when instructional training is aimed at organizational processes.

A fairly large number of techniques have been advanced over the years to promote organizational skills with the help of associative cues, categories, and mnemonics. Commonly employed systems of association include the topical system, grouping methods, the chain system, alphabetical arrangement, numerical methods, and the "hooks and pegs" system (Young and Gibson, 1975).

In the topical system (or method of loci), an individual first learns the names of several loci or locations in a familiar surrounding such as a room, house, building, or neighborhood. Once these locations are well learned, the individual forms a visual image connecting the first item of the list to be learned and the first location, then the second item and the second location, and so on.

In using a house for locations, one pictures a house with ten or more locations. Once these locations (bedroom, bathroom, kitchen, etc.) are well learned in a serial order, the list of items to be learned are visualized as being placed in each locations.

The grouping method of remembering involves categorizing items in appropriate categories (vegetables, fruits, bathroom items, etc.) The chain system may include linking related items such as a hat and a coat. One may also link unrelated items or a large number of items in the form of an imaginary story that may be easier to recall than discrete items. Similarly, use of acronyms, acrostics, and rhyming may help the retention and recall of some items.

Several association techniques have been suggested for remembering names and faces. All these techniques emphasize listening to the name carefully, repeating it verbally, studying the face of the person carefully, and making some association between the name and some features of the face or body and additional associations with the personality and mannerisms of the person.

Memory skill training has been criticized for being task specific and showing little or no transfer of training to day-to-day living. Furthermore, these training methods are of limited value in demented individuals who require more help in organizing and remembering their immediate environment. The elderly with primary degenerative disease need help in remembering daily care items such as personal hygiene, avoidance and disposal of dangerous items (such as matches, burning cigarette butts), and turning off stoves.

## C. PSYCHIATRIC TREATMENTS

A high level of anxiety is common in the elderly and it appears to be related to diminishing cognitive and motor functions. It has been suggested that the high anxiety levels of the elderly impair attention and consequently produce poor learning. Various relaxation techniques and hypnosis have been employed to reduce anxiety and improve learning.

Yesavage *et al*. (1982) trained 26 elderly subjects from local senior centers (age range 59 to 85) to use a standard relaxation technique. They were then tested for the effects of relaxation training on a performance task. In a single session, the subjects were first given a cognitive task (the memorizing and immediate recall of a list of common nouns); they then relaxed with the technique learned earlier. The cognitive task was repeated after the relaxation period. The results indicated that the amount of change in the performance after the relaxation period depended upon the initial level of the anxiety. The subjects with a high level of initial anxiety performed better on recall after relaxation, while the subjects with relatively low levels of initial anxiety showed an impairment of learning after relaxation.

The need for individual, group, and family therapy should be assessed. Appropriate therapy should be provided to help the elderly with personal, social, and family adaptations.

## D. ENVIRONMENTAL AND REALITY ORIENTATION PROGRAM

The reality orientation (RO) approach involves informing the patients about such things as the date, the time, the location, the patient's name, and staff names. Zepelin *et al*. (1977) carried out a yearlong study of RO program with a group of institutionalized elderly with varying degrees of disorientation and behavior deficits. They were compared with a control group that received routine institutional care. The effects of the program were evaluated at six-month intervals with the help of the Mental Status Questionnaire and a rating of Activities of Daily Living and interpersonal behaviors. The experimental group showed slight but statistically significant improvement on the mental status questionnaire after the first six months. There were no favorable effects on the Activities of Daily Living.

Eisdorfer *et al*. (1981) found that most of the studies evaluating RO program showed mixed results. They concluded that RO programs in the institutionalized elderly usually have no beneficial effects on social behavior or on self-care habits. It is to be expected, however, that RO programs would constitute only a small component of the total management of the demented elderly. Focusing on any narrow treatment approach to the exclusion of others in the present state of knowledge is certainly inappropriate.

## E. OTHER THERAPIES

Adjunct therapies such as art, music, and dance activities have a very important place in the institutional care of the elderly and demented individuals. They help keep their time occupied with meaningful activities. Although control studies are lacking and although it may be difficult to attribute specific behavior changes to adjunct therapy, there are many individuals in the institution who are more greatly benefited by these activities than by many other components of daily care.

## F. SUMMARY

Several studies (Plemore *et al.*, 1978; Sanders and Sanders, 1978) have shown that intellectual performance in old age is more modifiable through cognitive skill training than is traditionally assumed. When all the factors such as interest, motivation, anxiety, and depression are taken into consideration, improvement in the performance of the aged can be substantial with cognitive training.

Cognitive skill training, however, is not as effective in primary degenerative disease and only minor gains may be made with intensive efforts in specific areas. The gains may also be short-lasting due to the progressive nature of the disease. The primary hope for this group of individuals lies in the development of effective pharmacotherapy. None of the currently available drugs are able to halt or reverse cognitive deterioration. Mild to moderate improvement in cognitive functions are noticed in some patients with drugs, especially when they are treated in the early stages of the disease. However, these improvements have not been shown to last for a prolonged period of time. The total management of demented individuals at present requires careful attention to all physical and mental problems with multiple drug therapy, cognitive skill training, reality orientation, and adjunct therapies.

## G.   REFERENCES

Arrigo A, Braun P, Kauchtschischwili G, *et al*: Influence of treatment on symptomatology and correlated EEG changes in the aged. *Curr Ther Res* 1973; 15:417–426.

Abuzzahah F, Merwin G, Zimmerman R, *et al*: A double-blind investigation of piracetam (nootropic) versus placebo in the memory of geriatric inpatients. *Psychopharmacol Bull* 1978; 14:23–25.

Bajada S: A trial of choline chloride and physostigmine in Alzheimer's disease, in Corkin S, Davis K, Growden J (eds): *A Report of Progress in Research*, New York, Raven, 1982, pp 427–432.

Branconnier RJ: The efficacy of the central metabolic enhancers in the treatment of senile dementia. *Psychopharmacol Bull* 1983; 19:212–219.

Caltagirone C, Albanese A, Gainotti G: Oral administration of chronic physostigmine does not improve cognitive or amnesic performances in Alzheimer's presenile dementia. *Int J Neurosci* 1982; 16:247–249.

Caltagirone C, Albanese A, Gainotti G: Acute administration of individual optimal dose of physostigmine fails to improve amnesic performances in Alzheimer's presenile dementia. *Int J Neurosci* 1983; 18:143–147.

Cermak LS: Comments on imagery as a therapeutic mnemonic, in Poon L, Fozard J, Cermak L (eds): *New Directions in Memory and Aging: Proceedings of G Talland Memorial Conference* Hillside, NJ: Lawrence Erlbaum, 1980, pp 507–510.

Chase T, Durso R, Fedio P, *et al*: Vasopressin in treatment of cognitive deficits in Alzheimer's disease, in Corkin S, Davis K, Growdon J (eds): *Alzheimer's Disease: A Report of Progress in Research*. New York; Raven, 1982, pp 457–461.

Chouinard G, Annable L, Ross-Chouinard A, *et al*: Piracetam in elderly psychotic patients with mild diffuse cerebral impairment. *Psychopharmacology* 1983; 81:100–106.

Christie JE, Shering A, Ferguson J, *et al.*: Physostigmine and arecoline: Effects of intravenous infusions in Alzheimer presenile dementia. *Br J Psych* 1981; 138:46–50. Alzheimer's disease, in New York, Raven, 1982, pp 413–419.

Christie JE, Shering A, Ferguson J, *et al*: Physostigmine and arecoline: Effects of intravenous infusions in Alzheimer presenile dementia. *Brit J Psychiatry* 1981; 138:46–50.

Cohen E, Wurtman R: Brain acetylcholine: Increase after systemic choline administration. *Life Sci* 1975; 16:1095–1102.

Craik FI: Age differences in human memory, in Birren J, Schaie K (eds): *Handbook of the Psychology of the Aging*. New York, Van Nostrand Reinhold, 1977, pp 384–420.

Crook T, Ferris S, Sathananthan G, *et al*: The effect of methylphenidate on test performance in the cognitively impaired aged. *Psychopharmacology* 1977; 52:251–255.

Darvill FT: Double-blind evaluation of methylphenidate (Ritalin) hydrochloride—Its use in the management of institutionalized geriatric patients. *JAMA* 1959; 169:1739.

Davis K, Mohs R, Tinklenberg J, *et al*: Physostigmine: Improvement of long-term memory processes in normal humans. *Science* 1978; 201:272–274.

Davis K, Mohs R, Tinklenberg J, *et al*: Cholinomimetics and memory: The effect of choline chloride. *Arch Neurol* 1979a; 37:49–52.

Davis K, Mohs R, Tinklenberg J: Enhancement of memory by physostigmine. *N Engl J Med* 1979b; 301:946.

Denney NW: Clustering in middle and old age. *Dev Psychol* 1974; 10:471–475.

de Wied D: Behavioral actions of neurohypophysial peptides. *Proc R Soc (London) Ser B Biol Sci* 1980; 210:183–195.

Domino E, Minor L, Duff I, *et al*: Effects of oral lecithin on blood choline levels and memory tests in geriatric volunteers, in Corkin S, Davis K, Growdon J (eds): *Alzheimer's Disease: A Report of Progress in Research*. New York, Raven, 1982, pp 393–397.

Eisdorfer C: A double-blind, comparative study of Hydergine sublingual tablets vs placebo in hospitalized geriatrics. Data on file at Sandoz Inc, USA, 1975.

Eisdorfer C, Conner J, Wilkie F: The effects of magnesium pemoline on cognition and behavior. *J Gerontol* 1968; 23:283–288.

Eisdorfer C, Cohen D, Preston C: Behavioral and psychological therapies for the older patient with cognitive impairment, in Miller N, *et al* (eds): *Clinical Aspects of Alzheimer's Disease and Senile Dementia*. New York, Raven, 1981, pp 209–224.

Etienne P, Dastoor D, Gauthier S, *et al*: Lecithin in the treatment of Alzheimer's disease. In Corkin S, Davis K, Growdon J (eds): *Alzheimer's Disease: A Report of Progress in Research*. New York, Raven, 1982, pp 369–372.

Ferris S: Empirical studies in senile dementia with central nervous system stimulants and metabolic enhancers, in Crook T, Gershon S (eds): *Strategy for the Development of an Effective Treatment for Senile Dementia*. New Canaan, Conn, Mark Powderly, 1981, pp 173–188.

Ferris S, Reisberg S, Crook T, *et al*: Pharmacologic treatment of senile dementia: L-dopa, piracetam and choline plus piracetam, in Corkin S, *et al* (eds):*Alzheimer's Disease: A Report of Progress in Research*. New York, Raven, 1982, pp 475–481.

Gaitz C, Varner R, Overall J: Pharmacotherapy for organic brain syndrome in late life. Evaluation of an ergot derivative vs placebo. *Arch Gen Psychiatry* 1977; 34:839–845.

Gilbert J, Donnelly K, Zommer L, *et al*: Effects of magnesium pemoline and methylphenidate on memory improvement and mood in normal aging subjects. *Aging Hum Dev* 1973; 4:35–51.

Giurgea CE: The nootropic concept and its prospective implications. *Drug Dev Res* 1982; 2:463–474.

Glen A, Whalley L: *Alzheimer Disease: Early Recognition of Potentially Reversible Deficits*. Edinburgh, Churchill Livingston, 1979.

Gurland B, Fleiss J, Goldberg K, *et al*: The geriatric mental state schedule, II. Factor analysis. *Psychol Med* 1976; 6:451–459.

Haubrick D, Wang P, Clody D, *et al*: Increase in rat brain acetylcholine induced by choline or deanol. *Life Sci* 1975; 17:975–980.

Holliday A, Joffe J: A controlled evaluation of protriptyline compared to a placebo and to methylphenidate hydrochloride. J New Drugs 1965; 5:257 (abstr).

Hughes J, Williams J, Carrier R: An ergot alkaloid preparation (hydergine) in the treatment of dementia. Critical review of the clinical literature. *J Am Geriatr Soc* 1976; 24:490–497.

Itil T, Menon G, Bozak M, *et al*.: The effects of oxiracetam (ISF 2522) in patients with organic brain syndrome (a double-blind controlled study with piracetam). *Drug Dev Res* 1982; 2:447–461.

Kahn R: Psychological aspects of aging, in Rossmar I (ed): *Clinical Geriatrics*. Philadelphia, Lippincott, 1971.

Kahn R, Zarit S, Hilbert N, *et al*: Memory complaint and impairment in the aged: The effects of depression and altered brain function. *Arch Gen Psychiatry* 1975; 32:1569–1573.

Kaplitz S: Withdrawn, apathetic geriatric patient responsive to methylphenidate. *J Am Geriatr Soc* 1975; 23:71–76.

Mindus P, Cronholm B, Levander S, *et al*: Piracetam-induced improvement of mental performance: a controlled study on normally aging individuals. *Acta Psychiatr Scand* 1976; 54:150–160.

Mohs R, Davis K: Choline chloride effects on memory: Correlation with the effects of physostigmine. *Psychiatr Res* 1980; 2:149–156.

Mohs R, Davis K, Tinklenberg J, *et al*: Choline chloride effects on memory in the elderly. *Neurobiol Aging* 1980; 1:21–25.

Mohs R, Davis K, Johns C, *et al*: Oral physostigmine treatment of patients with Alzheimer's disease. *Am J Psychiatry* 1985; 142:28–33.

Peters B, Levin H: Chronic oral physostigmine and lecithin administration in memory disorders of aging, in Corkin S, Davis K, Growdon J (eds): *Alzheimer's Disease: A Report of Progress in Research*. New York, Raven, 1982, pp 421–426.

Plemor J, Willis S, Baltes P: Modifiability of fluid intelligence in aging: A short-term longitudinal training approach. *J Gerontol* 1978; 33:224–231.

Reisberg B, London E, Ferris S, *et al*: Novel pharmacologic approaches to the treatment of senile dementia of the Alzheimer type. *Psychopharmacol Bull* 1983; 19:220–225.

Rigter H, Hannan T, Messing R, *et al*: Enkephalins interfere with acquisition of an active avoidance response. *Life Sci* 1980; 26:337–345.

Sanders R, Sanders J: Long-term durability and transfer of enhanced conceptual performance in the elderly. *J Gerontol* 1978; 33:408–412.

Schmitt F, Murphy M, Sanders R: Training older adults. Free recall rehearsal strategies. *J Gerontol* 1981; 36:329–337.

Sitaram N, Weingartner H, Gillin J: Human serial learning: Enhancement with arecoline and impairment with scopolamine correlated with performance on placebo. *Science* 1978; 201:274–276.

Sullivan E, Shedlack K, Corkin S, *et al*: Physostigmine and lecithin in Alzheimer's disease, in Corkin S, Davis K, Growdon J (eds): *Alzheimer's Disease: A Report of Progress in Research*. New York, Raven, 1982, pp 361–367.

Tinklenberg J, Pigache R, Pfefferbaum A, *et al*: Vasopressin peptides and dementia, in Corkin S, Davis K, Growdon J (eds): *Alzheimer's Disease: A Report of Progress in Research*. New York, Raven, 1982, pp 463–468.

Venn RD: Review of clinical studies with ergots in gerontology. *Adv Biochem Psychopharmacol* 1980; 23:363–377.

Vroulis G, Smith R: Cholinergic drugs and memory disorders in Alzheimer's type dementia, in Enna SJ, Samorajski T, Beer B (eds): *Brain Neurotransmitters and Receptors in Aging and Age-related Disorders*. New York, Raven, 1981, pp 245–254.

Winograd E, Simon E: Visual memory and imagery in the aged, in Poon L, *et al* (eds): *New Directions in Memory and Aging: Proceedings of the George A Talland Memorial Conference*. Hillsdale, NJ, Lawrence Erlbaum, 1980, pp 487–506.

Yesavage JA: Imagery pretraining and memory training in the elderly. *Gerontology* 1983; 29:271–275.

Yesavage J, Tinklenberg J, Hollister L, *et al.*: Vasodilators in senile dementia: A review of the literature. *Arch Gen Psychiatr* 1979; 36:220–223.

Yesavage J, Rose T, Spiegel D: Relaxation training and memory improvement in elderly normals. Correlation of anxiety ratings and recall improvement. *Exp Aging Res* 1982; 8:195–198.

Young M, Gibson W: *How to Develop an Exceptional Memory*. Hollywood, Calif, Wilshire, 1975.

Zarit S, Kenneth D, Cole M, *et al*: Memory training strategies and subjective complaints of memory in the aged. *Gerontologist* 1981; 21:158–164.

Zepelin H, Wolfe C, Kleinplatz F: Evaluation of a year-long reality orientation program. *J Gerontol* 1977; 36:70–77.

# Author Index

Abuzzahah, F., 247, 253
Acker, W., 95, 98, 102
Adams, R., 99, 103, 169, 177
Adams, R. D., 166, 177
Agranoff, B. W., 69, 70, 71, 86
Aguilar, M. J., 137, 146
Aita, J. A., 182, 195
Akert, K., 21, 35
Albanese, A., 79, 86, 110, 117, 242, 254
Albert, M., 49, 64, 134, 145
Albert, M. L., 121, 132, 134, 139, 144
Albert, M. S., 49, 63
Aleksidze, N. G., 27, 35
Alexander, M. P., 153, 156
Alfrey, A. C., 168, 177
Alkana, R., 92, 102
Allen, S. R., 69, 86
Allweis, C., 15, 37
Alvord, E. C., Jr., 139, 144
Aminoff, M., 134, 144
Anders, T., 222, 236
Angel, L., 98, 102
Anisman, H., 110, 119
Annable, L., 247, 254
Arbuckle, T., 7, 35
Arrigo, A., 248, 253
Artunkal, S., 171, 177
Asher, R., 172, 177
Atkinson, R. C., 2, 11, 36
Austen, F. K., 166, 177

Babcock, H., 44, 63
Bacon, E., 74, 87
Bagley, C. R., 183, 195
Bajada, S., 244, 253

Balavadze, M. V., 27, 35
Baldwin, B., 13, 36
Baltes, P., 253, 255
Ban, T. A., 78, 81, 86
Banconnier, R. J., 247, 253
Bandle, E., 82, 86
Baratti, C. M., 109, 117
Barbizet, J., 42, 63, 220, 236
Barnes, D., 96, 103
Battig, W., 42, 65
Bauer, J. H., 18, 36
Bean, J., 109, 110, 119
Beard, A. W., 136, 144
Bearn, A. G., 136, 146
Beck, A. T., 200, 216
Beck, G., 174, 177
Beekhuis, M., 202, 218
Behan, P. O., 123, 144
Bellin, S., 98, 101
Belluzzi, J., 111, 117
Benson, D. F., 121, 145, 152, 156
Benton, A., 42, 47, 63, 64
Berg, L., 125, 145
Berger, R. J., 210, 216
Berry, R., 201, 217
Bettinger, L. A., 37
Bickford, R., 213, 218
Birnbaum, I., 92, 101, 102
Bisgrove, E., 90, 102
Bixler, E. O., 86
Bjork, R., 40
Blackwood, G., 109, 117
Blessed, G., 232, 237
Bloch, V., 37
Block, A. J., 166, 177
Bloom, F., 235, 237
Bloomfield, C. D., 124, 147

Bluestone, H., 171, 177
Blusewicz, M., 101
Bobillier, P., 30, 36
Bock, E., 24, 36
Bogoch, S., 23, 36
Boll, T. J., 139, 146
Boller, F., 139, 142, 145
Bolton, N., 127, 145
Bond, M., 183, 189, 196
Bond, M. R., 182, 195
Borg, S., 97, 101
Borisov, M. M., 97, 101
Borst, M., 231, 236
Botwinik, J., 221, 236
Boucher, J., 202, 217
Bourke, R., 182, 188, 193, 196
Bower, G., 7, 36
Boyd, W. E., 109, 117
Bozak, M., 247, 255
Braakman, R., 183, 196
Brady, J., 22, 36
Braham, J., 71, 87
Brandt, J., 134, 144
Bratgaard, S. O., 24, 36
Braun, P., 253
Breger, L., 29, 36
Brizzee, J. R., 231, 236
Broadbent, D., 57, 64, 222, 236
Brody, H., 230, 236
Bromley, D. B., 221, 236
Brooks, D. N., 186, 189, 190, 191, 192, 193, 195, 196
Brown, E., 51, 64
Brown, G., 140, 145, 155, 156
Brown, J., 8, 36
Brown, K., 109, 119

Brown, W. J., 137, 146
Bruetsch, W. L., 158, 163
Brutton, D. G., 127, 145
Buchhalter, J., 103
Bucy, P., 21, 38
Buell, S. J., 231, 236
Bures, J., 13, 36
Buresova, O., 13, 36
Burks, J., 168, 177
Burks, J. S., 168, 177
Burns, B. D., 14, 36, 230, 236
Burnsten, B., 171, 177
Burrell, H. R., 68, 86
Bursill, A. E., 76, 86
Butler, A., 90, 102
Butters, N., 40, 64, 90, 134,
    144, 145

Caine, E., 109, 119, 133, 134,
    135, 145, 147
Caird, W., 221, 237
Caird, W. K., 127, 145
Calahan, D., 94, 101
Caleve, A., 201, 202, 217
Caltagirone, C., 79, 86, 110,
    117, 242, 254
Campbell, B., 209, 217
Cany, E., 42, 63, 220, 236
Carey, R., 114, 118
Carlen, P., 98, 101
Carlton, P., 109, 118
Carmichael, M. W., 166, 177
Carrasco, M., 111, 118
Carrier, R., 248, 255
Cartwright, R., 211, 217
Celesia, G., 140, 145
Cerf, J., 13, 36
Cermak, L., 102, 134, 145
Cermak, L. S., 250, 254
Chaney, E., 99, 102
Chapman, J., 222, 237
Chase, T., 249, 254
Chow, K. L., 19, 36
Christensen, A., 52, 56, 64
Christiaasen, R., 12, 36
Christie, J. E., 241, 243, 254
Chubb, N. C., 87
Clark, L., 220, 236
Clark, W., 225, 237
Clarke, P. R., 73, 86
Cleeland, C. S., 191, 196
Cleghorn, R. A., 174, 177
Cleveland, S., 127, 145
Clifton, G., 182, 195

Clody, D., 243, 255
Cohen, D., 248, 254
Cohen, E., 166, 177, 243, 254
Cohen, M. R., 84, 86
Cohouinard, G., 247, 254
Cole, M., 169, 177, 250, 256
Coleman, P. D., 231, 236
Collins, G., 99, 103
Colquohoun, W., 89, 101
Conners, C. K., 76, 86
Connor, J., 254
Conrad, R., 223, 236
Cooper, P., 57, 64
Cooper, R. M., 18, 36
Corkin, S., 241, 255
Corsi, P. M., 22, 36
Craik, F. I., 11, 36, 221, 222,
    224, 227, 228, 236, 250, 254
Crapper, D. R., 123, 145
Crenshaw, D. A., 225, 236
Cronholm, B., 51, 64, 247,
    255
Crook, T., 245, 247, 254
Crossen, B., 56, 64
Crovitz, H., 188, 195
Crow, R. J., 76, 86
Crowell, R. M., 175, 177
Cuben, L., 125, 145
Cumin, R., 82, 86
Cummings, J., 133, 137, 146,
    147
Cummings, J. L., 121, 145,
    152, 156
Cury, L., 134, 146

Dalby, A., 128, 145
Dalby, M. A., 128, 145
Dallett, J., 20, 36
Damasio, A., 42, 63
D'Amour, M., 96, 101
Darvill, F. T., 245, 254
Dastoor, D., 244, 254
David, D., 109, 118
Davidson, E., 168, 169, 178
Davidson, K., 183, 195
Davies, D. L., 143, 145
Davies, P., 233, 237
Davis, B., 242, 255
Davis, B. M., 79, 86
Davis, K., 59, 65, 109, 118,
    241, 243, 254
Davis, K. L., 79, 86
Day, L., 102
Daye, C., 222, 237

Dawson, J. R., 159, 163
Dedicova, A., 112, 118
Degrell, I., 234, 236
Dejerine, J., 18, 36
de Leon, M., 60, 64
Delersea, R., 230, 238
Delgado, J. M., 21, 36
Del Rio, E., 112, 119
De Luca, D., 102
Denker, S. J., 189, 196
Denny, N. W., 250, 254
Denny-Brown, D., 181, 196
Denti, A., 30, 36
Depry, D., 89, 102
De Renzi, E., 154, 156
De Teresa, R., 124, 147
Deutsch, J., 109, 118
Deutsch, J. A., 27, 36
Dewan, E. M., 29, 36
Dewar, A., 233, 237
Dewhurst, K., 133, 145
deWied, D., 248, 254
DeWeid, H., 113, 119
Diamond, M., 39
Diamond, M. C., 26, 36, 230,
    236
Dias, R., 111, 112, 118
Digre, K., 42, 64
Diller, L., 140, 145
DiLolla, V., 3, 36
Dixon, D., 30, 38
Dixon, J. C., 128, 145
Dobias, B., 161, 162, 163
Dodrill, C., 56, 64
Dokas, L. A., 68, 86
Domhaff, B., 210, 217
Domino, E., 244, 254
Donnelly, K., 246, 255
Dooling, D., 12, 36
Dooling, E. C., 137, 145
Drachman, D., 223, 237
Drew, G., 89, 101
Drucker-Collin, R., 30, 36,
    115, 116, 118
Duara, R., 234, 237
Dudycha, G., 209, 217
Dudycha, M., 209, 217
Duff, I., 244, 254
Dundee, J., 73, 87
Dunn, A., 113, 118
Durso, R., 249, 254
Dustman, R., 101
Dyck, P. J., 234, 237
Dysinger, D., 127, 145

Ebert, M., 133, 134, 135, 145, 147
Eccersley, P. S., 73, 86
Edmonds, H., Jr., 98, 101
Egyhazi, E., 87
Eich, J. E., 91, 101
Eisdorfer, C., 246, 248, 252, 254
Eisenberg, L., 76, 86
Ekdahl, M., 44, 45, 65
Elizan, T. S., 141, 145
Elliott, J., 12, 37
Engel, G., 174, 177
Ensrud, K., 124, 147
Erber, J., 225, 237
Erickson, R., 50, 57, 64
Eriksen, C., 222, 237
Erlebacher, A. H., 6, 39
Ernst, B., 128, 145
Ervin, F., 28, 36
Eslinger, P., 42, 63
Eson, M. E., 182, 188, 193, 196
Essman, W. B., 71, 77, 86, 108, 118
Etienne, P., 244, 254
Evans, M., 89, 101
Ewert, J., 136, 145
Eysenck, M. W., 227, 237

Fedio, P., 22, 37, 249, 254
Feldman, R. G., 121, 123, 132, 144
Ferguson, J., 241, 254
Fernandez-Guardiola, A., 20, 37
Ferris, S., 60, 64, 65, 245, 247, 254
Fiedler, P., 19, 38
Fields, W. S., 152, 156
Finger, S., 39
Fischer, J. E., 169, 178
Fitz, T. E., 174, 177
Fitzgerald, P., 57, 64
Fleiss, J., 250, 255
Fleminger, J., 201, 218
Flexner, A., 8, 37
Flood, J., 106, 118
Fogarty, S., 200, 217
Folstein, M., 134, 146
Ford, J., 132, 146
Fortuny, L. A., 180, 196
Foulkes, D., 210, 217, 218
Fowler, R. S., Jr., 46, 64

Fox, C., 181, 197
Fozard, J., 222, 236
Frame, B., 174, 177
Frazer, D. C., 224, 237
Freud, S., 210, 217
Frieder, B., 15, 37
Friedman, A. S., 199, 217
Friedman, H., 221, 237
Friedman, J. H., 166, 177
Frisby, J. P., 73, 86
Fuld, P., 49, 64

Gainotti, G., 79, 86, 110, 117, 242, 254
Gaitz, C., 248, 255
Gajdusek, D. C., 160, 163
Gallagher, D., 200, 218
Gallbraith, S., 191, 196
Gamzu, E., 82, 86
Garralda, M., 201, 218
Garron, D. C., 150, 156
Gauthier, S., 244, 254
Gazzaniga, M. C., 18, 39
Gendelman, S., 176, 178
Gennavelli, T. A., 181, 196
Gerald, R., 13, 39
Gerstmann, J., 19, 37
Geschwind, N., 18, 37, 153, 156
Gibbons, J. L., 173, 177
Gibson, W., 251, 256
Gideon, D. A., 151, 156
Gilbert, J., 246, 255
Gililand, A. R., 77, 87
Gill, M., 43, 64
Gillin, J., 109, 119, 243, 255
Gilman, S., 143, 145
Ginn, H. E., 167, 177
Gispen, W., 113, 118
Giurgea, C. E., 246, 255
Glen, A., 110, 118, 242, 255
Glendenning, R. L., 17, 37
Glickman, S. E., 214, 217
Globus, A., 26, 37
Gold, M., 40
Gold, P., 107, 118
Goldberg, K., 250, 255
Golden, C. J., 56, 64
Goldman, H., 56, 65
Goldman, M., 93, 103
Goldman, S., 12, 37
Goldstein, N. D., 136, 145
Gomanko, M., 98, 103
Goochee, C., 234, 238

Goodell, H., 140, 146
Goodhardt, M., 130, 147, 233, 238
Goodwin, D., 93, 102
Gordon, S., 225, 237
Gorham, D., 60, 64
Graesser, A., 8, 37
Graham-White, J., 109, 117
Graves, R. J., 171, 177
Greekie, C., 95, 99, 102
Greenberg, R., 29, 37
Greenfield, J. G., 142, 142, 145
Greenough, W., 26, 37
Gregg, J. M., 73, 87
Gregory, M., 222, 236
Grinker, R., 202, 214, 217
Groat, R., 181, 197
Groat, R. A., 181, 182, 196
Groher, M., 189, 196
Gromova, E. A., 27, 37
Gross, M., 87
Gross, M. D., 74, 75, 87
Grossman, R., 182, 195
Grossman, R. G., 188, 190, 103, 196
Grossman, S., 109, 110, 119
Gruenberg, E., 123, 145
Gruesen, R., 21, 35
Gurland, B., 250, 255
Gustafson, L., 128, 145
Guthrie, A., 95, 99, 102
Guzikov, B., 98, 103

Haaland, K., 140, 146
Hachinski, V., 59, 64
Hadfield, J., 213, 217
Hagberg, B., 128, 145
Hagen, D., 127, 146
Hakim, S., 175, 177
Hall, C., 210, 217
Hallervorden, H., 145
Hallman, B. L., 174, 177
Halstead, W., 38, 48, 64
Hamlin, R., 222, 237
Hamsher, K. deS., 42, 63, 64
Hannah, F., 127, 145
Hannon, R., 90, 102
Hannover, A., 231, 237
Hansch, E. C., 139, 146
Hanson, W., 122, 146
harmatz, J., 65
Harris, J., Jr., 191, 196
Hartman, F. A., 174, 177

Haruda, F., 166, 177
Harwood, E., 225, 226, 237
Haubrick, D., 243, 255
Haxby, J., 234, 237
Haynes, C. D., 151, 156
Hebb, D. O., 14, 37
Hecaen, H., 18, 37
Heimstra, N. W., 83, 87
Hemsley, D., 200, 217
Hennevin, E., 29, 37
Henri, C., 209, 217
Henri, V., 209, 217
Henry, C. E., 167, 177
Henry, R., 191, 196
Henschen, S. E., 18, 37
Heron, A., 222, 236
Heston, L. L., 124, 145
Hilbert, N., 200, 217, 250, 255
Hilgard, E., 14, 37
Hill, S., 93, 102
Hille, B., 223, 236
Hiller, J., 98, 102
Hlasny, R., 211, 217
Hobson, J., 211, 217
Hobson, J. A., 210, 217
Hoehn-Saric, R., 74, 86
Holliday, A., 245, 255
Hollingshead, A., 94, 102
Hollister, L., 248, 256
Holloway, J., 103
Holloway, R., 26, 37
Hopper, S., 93, 102
Horel, J. A., 17, 37
Horn, R., 187, 195
Howell, S., 227, 237
Hubel, D., 32, 37
Huddlestone, J., 168, 177
Hughes, C., 125, 145
Hughes, J., 248, 255
Hughes, R., 12, 37, 134, 145
Huntington, G., 133, 146
Hunyadi, J., 115, 116, 118
Hurst, M., 57, 64
Hurst, P. M., 77, 87
Huston, A., 137, 146
Huston, J., 111, 119
Huygen, P., 109, 117
Hyden, H., 25, 26, 37, 87

Idzikowski, C., 69, 87
Iliff, L., 59, 64
Inglis, J., 127, 146, 221, 237
Inman, V., 227, 237

Iramain, C., 97, 102
Irwin, J., 10, 38
Itil, T., 247, 255
Izquierdo, I., 111, 112, 118

Jackson, J., 132, 146
Jacobs, G., 211, 217
Jakoubek, B., 112, 118
James, M., 46, 65
James, W., 1, 37
Jankovic, J., 132, 146
Jannett, B., 180, 183, 196
Jarvik, M., 106, 118, 199, 218
Javid, H., 150, 156
Jenkins, C., 57, 64
Jensen, R., 106, 118
Joffe, J., 245, 255
John, E. R., 14, 37
Johns, C., 242, 255
Johnson, J. H., 201, 217
Johnson, N., 90, 102
Johnson, W., 171, 177
Jones, B., 90, 92, 93, 102
Jones, G., 8, 37
Jones, M., 90, 92, 93, 102
Jongeward, R., 40
Joseassen, R., 134, 146
Jouvet, M., 20, 37
Judge, T. G., 170, 177

Kaada, B. R., 21, 37
Kahn, R., 200, 217, 250, 255
Kanner, L., 203, 217
Kaplan, D., 103
Kaplan, E., 153, 156
Kaplitz, S., 245, 255
Karlsberk, W. D., 179, 196
Karpati, G., 174, 177
Kasniak, A., 139, 147
Katz, J., 23, 38
Katz, W., 7, 35
Kauchtschischwili, G., 253
Kayton, L., 201, 217
Keet, J., 130, 147, 233, 238
Keiper, C. G., 77, 87
Kelley, M. P., 150, 156
Kelly, H. P., 3, 38
Kendrick, D., 128, 146
Kenneth, D., 250, 256
Kesner, R. P., 19, 28, 29, 30, 38
Keyes, J. B., 113, 118
Khan, A., vi, 31, 38
Kharlamov, A. N., 82, 87

Kiklusak, C., 103
Kimble, D. P., 45, 64
King, M. G., 106, 119
Kinsbourne, M., 224, 237
Kirby, R. J., 19, 38
Klawans, H., 139, 147
Klein, M., 213, 217
Kleinman, K., 56, 65
Kleinplatz, F., 252, 256
Klinger, D., 201, 217
Klove, H., 56, 64, 191, 196
Kluver, H., 21, 38
Knehr, C. A., 136, 146
Knowles, J., 220, 236
Koh, S., 201, 202, 217
Korboot, P., 201, 217
Kornetsky, C., 74, 87
Korsakoff, S. S., 1, 38
Kraiuchiunas, R., 222, 237
Kramer, M., 211, 217
Kremin, H., 18, 37
Krishnan, S. S., 123, 145
Krop, H. D., 166, 177
Krug, M., 25, 38
Kummer, P., 234, 236
Kuriyama, K., 97, 102
Kvande, H., 97, 101

Laczi, F., 114, 118
Laidlow, G., 169, 178
Landfield, P., 36
Larson, J., 210, 217
Lashley, K. S., 17, 38
Laszlo, F., 114, 118
Laurence, M. W., 225, 237
Lauria, A. R., 184, 196
Lawson, J., 222, 237
Leavitt, J., 223, 237
Leboucq, G., 230, 237
LeConte, P., 37
Lederman, R. J., 167, 177
Lee, C., 92, 103
Lehmann, D., 235, 237
Levander, S., 247, 255
Levin, H., 244, 255
Levin, K. H., 42, 47, 63
Levine, H. S., 188, 190, 193, 196
Levy, L., 44, 63
Levy, N., 214, 217
Lewis, V., 8, 36
Ley, R., 43, 64
Lezak, M., 41, 64
Lezak, M. D., 190, 196

Liedderman, P. H., 29, 37
Liljequist, R., 109, 118
Lilliquist, T., 222, 236
Lindboe, C., 103
Lindgren, A., 129, 146
Lindsay, A., 134, 146
Linnoila, M., 73, 87
Lishman, W., 95, 98, 102
Lishman, W. A., 125, 146
Lisman, S. A., 102
Liz, T., 171, 177
Locascio, D., 43, 64
Lockhart, T., 11, 36
Long, H., 89, 101
Lorente de No, R., 14, 38
Lorsbach, T. C., 223, 237
LoVerme, S., Jr., 121, 145

Macht, M. L., 223, 237
MacVane, J., 90, 102
Madden, D. J., 226, 237
Madill, M., 91, 102
Magoun, H., 181, 182, 196
Maguire, W. M., 2, 38
Makela, M., 182, 195
Mandleberg, I. A., 186, 196
Mandler, G., 8, 37, 38, 225,
  237
Margolin, S., 174, 177
Mark, V., 175, 177
Marquis, D., 14, 37
Marshall, J., 134, 144
Martinez, J., 106, 111, 118
Martz, R., 89, 101
Marusarz, T., 202, 217
Maslenilov, V., 152, 156
Matarazzo, J., 56, 64
Matarazzo, R., 56, 64
Mathan, D., 180, 196
Mathies, H., 25, 38, 109, 119
Matthews, C. G., 140, 146
Mattila, M., 87, 109, 118
Mayeux, R., 140, 146
McAllister, T., 160, 163
McCarley, R., 210, 217
McCarty, R., 106, 118
McDermott, L., 110, 119
McGaugh, J. L., 28, 38, 83,
  86, 106, 119
McGeer, E., 232, 237
McGeer, P., 232, 237
McGhie, A., 201, 217, 222,
  237
McHugh, P., 134, 146

McKay, A., 233, 237
McKinley, W. W., 189, 196
Meerloo, J., 205, 218
Meggison, D. L., 225, 238
Mello, N., 93, 102
Melton, A., 10, 38
Mendelson, J., 93, 102
Menon, G., 247, 255
Merwin, G., 247, 253
Messing, R., 106, 118
Metter, E. J., 122, 146
Meyer, G. E., 2, 38
Meyer, J., 152, 156
Michael, R. D., 173, 177
Miczek, K. A., 109, 119
Miller, E., 43, 64, 125, 126,
  127, 128, 146
Miller, G. A., 4, 38
Miller, M., 114, 118
Miller, R. R., 215, 218
Miller, W. R., 94, 102
Mills, K., 90, 102
Milner, B., 3, 21, 28, 38, 39,
  48, 49, 64
Milo, J., 109, 117
Mindus, P., 247, 255
Minor, L., 244, 254
Mishell, J. M., 168, 177
Mitchel, V. E., 77, 87
Mizutani, T., 139, 142, 145
Modan, M., 71, 87
Mohs, R., 59, 65, 109, 118,
  241, 242, 243, 254, 255
Molander, L., 51, 64
Mollenauer, S., 109, 110, 119
Mollgaard, K., 39
Monk, A., 8, 36, 202, 217
Monroe, L., 210, 218
Montgomery, K., 90, 102,
  145
Moor, B. W., 23, 38
Morgane, P. G., 116, 119
Morley, B., 109, 119
Mortimer, J. A., 139, 146
Moskowitz, H., 89, 92, 102
Murdock, B. B., Jr., 4, 38
Murphy, M., 251, 255
Murray, J., 89, 92, 102
Myers, R., 19, 39
Myers, R. E., 19, 38

Nandy, K., 123, 146
Nathan, P., 13, 39
Naus, M., 102

Nauta, W., 22, 36
Naylor, G., 225, 226, 237
Negishi, K., 39
Neisser, U., 226, 237
Nelson, T., 12, 38
Newcome, F., 45, 64
Noble, E., 92, 102
Nobles, C. E., 64
Norman, D. A., 3, 6, 10, 38
Nott, P., 201, 218

O'Brien, P., 234, 237
O'Connell, D., 214, 218
Oei, T. P., 106, 119
Olds, J., 22, 38
O'Leary, M., 99, 102
Olivarus, Bde, F., 172, 177
Oliver, J., 133, 145
Olsen, S., 167, 178
Olszewski, J., 131, 147
Ommaya, A., 181, 196
Orme, J. E., 128, 146
Orme, M., 214, 218
Orne, M. T., 212, 218
Osborne, D., 51, 64
Oswald, I., 69, 87
Otis, L., 13, 36
Ott, T., 109, 119
Ottoson, J., 51, 64
Overall, J., 60, 64, 248, 255
Overstreet, D. H., 109, 119
Owasoyo, J., 97, 102
Owens, W. A., 228, 237

Pandit, S. K., 73, 87
Park, D. C., 227, 237
Parker, E., 92, 101, 102
Parker, S. A., 189, 192, 196
Partington, M. W., 179, 196
Pate, J., 161, 162, 163
Pearlman, C., 29, 37
Peck, A., 124, 147, 230, 238
Pellegrino, J., 12, 37
Penfield, W., 22, 38
Perozzolo, F. J., 146
Perry, E., 232, 237
Perry, M., 111, 112, 118
Perry, R., 232, 237
Peters, B. H., 193, 196
Peters, B., 244, 255
Petersen, P., 175, 178
Petersen, R. C., 109, 119
Petkinovich, L. F., 83, 87
Pettit, M., 74, 87

Pfefferbaum, A., 249, 255
Pickett, D., 30, 38
Pigache, R., 249, 255
Pirozzolo, F. J., 139, 146
Plemor, J., 253, 255
Pless, J., 89, 103
Plotnick, R., 109, 110, 119
Popkin, S., 200, 218
Porov, V., 25, 38
Porter, A. L., 72, 87
Post, F., 128, 146
Postman, L., 9, 38
Prange, A. J., Jr., 171, 172, 178
Presley, A., 95, 99, 102
Preston, C., 248, 254
Price, T. R., 160, 163
Puglis, J., 227, 237
Puretz, S., 39

Quartron, G. C., 69, 72, 76, 86, 87
Quijo, J., 99, 102
Quittkat, S., 123, 145

Radford, L., 99, 102
Radlow, R., 87
Rado, S., 202, 218
Randall, R., 136, 145
Randall, W., 19, 36
Randt, D., 51, 64
Ransmeier, R., 13, 38
Rapaport, D., 43, 64
Rapoport, S. I., 234, 237
Rasch, E., 24, 39
Rasmussen, W., 213, 218
Rassmussen, T., 22, 38
Rauscher, G., 97, 102
Rawat, A. K., 97, 102
Rawson, R., 173, 178
Rayevsky, K. S., 82, 87
Rechtschaffen, A., 210, 218
Redlich, F., 94, 102
Reed, E., 169, 178
Reed, H., 134, 146
Regina, E. G., 77, 87
Reidman, D., 112, 119
Reiff, R., 213, 214, 218
Reige, W., 122, 146
Reisberg, B., 60, 64, 65, 249, 255
Reisberg, R. B., 97, 103
Reisberg, S., 247, 254
Reitan, R. M., 56, 65, 139,

146, 172, 178, 182, 195
Remington, G., 110, 119
Rezdilsky, B., 137, 146
Rice, E., 176, 178
Richardson, E., Jr., 137, 145
Richardson, J. C., 131, 147
Riege, W., 92, 95, 103, 226, 237
Riesen, A., 24, 38
Riezen, H., 113, 119
Rigter, H., 106, 111, 113, 118, 119, 249, 255
Riklan, M., 140, 145
Riley, J., 96, 103
Robbins, L., 171, 178
Robertson, B., 224, 238
Robinowitz, J. C., 225, 238
Rockford, G., 129, 146
Rodda, B., 89, 101
Roder, E., 172, 177
Roemer, R., 134, 146
Roessmann, V., 139, 142, 145
Rogde, S., 103
Rogers, J., 235, 237
Romanek, I., 211, 217
Ron, M., 95, 98, 102, 201, 218
Rose, J. E., 188, 190, 193, 196
Rose, R., 57, 64
Rose, T., 252, 256
Rosen, J., 140, 146
Rosen, L., 92, 103
Rosen, W., 59, 65
Rosenweig, M., 26, 39
Ross, J., 110, 119
Ross, S., 77, 87
Ross-Chouinard, A., 247, 254
Roth, M., 123, 146
Rowntree, L., 173, 178
Royce, G. J., 37
Rozin, P., 17, 39
Ruesch, J., 46, 65
Russell, E. W., 50, 65
Russell, M., 200, 218
Russell, P., 202, 218
Russell, W., 13, 39, 181, 196
Russell, W. R., 180, 185, 186, 196
Russin, R., 109, 119
Ryan, D. E., 73, 87
Ryback, R. S., 95, 103

Sacks, O. W., 137, 146
Sadeh, M., 71, 87

Saisy, T., 152, 156
Sakai, F., 30, 36
Sakitt, B., 2, 39
Salzman, C., 65
Sambursky, J., 161, 162, 163
Sanders, H., 49, 65
Sanders, J., 253, 255
Sanders, R., 251, 253, 255
Sathananthan, G., 245, 254
Saucedo, C., 92, 94, 102
Savage, R., 127, 145
Sax, D., 134, 145
Schafer, R., 43, 64
Schail, K., 229, 238
Scharf, M. B., 86
Scheerer, M., 213, 214, 218
Schenkenberg, T., 101
Schmitt, F., 251, 255
Schmitt, M. A., 153, 156
Schneck, M., 60, 65
Schneider, W., 4, 39
Schoene, W., 137, 145
Schon, M., 173, 178
Schonfield, D., 220, 224, 238
Schreiber, D., 56, 65
Schulman, H. G., 39
Schulster, J., 57, 65
Schultz, P., 234, 237
Schwarz, B., 213, 218
Scott, J., 112, 119
Scott, M., 50, 57, 64
Scotti, G., 154, 156
Scoville, W. S., 3, 21, 39
Sedvalle, G., 97, 101
Sell, S. H., 161, 162, 163
Semiginovsky, B., 112, 118
Sem-Jacobsen, C., 22, 39
Sequin, S., 30, 36
Serota, N., 214, 217
Serrats, A. F., 189, 192, 196
Shader, R., 65
Shahani, B., 96, 101
Sharpe, L., 76, 86
Shashoua, V. E., 26, 39
Shedlack, K., 241, 255
Shefer, V. F., 230, 238
Shering, A., 241, 254
Sherlock, S., 168, 169, 178
Shiffrin, R. M., 2, 3, 4, 11, 28, 36, 39
Shor, R., 214, 218
Sidell, F., 89, 103
Silversides, J. L., 134, 146
Silberstein, M., 49, 65, 226,

Silberstein, M. (*cont.*)
 238
Simon, E., 98, 102, 250, 256
Simons, D., 17, 39
Simpson, G. B., 223, 237
Singh, J. K., 109, 119
Sitaram, N., 79, 87, 109, 119, 243, 255
Sjogren, H., 129, 146
Sjogren, R., 129, 146
Slater, P., 57, 65, 127, 146
Sloane, M. C., 213, 218
Smit, G., 26, 39
Smith, A., 42, 52, 65
Smith, C., 109, 119
Smith, C. B., 234, 238
Smith, E., 134, 144, 189, 196
Smith, G., 106, 118
Smith, G. M., 77, 87
Smith, J., 191, 196
Smith, R., 244, 256
Snell, A., 173, 178
Soeters, P. B., 169, 178
Soldatos, C. R., 86
Soltysik, S., 13, 36
Sorenstein, S., 143, 145
Spanis, C., 30, 36, 115, 116, 118
Spatz, M., 145
Spear, N., 209, 217
Sperry, R. W., 18, 39
Spiegel, D., 252, 256
Spiliotis, P. H., 17, 19, 39
Spinnler, H., 154, 156
Springer, A. D., 68, 69, 86
Springer, A. S., 215, 218
Squire, L., 57, 65, 127, 146
Squire, L. R., 46, 65, 68, 87
Stanbli, U., 111, 119
Steele, J. C., 131, 147
Stein, L., 111, 117
Steisel, A., 209, 218
Stern, W. C., 116, 119
Stern, Y., 140, 146
Sternberg, D., 106, 118, 199, 218
Sternberg, S., 222
Stoll, W. A., 174, 178
Storandt, M., 221, 236
Strother, C., 227, 238
Sullivan, E., 241, 255
Summerskill, W. H., 168, 169, 178
Sutherland, A., 173, 178

Swanson, E., 210, 217
Swash, M., 109, 119
Sweet, W., 36
Swigt, H., 24, 39
Sylinski, I., 98, 103
Symonds, C. P., 187, 196
Sylvester, D., 98, 101
Sze, P., 97, 102

Tagliente, T., 72, 87
Talland, G., 221, 238
Talland, G. A., 44, 45, 57, 65, 72, 76, 87, 103
Taub, H. A., 221, 238
Taylor, F., 205, 218
Taylor, P., 191, 196
Teasdale, G., 180, 183, 196
Teasdale, J., 200, 218
Tejani, A., 161, 162, 163
Tennent, T., 183, 196
Terry, R. D., 124, 147, 230, 238
Tew, J. M., 175, 177
Thibault, L., 181, 196
Thomas, G., 19, 38
Thompson, L., 200, 218, 220, 238
Thompson, R., 17, 18, 19, 39
Thorn, S., 174, 177
Thorn, W. A., 212, 218
Tinklenberg, J., 79, 86, 109, 118, 241, 243, 248, 249, 354
Toglia, M. P., 42, 65
Togrol, B., 171, 177
Tomlinson, B. E., 124, 147
Toone, B., 201, 218
Tooth, G., 191, 197
Torvik, A., 98, 103
Treadway, C. R., 171, 172, 178
Trick, K., 133, 145
Trimble, M. R., 133, 147
Troupin, A., 56, 64
Tulving, E., 6, 7, 8, 9, 37, 39, 227, 236
Turner, D., 73, 87

Underwood, B. J., 6, 39
Uylings, H. B., 26, 39

Valchar, M., 97, 103
Valkusz, Z., 114, 118
Van Allen, M., 42, 47, 63
Van Buren, J., 22, 37

Van Buskirk, R., 106, 118
Van der Poel, A. M., 109, 119
Van Riezin, H., 113, 119
Varner, R., 248, 255
Varney, M., 42, 63
Vasquez, B., 106, 118
Velten, E., 200, 218
Venables, P., 202, 217
Venn, R. D., 248, 256
Verzeano, M., 14, 39
Victor, M., 99, 103
Vinson, D., 171, 178
Volkmar, F., 26, 37
Von Forester, H., 39
Vroulis, G., 244, 256

Waldfogel, S., 209, 218
Walker, D. W., 96, 103
Walsh, S., 220, 238
Walter, D., 187, 195
Walton, D., 199, 218
Wanamaker, W., 140, 145
Wang, P., 243, 255
Warburton, D., 109, 119
Warren, R., 56, 64
Warrington, E., 46, 49, 65, 147, 226, 238
Watkins, M., 9, 40
Watkins, M. J., 4, 39
Watkins, O., 7, 39
Webb, W., 161, 162, 163
Wechsler, D., 50, 65
Weiland, I., 209, 218
Weingartner, H., 79, 84, 86, 87, 109, 119, 133, 134, 135, 145, 147, 243, 255
Weiskrantz, L., 147
Wells, F. L., 46, 65
Wenger, L., 220, 238
Wetzel, C., 127, 146
Whalley, L., 110, 118, 242, 255
Whalley, L. J., 94, 103
White, P., 130, 147, 233, 238
White, W., 99, 103
Whitehorn, J., 171
Whybrow, P. C., 171, 172, 178
Wiesel, T., 32, 37
Wilcox, K. W., 214, 215, 218
Wilkenson, D., 98, 101
Wilkie, F., 254
Williams, D., 93, 103

Williams, J., 248, 255
Williams, M., 43, 65, 187, 197
Williams, R., 93, 103
Williams, T., 201, 217
Willis, A. L., 121, 132, 144
Wilson, J., 73, 87
Wilson, R. S., 139, 147
Wilson, S. A., 135, 136, 147
Wilson, W., 140, 145, 155
Wilson, W. P., 156
Windle, W., 181, 182, 196
Windle, W. F., 181, 197
Winograd, E., 150, 156

Wolfe, C., 252, 256
Woodward, A., Jr., 11, 40
Woolley, D. W., 107, 119
Woolsey, C., 21, 35
Worden, P. E., 225, 238
Wortzman, G., 98, 101
Wrens, A., 56, 64
Wurtman, R., 243, 254
Wynne, R., 74, 87

Yamamura, H., 109, 118
Yates, A., 201, 217
Yen, J., 188, 193, 196
Yesavage, J., 248, 252, 256
Yesavage, J. A., 250, 256

Young, L. D., 91, 103
Young, M., 251, 256
Young, R., 96, 101
Yunix, J. Y., 124, 147

Zangwill, O. L., 6, 40
Zarit, S., 200, 217, 250, 255
Zenner, K., 243, 236
Zepelin, H., 252, 256
Zilhka, E., 59, 64
Zimmerman, R., 247, 253
Zommer, L., 246, 255
Zornetzer, S., 235, 237
Zornetzer, S. F., 20, 40, 71, 87

# Subject Index

Acalculia
  angular gyrus syndrome, 152
  localization of lesions, 18, 19
Acetylcholine, 108, 116, 240, 241, 244, 245
Acute alcoholic intoxication, 91–94, 100
  alcoholic blackouts, 93, 94
  memory storage and retrieval, 91–93
  state-dependent learning, 91
Addison's disease, 173, 174, 177
Adrenocorticotropic hormones, 112–114, 170,
    248
Age regression, hypnosis, 213, 214
Agnosia, 144
  Alzheimer's disease, 129
  Pick's disease, 130
Agraphia
  alexia and, localization of lesions, 18
  angular gyrus syndrome, 152
Alexia, localization of lesions, 18
Alcohol abuse, memory disorders, 239
Alcohol blackouts, 93, 94
Alcohol dementia, 99
Alcohol and memory impairment, 89–101
Alcohol state-dependent learning, 91, 100
Alzheimer's disease, 121–129, 144
  cholinergic system, 109, 110, 116, 117, 124
  cognitive and emotional changes, 125–129
  comparison with angular gyrus syndrome,
    152–154, 156
  etiology, 123, 124
  memory disorders, 239
  memory scales, 59, 60
  neuropathology, 124
  treatment
    cholinergic drugs, 240–245
    neuropeptides, 249
    nootropic drugs, 247
Alzheimer's disease assessment scale, 59, 60
Amnesia; see also Anterograde and retrograde
    amnesia of childhood memories, 209

Amok and latah, 207
Amphetamine and memory, 75, 76
Amygdala stimulation and localization of
    memory, 21
Amyotrophic lateral sclerosis of Guam,
    141
Anabolic agents and memory, 81
Anemias and memory, 166
Anesthetics and memory, 72, 37
Angular gyrus syndrome, 152–154, 156
Anterograde amnesia, bilateral temporal lobe
    ablation, 21
Anticholinergic agents and memory, 71
Antipsychotic drugs, 73, 74
Aphasia
  angular gyrus syndrome, 152, 153
  central nervous system syphilis, 157
  chronic ischemia, 151
  cortical dementia, 122, 144, 156
  head trauma, 183
  Pick's disease, 130
  screening test, 55, 56
Apraxia, 156
  Alzheimer's disease, 129
  central nervous system syphilis, 157
Arecoline treatment, 243
Association cortex and memory, 18, 32
Ataxia
  central nervous system syphilis, 157
  head trauma, 182, 183
Attitude and memory skill, 250
Auditory sensory memory, 2, 3
Autistic children, memory dysfunction, 202,
    203

Babcock story recall test, 44
Bacterial meningitis in children, long-term
    sequelae, 161, 162
Barbiturates and memory, 71, 72, 85,
    91

Basal ganglia lesions and localization of memory, 19

Bemegride and memory, 78

Benton visual retention tests, 47

Benzodiazepines and memory, 73, 85

Binswanger's disease, 155

Biological aspects of memory and aging, 229–235

Blood flow
  brain activity and, 149, 150
  brain metabolism and aging, 233, 234

Brain atrophy and chronic alcoholism, 98, 99, 101

Brain damage and head trauma, focal versus diffuse, 180–182, 189, 190, 194

Brain growth and neuronal loss, aging, 230

Brain lesions and localization of memory, 16–21

Brain metabolism and aging, 229, 233, 234

Brain-specific proteins, 23, 24

Brain stem reticular formation, lesions and localization of memory, 19

Brief cognitive rating scale, Alzheimer's disease, 60–63

Brief psychiatric rating scale, 60

Brief word learning tests, 43

Caffeine and memory, 77

Cardiac diseases and memory, 165, 176

Catecholamines, learning and memory, 106, 112

Category-recall relationship and aging, 225, 226

Cell death (neuronal) and aging, 228, 230

Central nervous system stimulants
  memory and, 75–77
  treatment of memory disorders, 245, 246

Central nervous system syphilis and memory, 157, 158

Cerebral cortex lesions and localization of memory, 17–19

Cerebrovascular disorders and memory, 149–156
  chronic ischemia of the brain, 150, 151
  large cerebral infarctions, 152–154
  multi-infarct dementia, 154, 155
  transient ischemic disorders, 151, 152

Choline acetyltransferase (ChAT)
  aging and, 232, 233
  treatment, 240

Choline treatment, 243–245

Cholinergic drugs
  memory and, 78, 79, 85
  treatment, 240–245; see also specific drugs

Cholinergic system, 109–110, 116, 117

Cholinesterase inhibitors and memory, 79

Chronic alcoholism, 94–99
  brain atrophy, 98, 99
  cognitive changes, 94, 95
  memory deficits, 95, 96
  neurochemistry, 97, 98
  neuropathology, 96
  reversibility, 99

Chronic anoxia of brain, 165, 176

Chronic central nervous system infections and memory, 157–163
  bacterial meningitis in children, 161–162
  central nervous system syphilis, 157–158
  chronic viral infections, 158–159
  progressive multifocal leukoencephalopathy, 159–160
  subacute sclerosing panencephalitis, 159
  transmissible spongiform encephalopathies, 160–161

Chronic diseases and memory, 165–177
  anemias, 166
  cardiac diseases, 165
  chronic anoxia, 165
  chronic liver diseases, 168, 169
  chronic renal failure, 166–168
  endocrine disorders, 170–176
  fluid and electrolyte disturbances, 169, 170
  lung diseases, 166

Chronic ischemia of the brain, 150, 151

Chronic liver diseases, 168, 169, 176

Chronic renal failure, 166–168, 176

Chronic viral infections, 158, 159

Clinical examination of memory, 57, 58

Cognitive changes
  chronic alcoholism, 94, 95, 100, 101
  head trauma, 182

Cognitive deficits during posttraumatic amnesia, 186, 187
  Addison's disease, 173
  Alzheimer's disease, 125–129
  amyotrophic lateral sclerosis and parkinsonian dementia complex of Guam, 141
  central nervous system syphilis, 158
  chronic ischemia, 150, 151
  chronic renal failure, 167
  fluid and electrolyte disturbances, 169, 170
  Hallervorden–Spatz syndrome, 137
  Huntington's disease, 132–135
  hydrocephalus, 175
  hyperparathyroidism, 174
  hyperthyroidism, 171, 172
  hypothyroidism, 172, 173

Cognitive deficits (*cont.*)
    idiopathic calcification of basal ganglia, 142
    multi-infarct dementia, 154, 155
    Parkinson's disease, 137–141
    Pick's disease, 130
    progressive supranuclear palsy, 132
    spinocerebellar degenerations, 143
    transient ischemic disorders, 151, 152
    Wilson's disease, 135–137
Cognitive function
    head trauma, 180, 182–184
    in the elderly, 228
    treatment, 245, 246
Cognitive impairment and social drinking,
    90, 91
Communication disorders and head trauma,
    184
Concussion, 181, 182, 186
Confabulation, 207
    hypnosis, 212
    posttraumatic amnesia, 185, 186
Consolidation and long-term memory
    adrenocorticotropic hormone, 112, 113
    alcohol, 93
    growth hormone, 115
Consolidation theory, memory, 29
Convulsant stimulants and memory, 77, 78
Corsis block-tapping test, 48
Cowboy story, memory test, 48
Creutzfeldt–Jakob disease, 160, 161
Cushing's syndrome, 173, 177
Cycloheximide and memory, 68–70, 75

Decay theory, forgetting, 9, 10, 29
Degenerative diseases of the nervous system
    and memory, 121–144
Deja vu, 206, 207
Delayed posttraumatic amnesia, 185
Dementia
    central nervous system syphilis, 158
    chronic anoxia of brain, 165
    Creutzfeldt–Jakob disease, 161
    Kuru, 160
Dementia, cortical versus subcortical, 121,
    122, 144
Dementia score scale, 59
Dendritic spines, changes with age, 230, 231
Depersonalization, 203, 204
Depression
    dreams, 211
    memory disorders, 239
    memory impairment, 199, 200, 215
Design reproduction tests, 47
Dialysis dementia, 168

Digit span tests, 41, 42, 58, 61
Dissociative disorders
    memory disorders, 239
    memory impairment, 203–209, 215, 216
Dissociative trance states, 205
Divided attention conditions and the elderly,
    221, 222, 235
Dopamine system and memory, 105–107
Dream amnesia, 209–211
Dream memory, 209–211
Drugs
    facilitating memory, 74–85
    impairing memory, 68–74, 84, 85
    influencing learning and memory, 67–86
Dual-process theory and memory, 11, 12

Echoic memory, 2, 3
Electrical stimulation, 21–23
Electroconvulsive therapy, memory loss, 214,
    215
Emotional changes, head trauma, 182, 194
Encoding, 6, 7, 12
    Alzheimer's disease, 125–127
    Huntington's disease, 135
    schizophrenia, 202
Endocrine disorders and memory, 170–176
Engram sites, 16, 17
Enkephalin, 110, 111
Enzymes, ChAT, GAD and aging, 232, 233
Epilepsy and memory localization, 20, 21

Fleeting thought, 208
Fluid and electrolyte disturbances and mem-
    ory, 169, 170, 176
Forgetting, 9–11, 29, 34
Forgetting a name, 207, 208
Four-phase model, memory, 15, 16
Frontal lobe stimulation and localization of
    memory, 22, 23
Fuld object-memory evaluation, 49
Functional disorders of memory, 199–216
    autistic children, 202, 203
    dissociative disorders, 203–209
    dream memory and dream amnesia, 209–
    211
    electroconvulsive therapy, 214, 215
    hypnosis, 212–214
    schizophrenia, 201, 202

GABA-ergic drugs and memory, 82
Ganser's syndrome, 206
Genetic–evolutionary theory of memory, 31,
    32
Gerstmann's syndrome, 152

Glial cells and aging, 231
Global deterioration scale, 60
Glutamic acid decarboxylase (GAD) and
  aging, 232, 233
Gonadotropin-releasing hormone, 170
Growth hormone and memory and learning,
  115, 116

Hallervorden–Spatz syndrome, 137
Halstead–Reitan neuropsychological battery,
  52–54, 61
Head injury, retrograde amnesia, 13
Head trauma and memory, 179–195
  disability, 182, 183
  focal versus diffuse damage, 180–182
  impairment, 192–194
  memory disorders, 184–188
  recovery, 183, 184
  recovery of memory, 188–192
  severity of injury, 180
Highway hypnosis, 205
Hippocampus
  memory retrieval, 30
  remote long-term memory, 28
Hormones and memory and learning, 111–117
Huntington's chorea, cholinergic system, 109,
  116
Huntington's disease, 132–135, 144
Hydergine
  memory and, 80, 85
  treatment, 247, 248
Hydrocephalus, 175, 176
Hyperamnesia, 207
  hypnosis and, 212, 213
Hyperbaric oxygenation and memory, 84
Hyperparathyroidism, 174, 175
Hyperthyroidism and memory, 171, 172, 176
Hypnosis and memory dysfunctions, 212–
  214, 216
Hypothyroidism, 172, 173

Iconic memory, 2, 3
Idiopathic calcification of basal ganglia, 141,
  142
Impaired memory and head trauma, 192–194
Intellectual functions and aging, 228, 229
Intelligence
  autistic children, 203
  head trauma, 190
Interference theory of memory and forget-
  ting, 10, 29, 34
Intracellular changes with age, 231, 232
Intracranial hematoma and recovery of mem-
  ory, 191

Intracranial pathology and memory disor-
  ders, 239
IQ changes, 144
  Alzheimer's disease, 127, 128
  Huntington's disease, 134
  Parkinson's disease, 140
Islands of memory, posttraumatic amnesia,
  184, 185, 188

Jamais vu, 206, 207

Kinesthetic memory, 2
Knox cube imitation test, 48
Korsakoff's syndrome, 207
  chronic alcoholism, 95, 99, 100, 101
Kuru, 158, 160

Labile memory, 13–15, 35
Lacunar state, 154, 155
Language impairment, 143, 144
  Alzheimer's disease, 128, 129, 144
  Pick's disease, 13, 144
  progressive multifocal leukoencephalopa-
    thy, 159
Large cerebral infarctions, 152–154, 156
Learning, 67–86
  memory and, 1, 2, 7, 10, 13, 58
  RNA metabolism and, 24–26
  synaptic function, 26, 27
Lecithin treatment, 243–245
Letter span tests, 42
Level of processing model and aging, 227
Levels of processing theory of memory, 11,
  12, 34
Limbic system lesions and localization of
  memory, 20
Localization of memory, 16–28
  electrical stimulation, 21–23
  lesions, 16–21
Locus coeruleus lesion and localization of
  memory, 19, 20
Long-term memory (LTM), 2, 3, 5, 11, 20, 33,
  34, 58, 60, 91, 92
  aging, 219
  alcohol, 92, 93, 100
  Alzheimer's disease, 125, 127
  cholinergic drugs, 241, 244
  drugs influencing, 79
  elderly, 224–226, 235
  encoding, 6, 7
  forgetting, 9, 10
  hormones, 112
  neurobiology, 12, 15

Long-term memory (*cont.*)
  protein synthesis, 25, 68
  recall, elderly, 227
    schizophrenia, 201, 202, 215
  retrieval, 7, 28–30
Lung diseases and memory, 166
Luria's neuropsychological battery, 56

Memory
  definition, 2
  drugs influencing, 67–86
  head trauma, 179–195
    disability, 182, 183
    focal versus diffuse damage, 180–182
    impairment, 192–194
    memory disorders, 184–188
    recovery, 183, 184
    recovery of memory, 188–192
    severity of injury, 180
  learning, 1, 2, 7, 10
  lesions, 17, 18
  localization, 16–28
  neurobiology, 12–33
  psychology, 1–12
Memory assessment, 41–63
Memory changes with aging, 219–236
  biological aspects, 229–235
  other factors, 228, 229
  psychological aspects, 219–228
Memory consolidation
  electroconvulsive therapy, 215
  schizophrenia, 202, 215
Memory deficits, chronic alcoholism, 95, 96,
    100, 101
Memory disorders
  functional, 199–216
  head trauma, 184–188, 194
  treatment strategies, 239–253
    environmental and reality orientation,
      252
    memory skill training, 249–251
    pharmacological treatments, 240–249
    psychiatric treatment, 252
Memory impairment
  Alzheimer's disease, 125, 126
  depression, 199, 200
  head trauma, 192–194
  Huntington's disease, 134
  multi-infarct dementia, 154
  Parkinson's disease, 140
Memory loss, electroconvulsive therapy, 214,
    215
Memory skill training, 249–251
  improving attitudes, 250

Memory skill training (*cont.*)
  improving organization and use of mne-
    monics, 250, 251
  improving visual imagery, 250
Memory span tests in the elderly, 220, 221
Memory storage problems and alcohol, 91, 92
Memory trace sites, 16
Metabolic disturbances and memory disor-
    ders, 239
Methylphenidate treatment (Ritalin), 245, 246
Modified Halstead–Wepman aphasia screen-
    ing test, 55, 56
Molecular and structural changes, localization
    of memory, 23–33
Motor cortex stimulation and localization of
    memory, 22
Motor memory, 2
Multi-infarct dementia, 58, 154–156
Multiple personality, 203–205

Naloxone, 249
  memory and, 84
Neurobiology of memory, 12–33
Neurochemistry, chronic alcoholism, 97
Neuronal activity and memory theories, 14,
    15, 35
Neuronal communication and aging, 229
Neuropathology
  Alzheimer's disease, 124
  central nervous system syphilis, 158
  chronic alcoholism, 96
  chronic liver diseases, 169
  head injury, 182
  Huntington's disease, 133
  Parkinson's disease, 137
  Pick's disease, 130
  progressive multifocal leukoencephalopa-
    thy, 159
  progressive supranuclear palsy, 131
  subacute sclerosing panencephalitis, 159
  Wilson's disease, 135
Neuropeptides
  role in memory, 105–117
    cholinergic system, 108–110
    hormones, 111–116
    noradrenaline and dopamine system, 105–107
    opioid peptides, 110, 111
    serotonergic system, 107, 108
    treatment of memory disorders, 248, 249
Neurophysiology and aging, 234, 235
Neuropsychological allied procedures, 54, 55
Neuropsychological test batteries, 51–56
Neurotransmitters
  aging and, 232

Neurotransmitters (*cont.*)
  chronic alcoholism and, 97, 98, 101
  memory and, 26–28, 35
Nicotine, 83
Nonlanguage paired-associate learning test, 46
Nonverbal memory and aging, 226, 227, 235
Nootropic drug, treatment of memory disorders, 246, 247
Noradrenaline system and memory, 105–107, 116

Object and picture memory span test, 46
Opioid antagonist treatment of memory disorders, 249
Opioid peptides, memory and learning, 110, 111, 116, 117
Organization and use of mnemonics, memory skill, 250, 251

Paragraph and story memory tests, 43, 44
Paramnesia, 187, 207
Parapraxes, 209
Parkinsonian dementia complex of Guam, 141
Parkinson's disease, 105, 137–141
  anticholinergic agents and memory, 71
  cholinergic system, 108
  pseudodementia, 201
Pentylenetetrazol and memory, 78
Personality changes
  Alzheimer's disease, 129
  chronic ischemia, 150, 151
  Huntington's disease, 133
  Pick's disease, 130, 131
  progressive supranuclear palsy, 132
Pharmacological treatment of memory disorders, 240–249
  central nervous system stimulants, 245, 246
  cholinergic drugs, 240–245
  neuropeptides, 248, 249
  nootropic drugs, 246, 247
  vasodilators, 247, 248
Physostigmine treatment, 241, 242
Pick's disease, 121, 129–131, 144
Picrotoxin and memory, 78
Piracetam and memory, 81
Plagiarism and cryptomnesia, 205, 206
Posthypnotic amnesia, 212
Posttraumatic amnesia, 184, 185, 189–195
Posttraumatic disorientation, 189, 192, 195
Posttraumatic psychosis, 183
Processing rate, short-term memory and the elderly, 222, 223

Progressive multifocal leukoencephalopathy, 159, 160, 162
Progressive supranuclear palsy, 131, 132, 144
Protein synthesis
  adrenocorticotropic hormone, 112–114
  learning and, 24–27, 30
  memory theory, 30, 35
  vasopressin, 114
Protein synthesis inhibitors and memory, 68–70
Pseudodementia, 201
Psychiatric treatment, memory disorders, 252
Psychogenic amnesia, 203, 204, 216
Psychogenic fugue, 203, 204, 216
Psychological aspects of memory changes with aging, 219–228
  level of processing model, 227, 228
  long-term memory, 224–226
  nonverbal memory, 226, 227
  sensory memory, 219, 220
  short-term memory, 220–224
Psychological theories of memory, 10–12
Psychology of memory, 1–12
Puromycin and memory, 68–70, 75
Pyrrolidinone derivatives and memory, 81, 82, 85

Questionnaires to assess memory, 56, 57

Randt memory test battery, 51
Raphe nuclei lesions and localization of memory, 19
Rapid-eye-movement (REM) sleep and memory processing, 20, 29, 30, 115, 116, 209–211
Rating scales and inventories, 58–60
Reality orientation program, memory disorders, 252
Recall
  Alzheimer's disease, 125–127
  dreams, 211
  head trauma, 192, 195
  Huntington's disease, 134, 135
  long-term memory, 6
  memory tests, 41, 44, 47–51
  retrieval and, 8, 9, 10, 34
  short-term memory, 4, 5
Recall amnesia, 212
Recall versus recognition, long-term memory in the elderly, 224, 225, 227, 228, 235, 236
Recent experience, interference with registration, 13

Recent memory disturbances and serotonin, 108
Receptors and aging, 233
Recognition
recall and, 227, 228, 235, 236
retrieval and, 8, 9, 34
Recovery of memory
factors complicating recovery, 189–192
head trauma, 188–192, 195
Recurring figures test, 45
Registration, 199
Rehearsal, 10, 11, 29
Relaxation technique training, memory disorders treatment, 252
Remote memory tests, 49, 58, 60, 61
Research methods, short-term memory, 4, 5
Residual memory impairment, head trauma, 184
Retention, 199
Retrieval, 7–9, 28, 29, 34
alcoholic intoxication, 92
Alzheimer's disease, 127
electroconvulsive therapy, 215
hormones, 113
Huntington's disease, 135
Retrieval, long-term memory in the elderly, 226
Retrieval problems and alcohol, 91–93
Retrograde amnesia
electroconvulsive therapy, 214, 215
head injury, 13, 184, 187, 188
operations, 28
shrinkage, 187, 188
Reverberation hypothesis, 14, 15, 31
Reversibility of effects, chronic alcoholism, 99, 101
Ritalin, 245, 246
RNA metabolism and learning, 24–26
RNA synthesis inhibitors and memory, 70, 71

Sandoz clinical assessment, geriatric, 59, 61
Schizophrenia and memory function, 201, 215
Screen memories, 207
Senile dementia, 123
Senquin formboard, 48
Sensory memory, 2, 11, 33, 91
Sensory memory in the elderly, 219, 220
Serotonergic system, learning and memory, 107, 108, 116
Short-term forgetting and the elderly, 223, 224
Short-term memory (STM), 2–5, 11, 33, 58, 60, 91, 92
aging, 219

Short-term memory (cont.)
alcohol, 92, 93, 100
Alzheimer's disease, 125–127
autistic children, 203
brain stimulation, 22
cholinergic drugs, 241
consolidation, 28, 30, 70
drug influencing, 76, 79
in the elderly, 220–224, 235
forgetting, 9
long-term memory and, 6, 7
neurotransmitters, 27, 35
recall, 199
research methods, 4, 5
schizophrenia, 201, 202, 215
Single tests of memory
nonverbal, 45–49
verbal, 41–45
Skull fracture and recovery of memory, 191
Sleep influence on memory, 29, 30
Social drinking, 89–91
Spinocerebellar degenerations, 142, 143
Spreading depression, 13
Stable phase of memory, 15, 35
State-dependent learning, 91, 100
Structural changes and memory, 26, 35
Strychnine and memory, 78
Subacute sclerosing panencephalitis, 159, 162
Syllable span tests, 42

Tardive dyskinesia, cholinergic system, 109, 116
Temporal lobe, lesions and localization of memory, 20, 21
stimulation, 22, 23
Test batteries for memory, 50, 51
Theories of memory, 30, 31; see also specific theories
Thyroid hormone, 170
Trace decay theory of forgetting, 9, 10, 34
Transient ischemic disorders, 151, 152, 156
Transmissible spongioform encephalopathies, 160, 161, 162
Traumatic automatism, 186
Treatment strategies for memory disorders, 239–253
environmental and reality orientation, 252
memory skill training, 249–251
pharmacological treatment, 240–249
psychiatric treatment, 252
Tricyanoaminopropene, 83
Two-phase model of memory, 13–15

Vasodilators and memory, 80, 81, 85
treatment of memory disorders, 247, 248

Vasopressin, 112, 113, 248
Very-short-term memory, 16
Visual agnosia, temporal lobe ablation,
    21
Visual imagery and memory skill, 250
Visual memory tests, 45–49
Visual retention test, 46
Visual sensory memory, 2, 3

Visual sequence recall tests, 47

Wechsler memory scale, 50, 51, 61
Wilson's disease, 135–137
Word span tests, 42, 43
Working memory, 4

Yeast RNA and memory, 82